AF830613

LATE EFFECTS OF RADIATION

LATE EFFECTS OF RADIATION

Proceedings of the Colloquium

held at the Center for Continuing Education,
The University of Chicago, Illinois

May 1969

Edited by

R. J. M. Fry and Douglas Grahn,
Biological and Medical Research Division,
Argonne National Laboratory, Argonne, Illinois

and

Melvin L. Griem and John H. Rust,
Department of Radiology, The University
of Chicago, Chicago, Illinois

TAYLOR & FRANCIS LTD
London

VNR VAN NOSTRAND REINHOLD
New York Cincinnati Toronto London Melbourne

First Published 1970 by Taylor & Francis Ltd., 10–14 Macklin Street, London, WC2B 5NF

Printed and bound in Great Britain by Warren & Son Ltd. (a member of the Taylor & Francis Group), The Wykeham Press, Winchester, Hampshire.

Library of Congress Catalog Card Number 72–128178

Distributed in the U.S.A. and its territories by Van Nostrand Reinhold Company,
450 West 33rd Street, New York, New York, 10001

List of participants

Chairmen of Sessions

MELVIN L. GRIEM
Department of Radiology,
The University of Chicago,
Chicago, Illinois.

JAMES J. NICKSON
Department of Radiology,
The University of Chicago and Department of Radiation Therapy,
Michael Reese Hospital and Medical Center,
Chicago, Illinois.

JOHN H. RUST
Departments of Pharmacology and Radiology,
The University of Chicago,
Chicago, Illinois.

Speakers

A. BERTRAND BRILL
Division of Nuclear Medicine and Biophysics,
Vanderbilt University,
Nashville, Tennessee.

ROBERT L. BRENT
Stein Research Center,
Jefferson Medical College and Medical Center,
Philadelphia, Pensylvania.

HENRY I. KOHN
Shields Warren Radiation Laboratory,
Harvard Medical School,
Boston, Massachusetts.

JACK F. FOWLER
Medical Physics Department,
Royal Postgraduate Medical School,
Hammersmith Hospital,
London.

PATRICIA J. LINDOP
Sub-Department of Radiobiology,
The Medical College of St. Bartholomew's Hospital,
London.

George W. Casarett
Department of Radiation Biology and Biophysics,
The University of Rochester School of Medicine,
Rochester, New York.

Douglas Grahn
Biological and Medical Research Division,
Argonne National Laboratory,
Argonne, Illinois.

Leonard F. Lamerton
Biophysics Department,
Institute of Cancer Research,
Sutton, England.

Michael A. Bender
Biology Division,
Oak Ridge National Laboratory,
Oak Ridge, Tennessee.

William J. Schull
Department of Human Genetics,
The University of Michigan Medical School,
Ann Arbor, Michigan.

Arthur D. Bloom
Department of Human Genetics,
The University of Michigan Medical School,
Ann Arbor, Michigan.

Robert J. Hasterlik
Department of Medicine,
The University of Chicago,
Chicago, Illinois.

Arne Nelson
Research Institute of National Defence,
Sundyberg, Sweden.

Charles W. Mays
Department of Anatomy,
The University of Utah School of Medicine,
Salt Lake City, Utah.

Marvin Goldman
Radiobiology Laboratory,
The University of California,
Davis, California.

ROGER McCLELLAN
Lovelace Foundation,
Albuquerque, New Mexico.

GEORGE A. SACHER
Biological and Medical Research Division,
Argonne National Laboratory,
Argonne, Illinois.

ROBERT W. MILLER
Epidemiology Branch,
National Cancer Institute,
Bethesda, Maryland.

VICTOR P. BOND
Medical Division,
Brookhaven National Laboratory,
Upton, Long Island, New York.

ALICE M. STEWART
Department of Social Medicine,
Oxford University,
Oxford, England.

AUSTIN M. BRUES
Biological and Medical Research Division,
Argonne National Laboratory,
Argonne, Illinois.

THE LORD RITCHIE-CALDER OF BALMASHANNAR
Professor of International Relations,
University of Edinburgh,
Edinburgh.

Editors

R. J. M. FRY, Senior Editor,
Biological and Medical Research Division,
Argonne National Laboratory,
Argonne, Illinois.

DOUGLAS GRAHN

MELVIN L. GRIEM

JOHN H. RUST

Preface

Almost 27 years ago the controlled release of atomic energy was first achieved under the West Stands at the University of Chicago, December 2, 1942. This stimulated the investigation of the biological effects of radiation in both animal and man.

Ten years ago Dr. John H. Rust received a grant from the Rockefeller Foundation to develop a center of inquiry, criticism, and education to deal broadly with the impact of the peaceful uses of atomic energy on the public health. " In a free society the public interest is best served when the affairs are directed by an informed and enlightened public opinion. The task is primarily educational but the direction of the educational program should be independent of government and industry and should be sensitive to public opinion." These last two statements are taken directly from the preface of a book *Living with the Atom* by Lord Ritchie-Calder and a statement of the problem by Dr. Rust as it was seen approximately ten years ago.

In the ten-year period series of lectures and colloquia have been held and books have been published. This colloquium is a climax of this ten-year effort. From our knowledge of the late and subtle affect of radiation on man and animals, it may be possible to draw conclusions and build models. With some of these models one may be able to predict the effects of environmental pollutants on the health and well being of those so exposed.

Lord Ritchie-Calder accepted the task of placing the knowledge of the Late Effects of Radiation in a framework of some of the other problems we face in related fields today. It was most fitting that he participated in the first and last of the colloquia thus giving continuity. This colloquium represents a fitting climax to Dr. Rust's efforts over the past ten years.

Finally, thanks are due to the Rockefeller Foundation for their generous support of this colloquium. We also thank the U.S. Public Health Service, and the Chicago Tumor Institute for their contributions.

We should also like to thank Mrs. Shirley Danner, Mrs. Myrtle Tuzar, Mr. Claude Weil, and Mrs. Ruth Letvinchik for their help in the arrangements that were necessary to organize and conduct this colloquium at the University of Chicago.

Contents

CHAPTER I

EXPOSURE OF MAN TO RADIATION

A.B. Brill and R.E. Johnston

Introduction

The major worries concerning exposures of populations to ionizing radiation are directed toward gonadal rather than somatic effects. This reflects a deep concern that future generations of man should not be penalized for errors in judgment we made of tolerable risk levels. The genetic effects have a continuity and amplification which involves more than a single individual and compounds the problem. Most of the information on radiation hazards to man involves somatic effects and has been derived from the study of unusual groups of people who received unusual exposures. When we postulate the magnitude of potential hazards from average population exposures, we are forced to extrapolate from effects observed at relatively high doses and dose rates to lower dose regions at which level no effects can be documented with certainty. Without knowledge of mechanisms of induction, one is forced to assume some shape for the dose-response curve in the low dose region, often several orders of magnitude below observed effects. Such extrapolations obviously are subject to great uncertainty. Regulatory bodies use quantitative estimates of radiation effects at high dose levels to determine proportional extrapolations of these risks to lower dose exposures. Thus, information on the magnitude of exposures received by the general population, and in particular estimates of gonadal dose, have become important in assessing the magnitude of risk from exposures to the lower doses that are generally encountered.

The biologically significant dose is the absorbed dose received by the organ of interest. Absorbed dose received by individuals exposed to ionizing radiation is best expressed in rems or mrems per unit of time. These units are additive and the amounts of radiation absorbed by the gonads, for example, from different sources can be summated. Assuming that effects are independent of dose rate, one can add the different exposures and determine average rates over relevant time periods. For the purpose of assessing the overall level of hazard within a definable population, the concept of genetically significant dose (GSD) was developed. The average annual genetically significant dose GSD is defined as

DEFINITION OF GENETICALLY SIGNIFICANT DOSE

AVERAGE ANNUAL GENETICALLY SIGNIFICANT DOSE (GSD) $= \sum D_i N_i P_i \;/\; \sum \hat{N}_i . P_i$

WHERE .... D_i is the average gonad dose for a specified type of exposure for a person in age-sex class (i);

N_i is the number of persons in age-sex class (i) who had the specified type of exposure during a year;

P_i is the expected number of future children to an individual in age-sex class (i);

and $\hat{N}_i$ is the number of persons in age-sex class (i) in the total population.

The GSD is the average value of D (the gonad dose for a specified type of exposure), weighted by N_i (the number of persons exposed), and P_i (the expected number of progeny they may produce. The GSD represents the average dose which, if received by every member of the population, would result in the same total genetic effect to the population as the doses which are in fact received by individuals within the population (UNSCEAR, 1958).

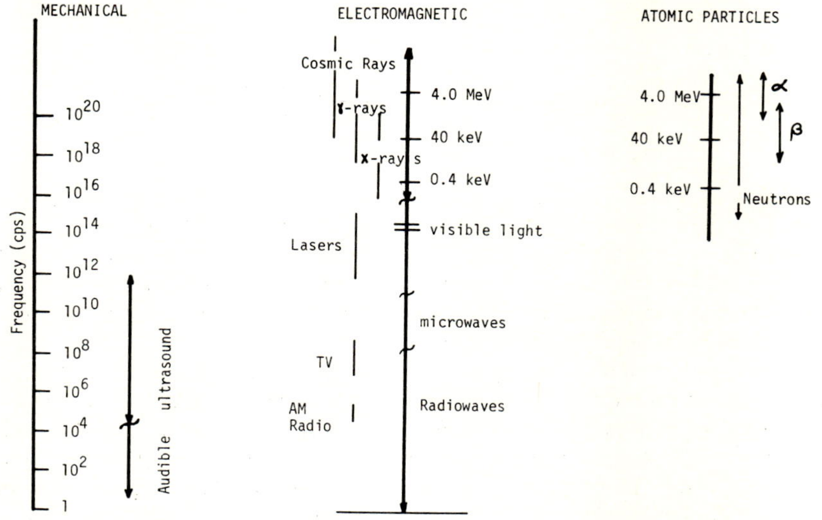

Fig. 1. Nature of radiation.

This report is directed toward summarizing information on the kinds and amounts of exposures currently being received by man and animals. Apart from medical exposure, we will assume that man and animals receive the same amounts of radiation exposure; recognizing that this is untrue in unusual ecological situations such as where animals live in or near such places as weapons test sites, for example. A brief review is presented in fig. 1 of the different types of radiation.

Mechanical, electromagnetic and atomic processes can give rise to radiation, each with a characteristic frequency. The mechanical radiations with which we are most concerned are in the sonic and ultrasonic frequencies. The audible region extends from 30 to 20,000 cycles per second. Above this frequency, we are in the ultrasonic region. Diagnostic studies with ultrasound have been confined to the 1 to 10 megacycle region, although the ultrasonic region extends up to 10^{12} cycles per second. At the power levels and duty cycles used diagnostically, no biolgical hazards have been observed as yet in animals or man.

The low frequency end of the electromagnetic spectrum includes radio, TV, and microwaves. Exposures to microwaves constitute a known hazard. TV constitutes a hazard, not only to the eye, ear, and mind, but also may emit even more penetrating ionizing radiation. Lasers generate extremely intense beams of electromagnetic radiation with a characteristic frequency some place between the infrared and the X-ray region. Some laser applications may be hazardous and result in burns. In this same region of the spectrum are the ultraviolet, infrared and visible radiations - which are not included in this review. These are superceded in frequency and energy by X and gamma rays and finally by cosmic radiations. The last source of radiation shown on the figure are the particulate radiations, examples of which are alphas, betas, and neutrons, as well as mesons, protons, and heavy nuclei.

Of all the sources of radiation exposure to which man is heir, we know more about the ionizing radiations than any other portion of the electromagnetic spectrum or for that matter any other environmental pollution, drug, or food additive known. This knowledge comes from extensive experience with medical uses and from the great impetus provided by research on the effects of atomic radiations since World War II. The non-ionizing radiations have received less attention in the past, although current increases in the use of microwaves, lasers and other radiation emitting systems will require the development of additional information on their effects, as well as on ways of monitoring exposure levels.

Irradiation from Natural Sources

Cosmic rays

The radiation from cosmic rays at any specific location remains relatively constant with time; but varies according to latitude and altitude. A distinguishing characteristic of cosmic radiation is that the entire world population has been so exposed from the beginning of time and these exposures will continue. Because of technological advances in space travel, cosmic ray contributions to the population GSD may increase in the future.

Primary cosmic radiation is usually grouped into three categories: galactic cosmic rays, geomagnetically trapped charged particles, and solar cosmic radiation.

Galactic cosmic radiation is derived from a more or less constant complement of particles. Outside the atmosphere at latitudes of $>55^{\circ}$, primary galactic cosmic rays consist of protons, alpha particles and heavier nuclei, in the ratio of 87:12:1 (UNSCEAR, para. 4, Annex E, 1962). The primary galactic cosmic particles interact with nuclei in the upper atmosphere producing secondary radiation which consists of mesons, electrons, photons, protons, and neutrons - all with very wide ranges of energies (Snyder, 1968). The primary radiation intensity gradually decreases with altitude and below 20 km the cosmic radiation is almost entirely secondary. Above 50 km cosmic radiation is essentially primary.

Since relative biological effectiveness (RBE) is a function of different types of radiation and energy, and because of the wide variations of particle composition and energy spectra of the cosmic radiation, it is difficult to arrive at an accurate single estimate for the radiation dose from the cosmic radiation. It is generally accepted that a typical value for tissue dose rate at sea level and middle latitudes is 50 mrem per year (UNSCEAR, para. 7, 8, Annex E, 1962).

Geomagnetically-trapped radiations, such as in the Van Allen belts, consists of electrons and protons captured by the earth's magnetic fields. The inner belt reaches a maximum intensity at about 2,000 miles and extends from 30° N to 30° S; the outer belt has a maximum intensity at about 10,000 miles and extends from 60° N to 60° S. It is difficult to estimate a radiation dose rate in these regions because it is highly dependent upon the amount of shielding assumed around the space traveller, but for the inner radiation belt, values of 10 to 120 rads/hour have been suggested. Dose rates in the outer belt may be as high as 10^{4} rads/hour but can be reduced considerably with shielding because of the large component of soft electron bremsstrahlung (UNSCEAR, para. 4, Annex E, 1962).

Solar radiation is the third major source of cosmic radiation. Large fluxes of protons are observed to reach the earth following severe solar flares which occur on the surface of the sun. Solar cosmic flares are either "high energy" or "low energy" events. The "high energy" events produce particles with energies high enough to be observed at ground level, whereas high altitude measurements are necessary to detect "low energy" events. The low energy phenomena appear to occur most frequently. Unlike the radiation belts, solar particles are not restricted to a small region of space that could be avoided or traversed rapidly, but apparently are distributed throughout the solar system (UNSCEAR, para. 4, Annex E, 1962).

Over the last few years, the possibility of human supersonic transportation has stimulated the report of a task group of the ICRP directed towards an appraisal of the radiation hazard that might be encountered by passengers on such commercial air craft travelling at 60,000 to 80,000 feet, or 12 to 16 miles (ICRP, 1966). The intensity of cosmic radiation in relation to altitude is shown in fig. 2.

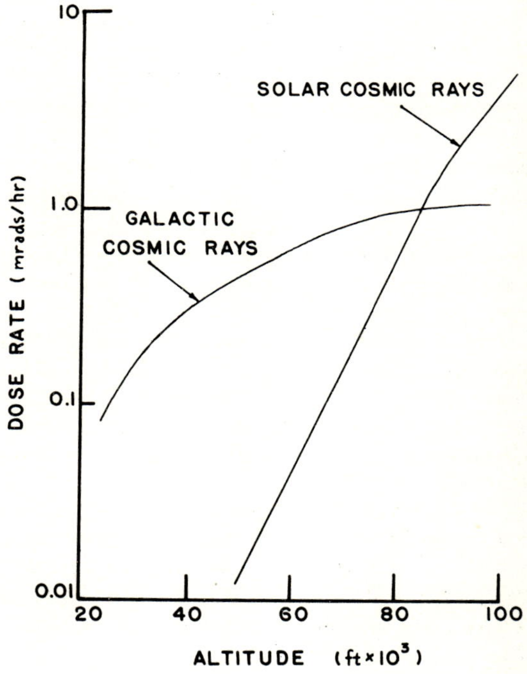

Fig. 2. Intensity of cosmic radiation vs altitude (Snyder, 1968).

The total radiation dose rate (galactic and solar) at 40,000 feet is 0.31 mrad/hour or 0.54 mrem/hour. This is a dose rate 100 times that experienced at sea level. At 80,000 feet it goes up to 3.1 mrem/hour, or 500 times sea level dose rates. Above 90,000 feet, the major cosmic source of radiation exposure is solar in origin, while below that height it is galactic (Snyder, 1968).

On rare occasions, perhaps once or twice during an 11-year period, a severe solar cosmic ray outburst may be expected to deliver a dose at peak rates as much as 2 to 20 rads/hour (Snyder, 1968). Exposures at these levels might be incurred by persons flying at 80,000 feet on future SST flights and thus measures are needed to detect such events in time so that they can be avoided.

Naturally Occurring Radioactive Nuclides

Radioactivity in the earth's crust

Naturally occurring radioactive materials are widely distributed throughout the earth's crust and contribute to mankind's radiation exposure from a value somewhat less than that due to cosmic rays to values in some regions which are many times greater (table 1). The major contributors are uranium-238, thorium-232, radium-226 and their daughter products, along with potassium-40 and cosmic ray produced radioisotopes of carbon and hydrogen. Many other radioactive materials exist but in low abundance and of negligible consequence.

Table 1

Exposure of man to naturally occurring radionuclides
(Morgan et al., 1967.)

TYPE OF EXPOSURE	MEAN DOSE TO GONADS mrad/yr	MEAN DOSE TO BONE mrad/yr	MEAN DOSE TO LUNGS mrad/yr
Internal			
^{40}K	18 - 22	7 - 11	15
^{226}Ra + daughter products		3 - 7	0.5
^{14}C	0.7 - 1.8	1.5	
$^{220,222}Rn$ wooden house			45
brick house			104
concrete house			158
TOTAL	22	16	100
External			
Normal Regions	47	(approximately the same as for gonads)	
Granite Regions in France	162		
Monazite Regions in India	802		
Monazite Regions in Brazil	287		
TOTAL FOR NORMAL REGIONS (GSD) = 69 mrem/yr.			

With the exception of certain areas in the world where radionuclide concentrations are unusually high (monazite sands), the mean dose rate to the gonads and bone received by the world population from external exposure to terrestrial gamma radiation is about 47 mrads/year. Persons living in certain granite-rich areas of France receive mean gonadal doses of 162 mrads/year, while persons living on monazite sands in Brazil and Karala, India, are exposed respectively to 287 and 802 mrads/year on the average. In addition, the lung is exposed to radon-220 and radon-222 released from different building materials. Living in a wooden house results in a lung exposure of approximately 45 mrads/year as opposed to 104 mrads/year from brick houses, and 158 mrads/year from concrete houses on the average (Morgan and Turner, p. 10, 1967).

Radioactivity in food and water

Drinking water and food contain variable amounts of radioactive material of natural origin which may be retained in the body after ingestion. Elements of the uranium and thorium series, potassium-40 and carbon-14, are the main natural sources of radioactivity deposited in the body. Potassium and carbon are distributed throughout the whole body and hence contribute to the gonadal as well as to the bone dose. Radium taken internally through food and water contributes primarily to bone dose. The mean dose to the gonads from these internal exposures is between 19 and 24 mrads/year. The mean dose to the bone is between 16 and 24 mrads/year, the average value being about 20, and comes primarily from potassium-40 and not from radium as might have been expected. The dose received by the lung tissue is derived in part from potassium-40 but mostly from the radon-daughters of radium from dietary sources. For normal regions, the mean dose to the gonads from naturally occurring radionuclides is 69 mrem/year, which is 38.5% of the GSD estimated for the U.S.A. (Morgan and Turner, p. 10, 1967).

Irradiation from Radioactive Contamination of the Environment Due to Explosions of Nuclear Weapons

Considerable data are available in the literature concerning the contamination of the environment with radioactivity resulting from nuclear weapons testing (table 2). Since almost all atmospheric weapons testing ceased in 1962, fall-out now results in a proportionally small contribution to population exposure.

Table 2

Dose commitments in mrad for testing 1954-1962
(Spiers, 1968, p.293.)

ISOTOPE	GONADS	CELLS LINING BONE SURFACES	BONE MARROW	THYROID OF A 0-1 YEAR OLD
External	50	50	50	50
Internal				
^{90}Sr	-	174	87	-
^{137}Cs	13	13	13	13
^{14}C	13	20	13	13
^{131}I	-	-	-	330
Total to Year 2000	76	257	163	406
Avg. Dose Rate / year	1.6	5.6	3.5	8.8
Dose from ^{14}C after year 2000	167	270	167	167

The major sources of external exposures from fall-out are from the short-lived gamma-emitting radionuclides, zirconium-95, niobium-95, and the longer-lived caesium-137. The tissue dose delivered from deposited fall-out not incorporated into the body depends upon the shielding effect of buildings, the fraction of time individuals spend outdoors, and the rate at which the radioactive debris settles onto the land.

Internal exposure is primarily from strontium-90, caesium-137, iodine-131, and carbon-14 (table 2). Diet, including both plant and animal foods, is the principal source of intake. The distribution of strontium in the body follows closely that of calcium. It is, therefore, deposited in the skeleton and retained for a period of years. The beta radiation from strontium-90 irradiates not only the bone itself, but also the bone forming and blood forming cells contained in the bone cavities. Caesium-137 is uniformly distributed throughout the body and has a considerably shorter biological half-life than strontium-90.

The explosions of nuclear weapons has added considerably to the amount of naturally-occurring cosmic ray produced carbon-14 in the atmosphere. By 1959, there was an increase of about 30% above background (UNSCEAR, para. 116, Annex E, 1962) and, by 1963, carbon-14 levels had increased by 80% over pre-1952 values (Spiers, p. 280, 1968). The dose rate from carbon-14 is small compared to that from other radionuclides produced by nuclear explosions. Carbon-14, because of its very long residence time in the biosphere, and its 5,760 year radioactive half-life, will continue to contaminate the environment for thousands of years to come. This constitutes a potential genetic hazard, because of the many generations which will be exposed to this radionuclide.

Iodine-131 is produced in relatively high yields by atomic explosions. It is short-lived (8-day physical half-life) but selectively concentrates in the thyroid gland. It is secreted in milk and reaches the body by the ingestion of fresh foods; milk being the principal source. The dose to the thyroid from uptake of iodine-131 varies with age. Because of the small size of the gland in infancy and the high milk consumption in this age group, the maximum dose rate from iodine-131 contamination of the environment occurs in the 0 to 1 year age group.

The accumulated dose in mrads from past nuclear weapons testing and extrapolations to the year 2000 and beyond is shown towards the bottom of table 2. Assuming no further weapons testing and based upon the measured dose rates from fall-out during the period from 1954 to 1962, the average gonadal dose rate is 1.6 mrads/year, and the average bone dose rate is between 3 and 5 mrads/year. The largest dose commitments are received from strontium-90 by the cells lining the bone surfaces, and from iodine-131 by the thyroid during the first year of life. The integral dose from carbon-14 after year 2000 is greater than that from all other fall-out products with the exception of the thyroid dose from iodine-131.

The cumulative radiation dose received by the bone marrow from natural background during the years 1954-2000 is shown as the hatched portion of fig. 3, on top of which is added the dose commitment received during the same number of years from fall-out due to weapons testing during the years up to 1962. This shows the fall-out contribution to an average individual born in 1954. Individuals born before or after this date on the average receive a smaller proportion of their total exposure from fall-out. The increment in population exposure from fall-out from weapons testing is not impressive when compared to that received from natural background radiation.

Disposal of Radioactive Wastes

Environmental contamination by radioactive waste from nuclear reactors and their associated operations is carefully policed by well-trained health physicists. All modern nuclear power plants use closed cycle cooling systems and consequently the release of environmental contamination is far less today than from the early Oak Ridge National Laboratory and Hanford reactors, for example, which were not closed cycle systems. Analysis of the six major power reactors which have been in operation for sufficient time to provide good data indicate a maximum of 11 curies of liquid waste discharge per year

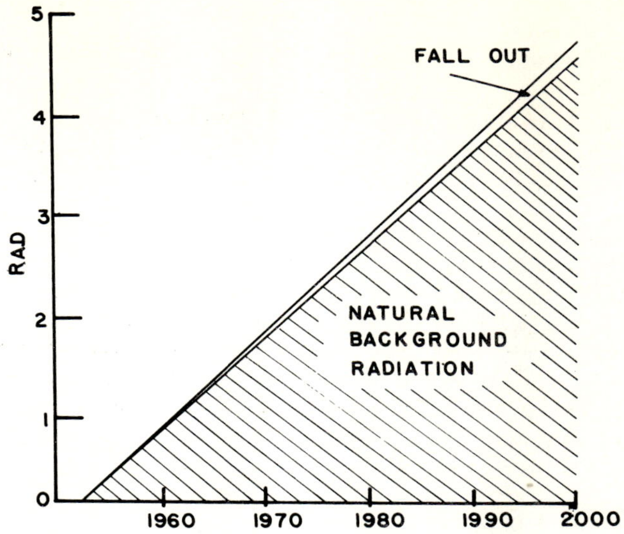

Fig. 3. Contributions of dose commitment to bone marrow from natural background and fall-out to the year 2000 (Ellis, 1965).

excluding tritium (Parker, 1967). If we include tritium, 1,300 curies is the maximum. Low and intermediate levels of radioactive waste from the chemical processing plants associated with reactor operations are chemically treated and discharged into basins from which there is slow seepage into nearby rivers, or they are diluted with large quantities of water and discharged directly into rivers, lakes, or the ocean. High-level radioactive waste for the most part is being stored in large underground holding tanks. At Idaho, high level wastes are stored in underground vaults, and at Hanford, in-tank solidification of the high level waste is being carried out. Other solutions are being investigated which require the presence of particular geologic conditions (Parker, 1969). Stream and air pollution, as well as biological samples, are carefully monitored around nuclear energy installations and in ports through which nuclear vessels pass.

At present, the contribution of wastes from reactor operations to the total dose received by the population-at-large is quite negligible. In the neighbourhood of the controlled areas of the large nuclear establishments, the radioactive waste is very carefully planned and kept under constant surveillance so that the maximum permissible levels suggested for the environment by the ICRP are not exceeded.

Repeated studies have shown that discharges of gaseous and liquid wastes have been less than 10% of the limits established for each reactor site. As the number of reactor installations increases, we will have to be careful to ensure that combined exposures or populations in the area are not in excess of present standards. The major fear of the general public concerning the siting of reactors in population centres relates to possible accidents.

Radiation Accidents

So far, only one radiation accident has occurred which resulted in significant contamination of the environment. This was the reactor incident at Windscale, England, which occurred in 1957 during a maintenance operation in which overheating occurred and some uranium fuel caught on fire and burned for two days. During this time, fission products escaped and contaminated the environs. The primary concern was iodine-131 in milk, and thousands of gallons of contaminated milk were destroyed. Hundreds, perhaps thousands, of people received an absorbed dose of a few rads to the thyroid, with the highest measured concentration of iodine-131 in a child's thyroid found to be 0.28 μCi. If maintained at this level by continued ingestion, this could have resulted in a maximum thyroid dose of 16 rem (Morgan and Turner, p. 46, 1967), with whole-body or gonadal doses of about 16 mrem.

The hazards to the population from properly sited, carefully designed nuclear installations is less than from the more common types of industrial plants to which we have become accustomed.

Irradiation from Man-made Sources (Non-Medical)

Occupational exposure to ionizing radiations

Data from industrialized countries indicate that about 0.3 to 0.8 individuals/ thousand of total population are occupationally exposed to ionizing radiations. The United Nation's Scientific Committee reports indicate that the genetically significant dose received by the general population from all occupational exposure (that is, both research and production) is very small. For example, it was estimated to be 0.2 mrem/year in 1955 in Austria, 0.3 mrem/year in 1960 in the Netherlands, and 0.4 mrem/year in 1959 in the United Kingdom. Perhaps in most countries the occupational exposure is even less. In the United Kingdom it was estimated that 40% of the occupational contribution to the population GSD came from workers in the Atomic Energy Industry. This includes exposure to radiation due to neutrons and gamma rays from nuclear reactors as well as exposures from associated chemical and engineering operations in the fabrication of fuel elements, separation of the fission products, and transuranic elements, and a wide variety of research operations. The contribution to population exposure from high-voltage accelerators is less than that from nuclear reactors by several orders of magnitude (Morgan and Turner, p. 29, 1967).

Industrial uses of radiographic equipment for flaw detection require high energy sources and are now extending into neutron radiography, as well as X rays. Currently, 5% of the X-ray units in the United States are in industrial and research areas (PHS, CCB 67-2, 1967). Exposures received by personnel are not significantly different from those received by X-ray technicians in medical installations. In view of the smaller number of people involved with industrial radiography, however, this results in a small contribution to the population GSD.

Table 3 shows the mean annual dose received by different categories of occupationally exposed workers in the United Kingdom in 1959 (UNSCEAR, p. 409, 1962). Persons conducting medical diagnostic studies received 470 mrem/year, while therapists received doses three times higher. Personnel exposed to industrial X-ray sources received intermediate exposures. Low levels were recorded in research and educational situations. Atomic energy establishment personnel received exposures equivalent to those received by diagnostic X-ray workers. Due to increasing numbers of power reactors, as well as the wide spread industrial use of isotopes for thickness gauging, flaw detection, etc., the potential exists for much wider incidence of exposure than when the sources of ionizing radiation were more closely controlled. In view of the large sources of potential exposure in the atomic energy industry, the low occupational exposures received is a tribute to the health physics practices that have been developed.

There is a rapid increase in interest in low energy charged particle accelerators and neutron generators for on-site production of short-lived radionuclides for use in medicine.

Table 3

Mean annual doses to occupationally exposed persons
United Kingdom Survey, 1959.
(UNSCEAR, p. 409, 1962.)

TYPE OF WORK	mrem
Medical	
Diagnosis	470
Therapy	1750
Industrial	1100
Research and Education	33
Atomic Energy Industry	420

Small cyclotrons, Cockroft-Walton type neutron generators and californium-52 sources are likely to be found in universities and hospitals where great expertise in health physics and radiochemistry does not always exist. Careful monitoring of this programme as it develops will be essential to maintain the fine safety records which we have come to expect.

Population exposure from TV sets and non-ionizing radiation devices

The rapid growth of modern electron devices which are widely dispersed throughout the general population present a potential radiation hazard that until recently has received little attention. Microwaves are a form of electromagnetic radiation in the frequency range above ultra high frequency television and below the infrared region of the spectrum. Sources of microwaves include high output radar devices used in navigation and weather systems, as well as small boats and burglar alarms. The former operate at power levels in the kilowatt and megawatt range, while the latter operate at lower power levels, namely 100 milliwatts to 3 kilowatts. Laboratory experiments on animals have demonstrated that lens opacities, haematologic, endocrine and possibly genetic effects can be caused by microwave radiations. Hazards are dependent upon frequency, intensity, and duration of exposure (Donnelly, 1967; Michaelson et al., 1967). The relationship between time and power density for induction of lens opacities in the rabbit eye with single doses of irradiation is shown in fig. 4 (Carpenter, 1967). Clearly both time and intensity factors are important. Frequency also appears to be of great importance with greatest hazard from the lower frequency ranges between 1,000 and 10,000 megacycles/second. Experiments on rabbits suggest that there may be cumulative effects of repeated subthreshold doses. There is no question of the radiation hazard from microwaves; the question yet to be answered is whether the present limit of 10 mW/cm^2 is really "safe" or if it should be revised downward toward the more conservative level of 0.01 mW/cm^2 accepted in Russia.

Microwave ovens are becoming increasingly popular and available to the general public. These are available for both home use and in self-service food facilities. The United States Public Health Service (USPHS) has sponsored several radiation surveys of such ovens installed in commercial establishments and found, in general, that for about one-half of them there was detectable radiation leakage around the oven door. Of those showing measurable leakage, 60 to 70% had emission levels less than 10 mW/cm^2 and 30 to 40% had emission levels greater than 10 mW/cm^2 (Rentos, 1967). These devices carried no warning signs; most owners and operators were unaware of any radiation hazard, and many servicemen were not knowledgeable that a radiation hazard was associated with this type of equipment.

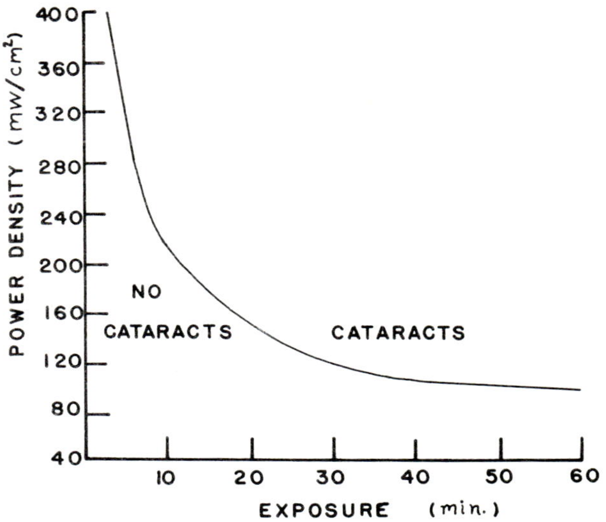

Fig. 4. Relationship of power density and esposure time to produce cataracts in the rabbit eye (Carpenter, 1967).

Thus, there are several factors regarding microwaves which are of current concern. One is that the sources of potential low-level exposure are increasing rapidly as a result of the proliferation of ultra high frequency television transmitters, radar devices, and microwave cookers; another is the lack of knowledge about the potential hazard from microwaves by those who use them; and lastly there is the possibility that the presently accepted exposure level of 10 mW/cm^2 may be subject to downward revision.

The laser represents a radiation hazard to the general population which must also be considered. The rapid growth of laser technology has produced a potentially valuable tool for communications engineering and industrial applications, as well as a novel research tool in biology and medicine.

Because of the focussing characteristics of the lens of the eye, the retina is the most vulnerable tissue to laser radiation. It is known that a power density of 6 W/cm^2 on the rabbit retina for a period of 3 minutes can produce a mild retinal burn. This corresponds to a retinal temperature rise of 17° above ambient during such exposure (Ham et al., 1968). It has been recommended that retinal exposure from continuous output lasers be kept well below 1 W/cm^2. Pulsed lasers operate at much high power levels and can cause retinal burns in times which are of the order of one microsecond or less. Thus, if an individual's eye is exposed to the primary beam of a high output laser, he will surely develop a retinal burn. Reflected beams can also be a hazard, depending on power level.

The USPHS recently conducted a survey of laser users in Massachusetts (Radiation Safety Act Hearings, Part II, p. 949). The findings of the study were reassuring and did not reveal any evidence of retinal damage from laser exposure. They did estimate, however, that 60% of laser workers in the scientific and instrument industry face potential risk unless careful control procedures are followed. Only one-half of the industrial establishments provided training in laser hazards to their employees, and only a few of the installations were marked so as to designate them as laser areas. This survey was conducted primarily in advanced industrial research laboratories and might not be typical of many of the laser installations in less sophisticated areas (Brown and Powell, 1968).

Occupational hazards to workers in and around laser laboratories is one category of risk. Inexpensive lasers of relatively low power are readily available to anyone at a very modest cost, and constitute a potential hazard to unskilled users. In addition, in situations such as ranging and communication applications, it is conceivable that the general public could be subjected unknowlingly to significant radiation hazards.

Ultrasound is another form of non-ionizing radiation that has found varied and expanding usage in industry and medicine. Ultrasound refers to mechanical vibrations at frequencies above human audibility (>20 Hz). At present, most ultrasound applications use the frequency range of 20 Hz to 10 MHz. At these frequencies, sound is fairly well absorbed by resonance phenomena at the molecular and structural level.

The principal industrial applications are for machining, cleaning, and emulsification. In these applications, relatively high power levels are used, usually at frequencies as low as is consistent with the absence of intolerable levels of audible noise.

Medical therapeutic uses of ultrasonics are primarily in the field of physical medicine where the radiation is applied to specific areas of the body through a water bath or contact grease at intensities up to 5 W/cm^2. These beams are applied either as continuous or as pulsed beams with duty factors between 0.2 and 1.0.

The common diagnostic application of ultrasound is a form of echo location in which 1.0 μsec pulses of radiation are sent every msec or more. The duty factor is thus on the order of 0.001. The peak intensities are about 1 W/cm^2. Some applications, particularly those involving the abdomen, employ moving beams which scan the area of interest. Some of the most successful applications of this technique have been in obstetrics. In this latter situation, and with out present state of knowledge concerning radiation hazards, the ultrasonics technique has been considered preferable to radiography from the point of view of radiation exposure (Baldes et al., 1958; Hill, 1968).

It is estimated that therapeutic and diagnostic applications of ultrasound may now occur at a rate of 1,000 cases per week in the United Kingdom (Hill, 1968). No detailed follow-up studies have yet been undertaken. However, no harmfull consequences of diagnostic uses have been reported.

Recently, much attention has been given to the problem of X-ray exposures from colour television sets. Investigations concerning the possible radiation hazards from television sets began in 1959 with a comprehensive laboratory study (Braestrup and Mooney, 1959). From their study and estimates of the general population's viewing habits in 1959, they calculated a mean yearly gonadal dose of less than 1 mrem, based on X-ray emissions from the face of the picture tube, and estimated population viewing habits.

More recently, in the spring of 1967, it was discovered that some colour television sets emitted excessive amounts of X rays from shunt regulator tubes in the high voltage supply, and studies were undertaken to evaluate their radiation output. Maximum exposure rates were found to be 0.6 R/hour at a distance of $33\frac{1}{2}$ in. below the anode of the tube after passing through a simulated apartement floor and ceiling, 83 R/hour at the surface of the floor

($12\frac{1}{4}$ in. below the tube anode), and 800 R/hour at 4 in. below the tube anode with no intervening shielding. A person lying underneath an operating set could receive upwards of 83 R/hour. Scattered radiation exposure rates near floor level were 1/50,000 of the maximum primary beam (1 to 2 mR/hour) (Terrill, 1967). The shunt regulator tubes were redesigned and local servicemen replaced them with new tubes in television sets already purchased. In the fall of 1967, the USPHS conducted a radiation survey of the corrected in-service television sets in Pinellas County, Florida (Smith et al., 1968). Replacement of the original shunt regulator tubes with the modified tubes significantly reduced the radiation levels from this source. Of the sets monitored, 29.2%, however, still had radiation output levels greater than 0.5 mR/hour.

The high voltage rectifier tube was found to be another source of radiation, due, most often, to operation at voltages above those recommended by the manufacturer. Since an extensive modification programme had been performed in Pinellas County, Florida, and instructions had been given to the repairman concerning the proper voltage setting, it was surprising to find that the majority of sets surveyed were being operated at excess voltages. Subsequent action resulted in correct adjustment of the voltage setting and replacement of the high voltage rectifier and shunt regulator tubes. This reduced X-ray levels in all cases to less than 0.5 mR/hour at all surfaces of the television sets. This is the maximum permissible radiation emission level at SCM from any accessible surface recommended by the National Council on Radiation Protection (NCRP) and the International Committee on Radiation Protection (ICRP).

Another USPHS survey was conducted in 1967 in the metropolitan Washington, D.C. area (PHS, TSB3, 1968). In this study, 1,124 colour television sets of a variety of brands and models were surveyed for X-ray emission. Of the sets surveyed, 72% emitted X radiation at levels less than 0.04 mR/hour, 18% emitted X radiation at levels between 0.04 mR/hour and 0.5 mR/hour. Radiation levels up to as high as 367 mR/hour were recorded in the remaining 8% of the sets surveyed. Again, in this survey the primary sources were identified as the high voltage shunt regulator tube, and the high voltage rectifier tube. Replacement of these tubes and reduction of the operating voltage reduced radiation levels to below the recommended 0.5 mR/hour level in all but one case. Additional shielding of the high voltage power supply tubes was needed to bring about the necessary reduction of radiation levels in that one special instance.

Thus it appears that the radiation levels from colour television sets can be made sufficiently small so as not to constitute an important addition to the GSD for the general population. What is strikingly obvious from the surveys is that improper operation and servicing of sets or even lack of service over a period of time can result in excessive levels of radiation exposure from some receivers. It seems reasonable to expect that manufacturers should construct sets with additional shielding in critical places so that even if the set is operated at higher voltages than recommended, and with defective regulator tubes, the radiation levels at accessible surfaces of the television set should not exceed the ICRP recommendation of 0.5 mR/hour.

Radiation from Man-made Sources (Medical)

This category includes those ionizing radiations which are administered to patients by physicians, dentists, etc. for diagnostic or therapeutic purposes. This type of exposure occurs more selectively than either natural background radiation or environmental contamination over which we have only limited control. Medical uses account for 95% of the GSD received by the general population from controllable sources. The GSD received from diagnostic X-ray studies in the United States relative to other advanced countries in the world is shown in table 4 (Penfil and Brown, 1968). Medical care in the United Kingdom is available to all the population and is of high quality. One might expect that their average radiation exposure would be higher than in the United States, but the opposite is true. In the United States, the GSD is 55 mrem/year, a figure which is approximately four times higher than reported for the United Kingdom. Lord Adrian, chairman of the committee responsible for the careful diagnostic X-ray exposure surveys made in England in 1957 suggests that if the techniques used by the best 25% of their hospitals were followed by all users in the United Kingdom, their exposure levels would fall to 2 mrem/year, a figure which is 25 times lower than that reported for the United States (Radiological Hazards to Patients, 1960). The big difference between practice in the United Kingdom and the United States reflects both the number of procedures performed per capita, and the dose delivered per procedure.

Table 4

Comparison of reported annual GSD from diagnostic roentgenology

STUDY	GSD (millirads)	EXAMINATIONS PER 100 POPULATION
United States (1964)	55	53
Sweden (1955)	38	29
Japan (1960)	39	41
Denmark (1956)	22	24
Great Britain (1957-58)	14	28
New Zealand (1963)	12	37

A careful survey of diagnostic X-ray exposures was conducted by the USPHS in 1964 (Gitlin and Lawrence, 1964). Table 5 shows the distribution of the genetically significant dose by sex, and by general type of X-ray procedure. Of the total dose, 82% resulted from examinations of males, about 16% from examinations of females, and only 2% from exposure to the foetus *in utero*. Radiography, using conventional X-ray film, contributes the greatest percentage of the total genetically significant dose, accounting for about 96%.

Table 5

Estimated distribution of GSD from diagnostic medical roentgenology, U.S., 1964

	Per cent of GSD			
	Total	Male	Female	Fetus
Total	100.0	82.0	16.0	2.0
Radiography	96.0	81.0	13.0	2.0
Fluoroscopy (including spot films)	4.0	1.0	3.0	1.0
Photofluorography	1.0	1.0	1.0	1.0

Fluoroscopy accounts for only 4% of the total, and photofluorography (the mass miniature chest-screening procedure) for less than 1%. The dose from dental examination is much smaller. It should not be concluded, however, that dental exposures are entirely benign since estimates as high as 1 rem/year to the thyroid of the general United States population have been made (Morgan, 1967).

The relative frequency of studies in different regions of the body is shown in table 6, as well as the exposure dose, for the testes and ovaries. 27% of all studies involve the abdominal region and contribute the largest gonadal doses. The testes due to their unshielded position receive a disproportionately large dose (Penfil and Brown, 1968).

Table 6

Estimated average gonad dose per examination (U.S. 1964)

EXAMINATION	DOSE IN mR TESTIS	OVARY	% OF ALL FILMS
Skull	1.	4.	7
Cervical spine	8.	2.	
Upper extremity (excluding shoulder)	2.	1.	8
Lower extremity (excluding hip)	96.	1.	8
Chest			50
Radiography	5.	8.	
Photofluorography	1.	8.	
Fluoroscopy	1.	71.	
Thoracic spine	196.	9.	
Shoulder	1.	1.	
Upper gastro-intestinal series			27
Total	137.	558.	
Radiography	130.	360.	
Fluoroscopy	7.	198.	
Barium Enema			
Total	1585.	805.	
Radiography	1535.	439.	
Fluoroscopy	50.	366.	
Cholecystography	2.	193.	
Intravenous or retrograde pyelography	2091.	407.	
Abdomen	254.	289.	
Lumbar spine	2268.	275.	
Pelvis	717.	41.	
Hip	1064.	309.	

The distribution of genetically significant dose by type of examination is shown in fig. 5. For purposes of comparison, the distribution of examinations performed in the United States during 1964 is also shown. It is obvious that the contribution to genetic dose is not proportional to the frequency with which examinations are performed. Although the thorax accounts for over 50% of the examinations performed in the United States during a one-year period, such examinations contributed only 4% to the genetic dose. Abdominal examinations amounted to only 25% of those reported in the X-ray exposure study, but because of field size and location, contributed over 90% of the genetic dose (Penfil and Brown, 1968).

ESTIMATED % DISTRIBUTION OF GSD BY TYPE OF MEDICAL ROENTGENOLOGIC EXAMINATION, US, 1964

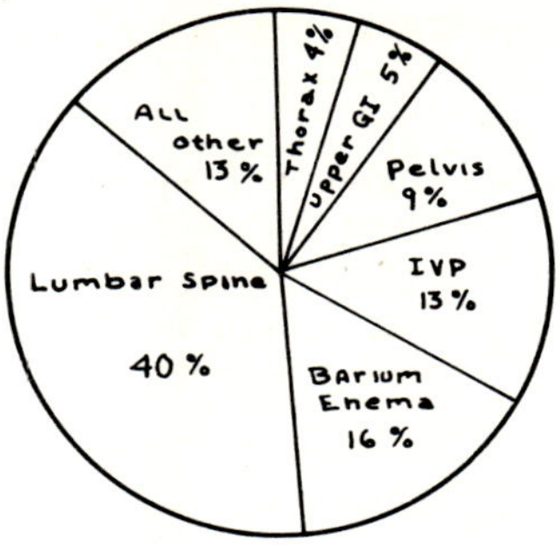

ESTIMATED % DISTRIBUTION OF RADIOGRAPHIC EXAMINATIONS BY BODY AREA EXAMINED, US, 1964

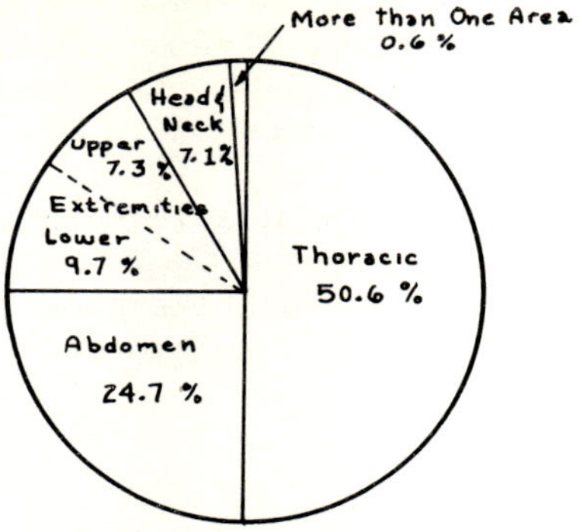

Fig. 5.

Reduction in radiation exposure per procedure can be achieved by the proper use of modern commercially available facilities and techniques. The most common causes of overexposure are listed in table 7 along with the magnitudes of the excess doses (Morgan, p. 29, 1967). Where abdominal radiography can substitute for fluoroscopy, a 100- to 300-fold reduction in gonadal dose can be achieved. Restriction of the X-ray beam to the field of interest can reduce exposure 2 to 100 times. Investigation of field sizes used by different types of X-ray users revealed that the use of beam areas four times as large as the film area were not at all uncommon. Restriction of these large fields can result in dramatic diminution of GSD. If film and beam size were the same, it has been estimated that the 55 mrem/year from medical diagnostic exposures would be reduced to 19 mrem/year (Penfil and Brown, 1968). The use of proper machine settings and positioning techniques can reduce dose 2- to 5-fold.

Table 7

Potential factors for gonadal dose reduction

Cause	Estimated excess dose (Multiples of optimum)
Fluoroscopy as substitute for radiography	100X to 300X
Excessive field or film size	2X to 100X
Improper technics	2X to 5X
Failure to use fast films	2X to 10X
Failure to use intensifying screens	2.5X to 100X
Improper film-processing materials or technics	2X to 5X
Use of screen type of film instead of screenless type when not using screens	2X

The use of proper films can result in 2- to 10-fold reductions, which can be further assisted by the use of properly matched intensifying screens. Correct film processing techniques can also result in 2- to 5-fold reductions in dose to the patient. All of these savings can be made without compromising the quality of the diagnostic information obtained, and in fact usually are associated with improved results. These savings, of course, can only be realized in those situations where poor techniques are being utilized.

The two other areas of medical uses include radiotherapy and radioisotopes. Radiotherapy procedures for malignant disease are most common in persons beyond the child-bearing age group. The majority of the GSD from radiotherapy, therefore, comes from the treatment of benign conditions and has been estimated at 7 mrem/year (Morgan, p. 48, 1967).

Radiation Dose from Internally-administered Radioisotopes

The growth of nuclear medicine and the administration of radioisotopes to people for diagnostic and therapeutic purposes has been very rapid over the past few years. The doubling time of X-ray procedures per capita is approximately 13 years, whereas it is close to 4 years for nuclear medicine procedures. Unfortunately, accurate current data of the type gathered for medical X-ray practices are not available for nuclear medicine.

The results of a survey made in the United Kingdom in 1957 indicated that the GSD from the clinical use of radioisotopes was 0.18 mrem/year (Radiological Hazards to Patients, 1960). At the time, the number of different clinical radioisotopic procedures was considerably less than today and reflects mainly the radiation dose from ^{131}I and ^{32}P.

Typical doses to different organs for a variety of diagnostic procedures in common use are given in table 8 as a function of age of the recipient (Seltzer et al., 1964).

Table 8

Average whole-body doses for various diagnostic tests employing radioactive isotopes

Radionuclide	Purpose of Procedure	Dose: Newborn mrads/μCi	Dose: Standard Man mrads/μCi	Dose: Standard Man mrads/procedure
$^{55}Fe_2Cl_6$	Plasma iron transport	120	5.9	147
$^{59}Fe_2Cl_6$	Degree and site of erythropoiesis	290	23.	115
$Na_2{}^{51}CrO_4$	Red-cell studies and splenic scan	2.3	.17	4.3
^{57}Co-Vit. B_{12}	Vitamin B absorption	54	5.3	2.6
^{58}Co-Vit. B_{12}	Vitamin B absorption	210	21	10
^{60}Co-Vit. B_{12}	Vitamin B absorption	2400	240	120
Colloidal ^{198}Au	Liver Blood Flow - Scan	5.4	0.54	54
^{197}Hg-Chlormerodrin	Kidney scan, brain scan	2.1	0.2	30
Na ^{131}I	Thyroid scan	10	0.45	27
R ^{131}ISA	Plasma Volume	28	1.7	17
Oleic acid ^{131}I	Lipid absorption	10	0.65	32.5
Rose Bengal ^{131}I	Liver function, Scan	3.7	0.36	36.
Hippuran ^{131}I	Liver function, Scan	.33	0.04	.6
$^{99}Tc^m$ pertechnetate	Brain scan	-	.01	100
$^{99}Tc^m$ Sul ur colloid	Liver scan	-	.015	30.

The limiting factor with internal emitting radionuclides is usually the specific organ dose. A radiopharmaceutical with the highest specific organ affinity is most desirable for organ visualization studies. This concentration also usually determines the upper boundary of the quantity of radioactivity that can be administered with safety. This table presents the average whole-body dose which in most cases is almost the same as the gonadal dose for various radioisotope procedures. The last column shows the total body dose for a standard man administered the amount of radioactivity commonly used for that procedure. The annual GSD from nuclear medicine studies has not been determined for the contemporary United States population. A questionnaire survey conducted by the USPHS in 1966, however, indicated a 4-fold increase in radioisotope administrations from 1959 to 1966 (Williams and Sutton, 1968). If one assumes a 10-fold increase from 1957-1969, and uses the GSD of 0.18 mrem/year from the 1957 survey of the United Kingdom, a value of 1.8 mrem/year can be estimated for the present day GSD. This may be an overestimate because although the number of radioisotopic procedures probably has increased more than ten times, the dose per procedure is diminishing as better equipment and radiopharmaceuticals become available.

The sources of radiation exposure and the associated contribution to the annual genetically significant dose for the United States population are summarized in table 9.

Table 9

Estimated annual GSD to the population

SOURCES	GSD mrem/yr	% OF TOTAL
NATURAL SOURCES		
EXTERNAL		
Cosmic Rays	50	
Terrestrial (Normal)	47	
INTERNAL		66.5
^{40}K	20	
Ra + daughters, Rn and ^{14}C	2	
ENVIRONMENTAL CONTAMINATION		
Nuclear weapons	1.5	
Waste disposal and accidental releases of radioactivity	0	0.8
MAN-MADE (NON-MEDICAL)		
Occupational	0.5	0.8
TV Sets	1.	
MAN-MADE (MEDICAL)		
Diagnostic Radiography	55	30.8
Radioisotopes	2	1.1
TOTAL	179. mrem/yr	100%

Natural background radiation is made up of external radiation from cosmic and terrestrial sources. These are approximately equal in magnitude in most places in the world and together add up to 97 mrem/year. Naturally-occurring internal emitters including potassium-40, members of the radium decay chain, and carbon-14 contribute an additional 22 mrem, bringing the total GSD contribution from natural sources to 119 mrem/year. This is 66% of the total GSD received by the general population. Less than 1% of the GSD is derived from fall-out from weapons testing. Even lower contributions are received from disposal of radioactive wastes and accidental releases of radioactivity. Occupational exposures and television viewing bring the total GSD to 122 mrem, which accounts for approximately 68% of the GSD received by the population in the United States. This leaves 57 mrem/year, or 32%, from medical uses, most of which are from diagnostic X rays. Of the categories of exposure that are subject to control, the medical exposures constitute 32/34 or 95%.

As medical care improves, the number of radiological procedures should increase. This could result in further elevation of the GSD from medical uses unless currently available technology is disseminated at a comparable rate.

In this report, we have attempted to outline the different sources of radiation to which the general population is exposed. Emphasis has been placed on general population genetic exposures for the reasons outlined earlier, and also because in studies of specific somatic or genetic effects, the relevant exposure depends on the sub-groups under study. These will be the subject of the discussions that follow.

References

Baldes, E.J., Herrick, J.F., and Stroebel, C.F. Biological effects of ultrasound. Am. J. Phys. Med., 37, 111-121, 1958.

Braestrup, C.B., and Mooney, R.T. X-ray emission from television sets. Science, 130, 1071-1074, 1959.

Brown, M.C., and Powell, C.H. Laser problems as related to the nations health. Hearings before the Committee on Commerce, U.S. Senate, 90th Congress, First session on S. 2067, S. 3211, and H.R. 10790. Radiation Control for Health and Safety Act of 1967. Part II. May 6, 1968. Serial No. 90-49, p. 1579.

Carpenter, R.L. An experimental study of the biological effects of microwave radiation in relation to the eye. RADC-TCR-62-131, February 28, 1967. Hearings before the Committee on Commerce, U.S. Senate, 90th Congress, First session on S. 2067. Radiation Control for Health and Safety Act of 1967, August 28, 29, 30, 1967. Serial No. 90-49, pp. 991-1049.

Donnelly, W.H. The spectrum of corpuscular and electromagnetic radiations: Their sources, uses, hazards and regulation. Hearings before the Committee on Commerce, U.S. Senate, 90th Congress, First session on S. 2067. Radiation Control for Health and Safety Act of 1967, August 28, 29, 30, 1967. Serial No. 90-49, pp. 344-372.

Ellis, R.E. An appraisal of the current fall-out levels and their biological significance. Phys. Med. Biol., 10, 153-176, 1965.

Gitlin, J.N., and Lawrence, P.S. Population exposure to X-rays. United States, 1964. Public Health Service Publication No. 1519, Sup. of Doc., U.S.G.P.O., Washington, D.C.

Ham, W.T., Jr., Geeraets, W.J., Williams, R.C., Guerry, D., and Mueller, H.A. Laser radiation protection. Proc. of the 1st Int. Cong. of Rad. Prot., 2, 933-946, 1968.

Hill, C.R. The possibility of hazard in medical and industrial applications of ultrasound. Br. J. Radiol., 41, 561-569, 1968.

ICRP. Radiobiological aspects of the supersonic transport (a report of the ICRP task group on the biological effects of high energy radiations). Hlth Phys., 12, 209, 1966.

Michaelson, S.M., Thomson, R.A.E., and Howland, J.W. Biological effects of microwaves. Hearings before the Committee on Commerce, U.S. Senate, 90th Congress, First session on S. 2067, S. 3211, and H.R. 10790, Radiation Control for Health and Safety Act of 1967. Part II, May 6, 1968. Serial No. 90-49, pp. 1443-1570.

Morgan, K.Z. Statement in hearings before the Committee on Commerce, U.S. Senate, 90th Congress, First session on S. 2067, Radiation Control for Health and Safety Act of 1967, August 28, 29, 30, 1967. Serial No. 90-49, p. 57.

Morgan, K.Z., and Turner, J.E. Principles of Radiation Protection. John Wiley & Sons, New York, 1967.

Parker, Frank L. Status of radioactive waste disposal in U.S.A. J.Sanit. Eng. Div., ASCE, Vol. 95, No. SA3, Proc. Paper 6597, June, 1969, pp. 439-464.

Parker, F. Recent developments in and future plans for radioactive waste management in the U.S.A. Atomic Energy Rev., 5, 93-121, 1967.

Penfil, R.L., and Brown, J.L. Genetically significant dose to the U.S. population from diagnostic medical roentgenology, 1964. Radiology, 90, 209-216, 1968.

PHS, 1967. Report of state and local radiological health programs. CCB 67-2, July, 1967. Bureau of Disease Prevention and Environment Control, NCRH, Rockville, Maryland.

Rentos, P.G. Microwave oven survey, Hearings before the Committee on Commerce, U.S. Senate, 90th Congress, First session on S. 2067. Radiation Control for Health and Safety Act of 1967, August 28, 29, 30, 1967. Serial No. 90-49, pp.344-372.

Seltzer, A.A., Kereiakes, J.G., and Saenger, E.L. Radiation exposure from isotopes in pediatrics. New Engl. J. Med., 271, 84, 1964.

Smith, D., Schneider, R., and Steiner, J. A pilot survey of X-radiation emissions from color television receivers. TSB No. 2, U.S. Department of HEW, PHS, NCRH, Rockville, Maryland, June, 1968. Also see PHS, TSB No. 3, 1968. A survey of X-radiation from color television sets in the Washington, D.C. metropolitan area. Technical Services Branch, NCRH, PHS, March 12, 1968.

Snyder, W.S. Health physics aspects of supersonic transport. Proceedings of First International Congress on Radiation Protection, 2, 863-869, 1968.

Spiers, F.W. Radioisotopes in the Human Body. Academic Press, New York, 1968.

Terrill, J.G., Jr. Statement in Hearings before the Committee on Commerce, U.S. Senate, 90th Congress, First session on S. 2067. Radiation Control for Health and

Safety Act of 1967, August 28, 29, 30, 1967. Serial No. 90-49, pp. 188-200.

UNSCEAR, 1958. Report of the United Nations Scientific Committee on the effects of atomic radiation. Supplement No. 17 (A/3838), United Nations, New York, 1958, para. 27, Chapter 2.

UNSCEAR, 1962. Report of the United Nations Scientific Committee on the effects of atomic radiation. Supplement No. 16 (A/5216), United Nations, New York, 1962.

Williams, K.D., and Sutton, J.D. Survey of the use of radionuclide in medicine: Preliminary report. MORP 68-10, USPHS, Washington, D.C., July, 1968.

Radiological Hazards to Patients. Second Report of the Committee, Her Majesty's Stationery Office, 1960.

CHAPTER II

EFFECTS OF RADIATION ON THE FOETUS, NEW-BORN AND CHILD*

Robert L. Brent

Introduction

Although there has been an increase in our understanding of the qualitative and quantitative aspects of radiation embryology, we are still not in a position to identify clearly the mechanism of the multiple effects of ionizing irradiation upon the developing mammalian embryo. In spite of this void in our knowledge, some important information has become available over the past 15 years that is important to the embryologist, health physicist, radiobiologist, and radiologist.

Acute Effects of X Irradiation at Various Gestation Stages

In the late 1940's and early 1950's, a great deal of information was published dealing with the effects of X irradiation on embryonic development. Because of the wealth of data available, a number of generalizations were made. Some of these generalizations have proven to be correct, others have proven to be wrong and some generalizations are still in doubt.

Generalizations that are obtained from Russell's work (1954) are that 200 R of acute radiation administered to the pregnant mouse on various days of gestation will have the following effects:

1. Very few or no congenital malformations will be produced in the pre-implantation period.
2. The peak incidence of malformations will occur following irradiation during the organogenetic period.
3. The pre-natal death rate (resorptions) will be highest following irradiation in the pre-implantation period and gradually will approach control levels in the early foetal stages.
4. The neonatal death rate is highest in the surviving embryos irradiated during the organogenetic period.
5. Few, if any, malformations will be observed in embryos irradiated during the foetal stages.

---

* Supported by AEC, NYO 2071-43.

At about the same time that Russell (1954) published her summary, we prepared a similar assessment in our laboratory (Wilson, 1954; Brent, 1960a) which also indicated that in rats malformations were more likely to occur in the organogenic period and that malformations were difficult to produce prior to the inner cell mass stage. These data differ in one respect from Russell's early data (1954) in that they indicate that malformations of the central nervous system can be produced throughout the entire period of gestation in the rat.

Over the past 15 years a number of other important changes have developed in the generalizations published in the early 1950's and important new information has now become available.

Pre-implantation period

Although the earlier observations were correct in saying that it is difficult to produce malformed embryos with irradiation at the pre-implantation stage of gestation, they were not absolutely correct in that in some species malformations have been reported but only with a low incidence. Russell reported (1963, 1966) that the sensitivity of the fertilized ovum to irradiation varies during the first few days of gestation (table 1).

Table 1

Effect of time of day on the stage of zygote development and sensitivity to irradiation on the first day of mouse gestation[a]

	Per Cent				
	No pronuclei	One pronucleus	Two pronuclei	Frequency of loss of sex chromatin following 100 R and 200 R	Fraction of control offspring per vaginal plug following 200 R
8.45 A.M.	86	3	11	...	....
11.00 A.M.	26	4	70	5.2	0
2.00 P.M.	0	7	93	4.5	....
3.30 P.M.	5	5	90	1.4	80.6
				No irradiation control 1.0%	

[a] Russell (1954).

Russell (1963, 1966) demonstrated that 200 R could produce an increase in the incidence of chromosome aberrations in the irradiated offspring. Just as lethality was dependent on the time of day that the embryos were irradiated, so too was the frequency of induction of non-dysjunction in chromatin material related to the time of irradiation.

The induction of mosaicism and mutations during the first 4 days of development were of interest because of the fact that a large percentage of the adult organism's cells will contain these defects. There is little quantitative data available for the human to evaluate the importance of these effects during the pre-implantation stage of development.

Post-implantation-pre-organogenetic period

Following implantation but before organogenesis begins, the embryo is less sensitive to the lethal effects of irradiation and has a low incidence of foetal malformations. On the other hand, growth retardation, which does not result from pre-implantation irradiation, can be produced in the implanted embryo even before organogenesis begins (table 2).

Table 2

The effect of irradiation on the 6-day-old rat embryo

	0 R	150 R
Zygotes	217	204
Term foetuses	201	159
Mortality	8%	28%
Term weight	4.87 g	4.38 g

It will be observed, in table 2, that 150 R delivered to the 6-day-old rat embryo results in a reduction in term foetal weight but will only produce a 28% mortality. In contrast, this same dose of irradiation when administered on the first day of rat gestation results in a term mortality of approximately 70% and no growth retardation will be observed at term.

Organogenetic period

Most of the studies in this field of radiation embryology have been concerned with teratogenesis. A high incidence of malformations can be induced with a relatively low dose of embryonic irradiation at the time that the germ layers and somites are being formed. This period of great susceptibility to the teratogenic effects of X irradiation occurs in the mouse in the $7\frac{1}{2}$ and $8\frac{1}{2}$-day-old embryos and in the rat in the $8\frac{1}{2}$ and $9\frac{1}{2}$-day-old embryos. The equivalent stages in human gestation would be approximately 12 to 22 days.

It is important to note that growth retardation can be induced with low dose irradiation prior to the induction of a high incidence of malformations. This observation is supported by data from our own laboratory which is presented in table 2. We noted that when 6-day-old rat embryos were exposed to 150 R, they exhibited growth retardation and an increase in mortality at term. Yet, the surviving embryos did not have a marked increase in the incidence of malformations. Skreb and co-workers (1963) have also demonstrated that the rat embryo is susceptible to the growth-retarding effects of X rays several days before the embryo can be malformed by X irradiation. Although growth retardation can be produced by X irradiation before the stages of differentiation, it should be noted that the stage most sensitive to the growth-retarding effects of X irradiation is during the period of differentiation which is the same as the stage for the maximum production of malformations.

There is a controversy about the lowest dose of irradiation which will cause non-reparable injury of the embryo and will have a deleterious effect. At the present time one country and a number of clinicians advise that therapeutic abortion be undertaken if a pregnant woman has received greater than 10 R of irradiation. In some circumstances, interruption of pregnancy is recommended when the exposure was less than 10 R. There is little information about the effect of irradiation on human embryos in this dose range. Not all the results from mouse and rat studies support the belief that 10 R delivered to the embryos causes significant permanent damage. This point is controversial.

There is other data which may be of some help in establishing threshold doses of irradiation at various periods of gestation. Brown (1964) reported that 2 R/day continuous irradiation did not alter any aspect of rat development or growth except a reduction of litter size after continuous irradiation for eleven generations. Havlena et al. (1964) irradiated the 36-hour rat embryo with as much as 100 R and reported no difference between the control and surviving irradiated animals with regard to learning and locomotor function as adults. Furthermore, they observed no congenital malformations in the surviving offspring. Meyer et al. (1968) examined the offspring of women, who themselves had been exposed to X-ray pelvimetry while in utero. There were no positive findings. Segal et al. (1964) studied the incidence of malformations in high and low dose radiation areas but found no evidence that malformation rates were related to background radiation. Tabuchi (1964) reported that diagnostic irradiation during pregnancy did not contribute to foetal disorders observed at term. Vorisek (1965) irradiated pregnant rats with 2.5 R/day and observed an increase in post-natal mortality in irradiated rats. The total exposure dose of continuous irradiation was 50 R. This observation does not agree with the results of Brown (1964).

On the other hand, Gentry et al. (1959), in a much criticized work, reported an association of increased malformation rates in humans in areas with higher background radiation. Jacobsen and Mellemgaard (1965, 1968) have reported an increase in abnormalities of the eyes of humans exposed to diagnostic irradiation while in utero. Rugh (1963), in his extensive investigation in mice, has reported that 10 R can increase the incidence of exencephalia in mice irradiated on the first day of pregnancy.

When the exposure dose is raised to 25 R, there have been reports of consistent morphological and histological alterations in the irradiated embryos. Russell (1957) reported that 25 R would alter the number of ribs and vertebrae in mice. Rugh and Grupp (1960) reported that the incidence of resorptions increased with as little as 25 R in the mouse, although Russell (1954) reported that a much higher dose was necessary to kill the pre-implanted embryo. Although 25 R produced some growth retardation in the 8 and 9-day-old rat embryos, the embryos that survived the irradiation were not stunted when they reached adulthood.

Rosette formation has been observed histologically in rat embryos irradiated after 9 days of gestation with 25 R, although all the rosettes disappear and are not seen in survivors at term.

In an early publication (Wilson et al., 1953) it was reported that 6% of rat foetuses irradiated after 9 days of gestation with 25 R were microphthalmic at term. If, however, we examine eye retardation data (table 3), it is clear that one must not confuse simple growth retardation with congenital malformations. Twelve-day-old rat foetuses described in table 3 received 100 R to 300 R. Although their eyes were small, they were no smaller than other structures in the stunted animals. Table 3 demonstrates the importance of analysing all the growth data before one says that an organ was preferentially retarded. In some instances, organ growth retardation is permanent and an organ remains small in the adult. This, then, may be considered a congenital malformation. One must differentiate between a small eye in a proportionately small animal and a small eye in a proportionately large animal. One should not label an eye microphthalmic unless the growth of the organism is evaluated as a whole and the eventual size and structures of the eye are determined.

Table 3

Per cent growth retardation of various organs and structures of term rat foetuses irradiated on the twelfth day of gestation[a]

Dose	Foetal weight reduction	(Occipital nasal length)^3	(Palate length)^3	(Eye diameter)^3	Liver weight
100 R	21.8	18.3	18.7	21.0	19.8
200 R	46.6	43.8	45.5	42.6	48.0
300 R	50.7	....	....	44.6	....

[a]Linear measurements were cubed in order to compare them with weight measurements. These data indicate that, although the eyes appeared small, they were no more retarded than other organs. Thus, microphthalmia may be a misnomer in this instance.

The effect of exposure to 50 R during the period of maximum sensitivity should be considered, without question, to be teratogenic. For example, though anophthalmia occurred in only 6% of irradiated rats, it is an irreversible effect. In practice, then, any embryo that has received 50 R during the organogenetic period should be considered to have been affected, although the incidence of grossly observable effects is low and the amount of growth retardation is relatively small.

Embryos that have been exposed to 100 R during the early organogenetic period will have a high incidence of congenital malformations, increased mortality, and permanent growth retardation.

Many malformations, involving all organ systems, have been observed in embryos irradiated during the period of organogenesis. The central nervous system and eye, however, are the organs most consistently observed to be malformed by X irradiation.

The periods of early and late organogenesis are the development stages when overall permanent growth retardation observed at term is produced. Doses which result in growth retardation at term also result in a reduction in the size of adult organisms. Permanent growth retardation can be produced by administering 100 R during the period of organogenesis and higher doses have resulted in growth retardation even when administered during the late foetal stages in mouse, rat, or the human. At the present time we do not know the lowest dose that will result in permanent growth retardation at various stages of gestation.

Our own work (Brent and Bolden, 1968) indicates that it is below 100 R. This may be one of the most radiosensitive effects of embryonic irradiation and one that should concern the health physicist.

Foetal stages

Over the past 20 years it has become increasingly apparent that the foetus is sensitive to the effects of X irradiation and that although grotesque abnormalities of major organ systems do not occur, permanent alterations can be produced in many organs and systems. Hicks (1958), Brizzee et al. (1961 a, b, 1967), Cowen and Geller (1960), Altman et al. (1968a, b), Dekaban (1968), and others have been interested in the selective ability of X irradiation to affect specific parts of the central nervous system. The specificity of the radiation effect is related to the stage of gestation when irradiation is administered. The severity is related to the magnitude of the dose of X radiation.

Hicks and D'Amato (1966) compared the gross size and structure of a normal adult rat brain in three animals that received 200 R on the thirteenth and seventeenth day of gestation and then on the first day after delivery. They determined that the degree of cortical atrophy varies with the stage of gestation when X irradiation was administered. A cross section of the most severely affected animals revealed marked atrophy, but reasonable gross organization. In fact, Hicks and co-workers (1966) originally reported that many of these adult animals with abnormal brains exhibited normal motor and behavioural activities. Microscopic examination of the irradiated brains exhibit irregular and bizarre neuron formation. There is no question that exposure of the foetus to 20 R produces discernible but subtle microscopic changes in the adult cortex (Hicks and D'Amato, 1963). It is interesting that these animals show no overt neurological anomalies. It is important to extend these studies to determine the extent to which some of the histological changes observed in the newborn are partially or wholly repaired by the time the animal reaches adult stage in development.

There have been some quantitative studies done by Brizzee and co-workers (1967) which demonstrate that the reduction in depth of the cortical plate is related to the dose and method of irradiation. It is interesting that protracted fractionation of the dose reduces drastically the effectiveness of the irradiation.

Other organ systems that have been affected specifically during the foetal stages are the thyroid and the diaphragm on the twelfth and thirteenth day of gestation in the rat (Brent, 1960a). Another interesting finding has been that testicular atrophy can be produced by two periods of irradiation of the foetus (Murphree and Pace, 1960; Brent 1960a). The effect is manifested following a relatively low dose of irradiation. As little as 50 R administered to 18-day-old rat embryos resulted in a reduction in the size of the adult testes. There exists another earlier peak for the induction of testicular atrophy during rat gestation. The same malformation occurs in the rat if the 9-day-old embryo is exposed to 100 R (Brent, 1960a). The fact that testicular atrophy can be induced by radiation exposure at two widely separate stages of embryonic and foetal development is a remarkable phenomenon and may indicate that although the result appears similar the mechanisms at each stage are quite different.

It is obvious from these observations that irradiation of the foetus can alter the structure of adult organs and tissues. In many instances it is difficult to evaluate the significance of these alterations, since they consist of cell and tissue depletions and, in some instances, organ hypoplasia. These subjects will be discussed in greater detail in another part of the paper.

In summary: (1) nondysjunction can be produced by X irradiation during the first day of development, (2) radiosensitivity of the zygote varies closely with the stages of cell division and, therefore, even the time of day during the first few days of development is critical, (3) the foetus is not resistant to the teratogenic effects of X rays, and (4) with low level (50 to 100 R) exposures effects of X irradiation are manifested at all stages of gestation, death during the pre-implantation period, malformations during the organogenetic period, and cell deletions (hypoplasia) during the foetal periods.

A recent publication (Yamazaki, 1966) listed the effects of low level exposures reported in the literature. The reported abnormalities occurred in embryos exposed to between 15 and 40 R. In many instances the abnormalities were observed before recovery processes were completed. In other instances, the experiments were performed poorly. The quantitative and qualitative effects of radiation in the range of 10 and 25 R should be investigated further with respect to their permanent and/or detrimental effects on the developing foetus.

Discrepancies in the Results of X Irradiating the Mouse and Rat Embryos

Exencephalia

Rugh and co-workers (1959, 1961, 1962, 1963, 1969) have reported that exencephalia can be induced in the pre-implanted embryo with as low an exposure dose as 15.0 R. The lesion is a familiar one and may appear in only one of the members of an irradiated litter or occasionally may affect more than one of the litter mates. Control litters, reported by Rugh (1959), had no animals with exencephalia. On the other hand, other publications of Rugh (1969) do mention the occurrence of exencephalia in non-irradiated embryos. We have observed exencephalia in non-irradiated mouse embryos in our own laboratory. Furthermore, Rugh et al. (1969) report the incidence of exencephalia following 50 R on the first day, and it does not differ greatly from the incidence following 15 R on the first day of pregnancy. This is unusual since one would expect a dose related response.

We have irradiated several thousand rat embryos during the pre-implantation period with exposure between 30 R and 150 R. With the exception of one control foetus, we have not observed exencephalia, although a significant number of embryos in the higher dose groups resorb after implantation (Brent and Bolden, 1967, 1968). Thus, there appears to be a marked discrepancy between the response of the pre-implanted mouse and rat embryo to irradiation.

Whole-litter resorptions

Another interesting occurrence that appears to be peculiar to the mouse is the phenomenon of whole-litter resorption following irradiation. Sometimes the response in the pregnant mouse is all or none; an entire litter may be resorbed very early in gestation. The phenomenon appears to be somewhat dose related. Russell (1965) postulated that whole-litter resorptions were due to maternal pituitary irradiation, but in our own studies we have always shielded the head and upper chest and yet we still observe whole-litter resorptions (Brent, 1968; Brent and Bolden, 1968).

Irradiation of the pregnant rat during the pre-implantation period does not result in whole-litter resorptions. In fact, as much as 150 R administered to inseminated females on the first day of pregnancy will result in the same incidence of pregnancy as in the unirradiated inseminated females. This is contrary to the findings in the mouse.

Thus, there is a species difference between the response of the mouse and rat embryo to X-ray "induced" exencephalia and whole-litter resorptions. These findings emphasize the difficulty in applying specific radiation findings from one species to another. These variations in species response must be explained before one can attempt to apply these data to the human.

Pathological Findings in Adult Organisms Resulting from Embryonic, Foetal, Neonatal, or Infant Irradiation

As indicated in the previous sections, the majority of investigations have been concerned with the pathological state of the irradiated embryo before the time or at the time of parturition. In recent years a greater interest has been exhibited in pathological alterations of adult organisms that have been irradiated in utero. The subject matter covered in this section will deal with pathological changes that may not be apparent at birth or would not even become manifest until later in life. Thus, the incidence and type of gross malformations, which can be recorded in term animals, will not be discussed except where necessary to support a particular point. The subjects that will be discussed are growth retardation, carcinogenesis, sterility, neuropathology, behaviour, neonatal mortality, eye defects, and longevity.

Growth retardation

There is ample evidence to indicate that growth retardation in new-born animals is a common and predictable consequence of *in utero* irradiation. Furthermore, the presence, absence, and degree of retardation are dependent on the dose of irradiation and the stage of gestation (Russell, 1954; Rugh, 1953, 1959; Russell and Russell, 1954; Brent, 1960a; Skreb et al., 1963; Brent and Bolden, 1968; Levy et al., 1953; Pobisch, 1960). The pre-implanted and undifferentiated mammalian embryo when it survives to term is not growth retarded by 150 R (Russell, 1954; Brent and Bolden, 1967, 1968). The early differentiating embryo is retarded in growth at term as is the late differentiating embryo. As the foetus proceeds through gestation, the 150 R dose is less effective in producing stunting at term but this may be due to a combination of factors in the rat and mouse: increasing radioresistance and increasing proximity of the irradiation time and parturition. There is ample evidence to indicate that the differentiating human embryo may be severely growth-retarded at term by high doses of irradiation (Murphy, 1929, 1952; Dekaban, 1968). There are also many case reports indicating both the obvious presence or absence of severe growth retardation when the human foetus is irradiated late in gestation (Dekaban, 1968; Glass, 1944; Ronderos, 1961; Murphy, 1929, 1952). There are not enough documented survivors of embryonic irradiation during the first week of gestation to determine whether the human foetus is not growth-retarded at term. Furthermore, if the dose of irradiation exceeds 200 R at this time, there is a reasonable probability that the zygote will not survive (Brent and Bolden, 1968; Russell, 1954).

Two obvious questions arise when considering the post-partum growth in irradiated embryos.

1. Is post-partum growth affected more or less than growth *in utero* when the embryo is irradiated?

2. Are the stages during which maximum *in utero* growth retardation is induced by irradiation the same stages when post partum growth is maximally affected?

3. Does irradiation during the pre-implantation period result in post-partum growth retardation in the survivors?

Rugh, Duhamel, Osborne and Varma (1964) and Rugh et al. (1966) examined the effect of intra-uterine irradiation on the post-partum growth of mice. They found that 100 R would produce growth retardation in 4-month-old mice if administered on any day from the eighth to the eighteenth day of gestation (fig. 1). Irradiation on the twelfth and thirteenth days of gestation resulted in the most retardation of growth at 4 months of age. This growth retardation was not only manifested by a decrease in body weight but also a decrease in measurements of the long bones and skull. It is interesting that the severest degree of in utero growth retardation occurs several days earlier but apparently the younger, "more sensitive" embryo has a greater capacity to approach its adult size than does the 12 to 13-day irradiated mouse embryo (Wilson, 1954; Wilson et al., 1953; Skreb et al., 1963). Rugh and his colleagues also demonstrated that the surviving pre-implanted embryo, which did not manifest growth retardation at term, also is capable of normal growth in the post-partum period.

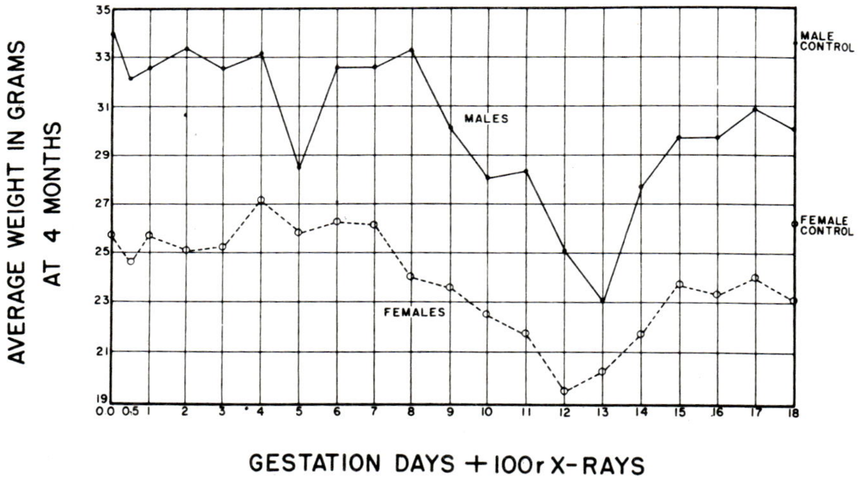

Fig. 1. Weight of control and irradiated male and female mice at 4 months of age following 100 R at gestational stages from conception to the eighteenth day. Note that permanent growth retardation is not produced until after implantation and is produced at every stage thereafter (Rugh et al., 1964, with permission from American Journal of Anatomy).

Although Rugh's data gives us an excellent profile of the growth-retarding effects of irradiation in the mouse, it does not indicate what the threshold dose is. Data from our own laboratory in the mouse indicate that the lowest dose that will produce growth retardation manifest at term is approximately 60 R. These data are summarized in table 4 and indicate that at term only the 12-day-old and 16-day-old embryos were retarded at birth after receiving 90 R. Yet, Rugh has shown that the 7-day-old and 8-day-old embryos exhibited growth retardation as adults following 100 R. In this instance, it appears that extra-uterine

Table 4

Mean birth weight in grammes (± Standard Deviation) of irradiated and control mice at term

Exposure dose Irradiation	Embryonic age (days)									
	0.5		7		8		12		16	
	N[a]	$\bar{X} \pm 1$ S.D.	N	$\bar{X} \pm 1$ S.D.	N	$\bar{X} \pm 1$ S.D.	N	$\bar{X} \pm 1$ S.D.	N	$\bar{X} \pm 1$ S.D.
0 R	31	1.5787 ± 0.2351	22	1.5749 ± 0.1766	19	1.6199 ± 0.1508	24	1.6251 ± 0.1532	18	1.6492 ± 0.2022
30 R	23	1.6300 ± 0.1857	18	1.6820 ± 0.1618	21	1.5767 ± 0.2317	19	1.6019 ± 0.2007	19	1.6448 ± 0.2553
60 R	21	1.7482 ± 0.2032	19	1.6089 ± 0.1315	22	1.6672 ± 0.2179	24	1.5969 ± 0.2222	21	1.5976 ± 0.1649
90 R	..	....	21	1.5745 ± 0.1652	22	1.6130 ± 0.1679	17	1.4901 ± 0.1571	19	1.5339 ± 0.1431

[a]N = number of litters; $\bar{X}$ = mean birth weight.

growth was a more sensitive parameter than intra-uterine growth. This is borne out by our own data in table 5 which indicate that at some stages in gestation the in utero threshold dose for growth retardation in adults may be between 30 R and 60 R. The stage when lower doses of irradiation had their greatest impact on post-partum growth was during the early foetal period of mouse gestation (table 5).

Table 5

Weight in grammes of irradiated and control female adult mice at 150 days of age following in utero irradiation

Exposure dose of irradiation	Stage of gestation irradiated			
	7	8	12	16
0 R	32.58[a]	29.38	30.99	30.04
30 R	29.78	30.56	30.38	28.43
60 R	29.28	27.80	24.28	28.47
90 R	28.46	27.58	23.55	28.12

[a]At least 70 animals in each group.

There are many other studies dealing with the effects of a single exposure of X irradiation on the post-partum growth of rodents (Levy et al., 1953; Murphree and Pace, 1960; Pobisch, 1960; Russell, 1954; Skreb et al., 1963) and goats (O'Brien et al., 1966). Murphree and Pace (1960) irradiated rats during the late foetal stages with exposures ranging from 110 R to 220 R. Rats irradiated on the twentieth day with 150 R were small as adults. All surviving rats irradiated in the late foetal stages with doses of greater than 110 R exhibited growth retardation.

In studies dealing with the indirect effect of irradiation on embryogenesis, Brent and McLaughlin (1960) demonstrated that 400 R could be administered to the pregnant mother or to the placenta (Brent, 1960b) without producing growth retardation of the foetus when the foetus or embryo was shielded. If the maternal organisms received 1,000 R or 1,400 R while shielding the embryos, then the foetuses showed retardation of growth but in these instances the mother lost considerable weight associated with radiation sickness.

The effects of chronic irradiation throughout gestation have been studied by a number of investigators. Russell, Badgett and Saylors (1959) administered a total dose of 200 R throughout mouse gestation and observed no effects on post-partum growth. Brown (1964) reported that 2 R/day given continuously for eleven generations, including the gestation periods, did result in a decrease in litter size, although the birth weight and weaning weights were normal. Coppenger and Brown (1967) reported that 50 R/day from conception to term had a marked effect on intra-uterine growth, as would be expected. Since two exposures to 50 R during the early foetal stages of rat gestation should produce growth retardation, these investigators also administered chronic irradiation (20 hours/day) to pregnant animals at the rate of 5 R, 10 R, and 20 R/day. These investigators were primarily interested in sterility, litter size, mortality, and malformations but their data indicate that the rat embryo can tolerate 5 and 10 R/day of chronic irradiation without exhibiting growth retardation.

There is ample evidence to indicate that retardation of growth occurs in the neonatal and infant mammal following irradiation. Billings et al. (1966) irradiated 4-day-old rats with 0, 5, 25, or 125 R and noted that growth retardation was only observed in the rats who received 125 R. Petrosyan and Pereslegin (1962) irradiated new-born rats with 50, 100, 200, 300, or 500 R. They noted marked growth retardation of the surviving animals given 300 or 500 R. There are numerous reports in the literature to indicate that the growth of the human neonate or infant can be retarded by the effects of irradiation (Conard and Hicking, 1965; Greulich et al., 1953; Miller, 1968; Murphy and Berens, 1952; Reynolds, 1954; Sutow et al., 1965). Following the exposure of children in Nagasaki, Hiroshima, and the Marshall Islands to the atomic bomb radiation or fall-out, there were many studies that not only indicated that infants and children were susceptible to the growth-retarding effects of irradiation but also that the younger children were more susceptible to these growth-retarding effects. Although there was definite growth retardation present in boys irradiated in the Marshall Islands, it is difficult to be certain if this is due to external irradiation plus thyroid irradiation, since an overall dose of 1,000 R to the thyroid, by radioactive iodine, was estimated to have been absorbed by some of the people (Conard and Hicking, 1965; Sutow et al., 1965). There is little doubt that dosages of 100 R or greater contributed to growth retardation in irradiated children in both Hiroshima and Nagasaki.

The extra-uterine growth of irradiated human embryos has been studied carefully by a number of investigators stationed in Hiroshima and Nagasaki after the atomic bomb explosions (Burrow et al., 1964; Tabuchi, 1964; Wood, Johnson and Omori, 1967; Wood, 1967c; Yamazaki et al., 1954; Burrow et al., 1965; Miller, 1956, 1968; Plummer, 1952). There were 86 children in Nagasaki who were followed until ages 13 to 15. There was a significant reduction in head circumference, height, and weight. The head circumference reduction was most significant in children who were believed to have received greater than 50 R irradiation. The presence of three factors were associated with the greatest reduction in head circumference: (1) symptoms of radiation sickness in the mother, (2) less than 1,500 metres from hypocentre, and (3) less than 15 weeks of gestation. It was also of interest to note that those children with a small head size at adolescence, had a small head size as infants. In other words, there was no "catch-up" growth since the smallness in head size was maintained through adolescence. The measurable retardation of growth in the group exposed <u>in utero</u> was not as severe as the growth retardation observed in children irradiated between 1 to 2 years of age (Tabuchi, 1964). This finding is not in agreement with the results of some animal experiments, but then the environment of the infant following the atomic bomb detonation might have contributed other factors that may have resulted in growth retardation.

Finally, there are scores of individual case reports in the medical literature describing the clinical status of children that were exposed to therapeutic doses of irradiation while <u>in utero</u> (Dekaban, 1968; Glass, 1944; Murphy, 1929; Ronderos, 1961; Scharer et al., 1968; Stettner, 1921). Many of these case reports are incomplete because either the exact time of gestation that the irradiation was given or the data on the growth of the child are inadequate. Dekaban (1968) collated the results from 26 cases and found them similar to those found in Hiroshima and Nagasaki. The most common finding following high doses of <u>in utero</u> irradiation is mild to severe growth retardation and the most likely time for this to be produced is during the third to the twentieth week of gestation (fig. 2) (Dekaban, 1968).

<u>Sterility following radiation of the embryo, foetus, neonate, or infant</u>

Laboratory investigations have been directed along two avenues. Some

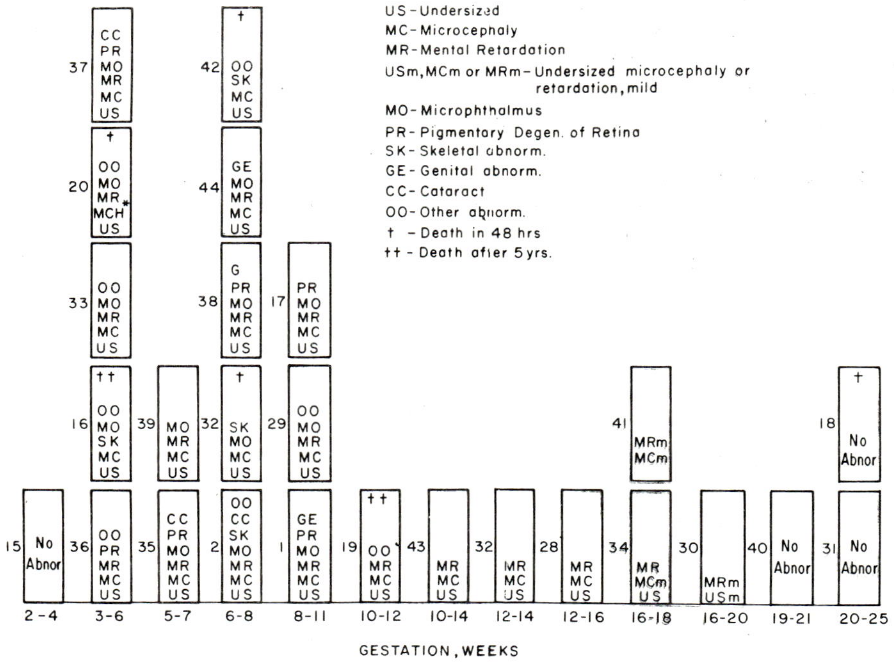

Fig. 2. The spectrum of malformations in 26 human infants irradiated in utero. Note that all infants receiving therapeutic doses of irradiation were growth retarded if they were irradiated between 3 and 20 weeks of gestation (Dekaban, 1968, with permission from Journal of Nuclear Medicine).

investigators have been interested primarily in the histological picture of the gonads following irradiation while others were interested in the functional capacity of an organism to sire or deliver offspring. In many instances, investigators have attempted to predict the presence or absence of sterility on the basis of histological interpretation, but it will be obvious that this cannot be done with any degree of certainty.

Because of the sex difference in the response of male and female, they will be discussed separately.

Male

Irradiation of the male rat embryo and foetus has yielded both interesting and unpredictable results. Irradiation of the 9-day-old rat embryo with 100 R results in a low incidence of severe testicular hypoplasia or aplasia. Only about 3% of the animals will be so affected but the animals are also sterile (Brent, 1960a). The mechanism of the testicular aplasia is unknown. Testicular hypoplasia or aplasia is not produced during the late organogenetic or early foetal period but begins to appear again following irradiation on the seventeenth through the twenty-second days of gestation (Hupp et al., 1960; Murphree and Pace, 1960). As little as 50 R on the twentieth day of rat gestation diminished testicular size from 3.5 g to 2.5 g, while 150 R resulted in testicles that weighed only 0.5 g. Although maximum reduction in testicular weight occurred from the nineteenth through the twenty-second day, minimal mating activity occurred in animals irradiated from the eighteenth through twentieth days. Male foetuses that received 150 R on the eighteenth, nineteenth, or twentieth day were sterile as adults and made no attempt to mate. Brown (1964) exposed pregnant rats to various doses of daily irradiation for 20 hours each day. The rats received 2, 5, 10, 20, or 50 R/day throughout their intra-uterine and extra-uterine life. All male animals receiving 10, 20, or 50 R/day were sterile. A second study performed by Brown (1964) limited the daily irradiation from the fifteenth day of pregnancy to the twenty-third post-partum day consisting of 1, 2, 5, 10, 20, and 40 R. The three highest dosage groups of male offspring were sterile from total doses of 300, 600, and 1,200 R protracted irradiation. Ershoff and Brat (1960) also noted significant testicular injury following 300 R of acute irradiation on the eighteenth day (17.92 R/min) and less damage from 300 R (0.03 R/min) administered from the thirteenth to the twentieth day.

Irradiation of neonatal male rats also resulted in permanent sterility, providing the dose of acute radiation was 300 R or greater (Petrosyan and Pereslegin, 1962). If the young rat is irradiated on the eighth or seventeenth day post-natally with 50, 150, 300, or 500 R (100 R/min) then testicular damage can be produced in 3% of the seminiferous tubules of 8-day animals given 300 R (Leonard et al., 1964). It is obvious that, following parturition, the rat testes rapidly lose the radiosensitivity demonstrated during the last few days of pregnancy.

Erickson et al. (1963) irradiated pregnant pigs at various stages of gestation with 400 R. Organization of the sex cords does not begin until the fiftieth day of gestation in the male pig foetus but yet 12% of male foetal pigs irradiated with 400 R were sterile as adults. After the fiftieth gestational day, the incidence of sterility rose sharply (animals irradiated at 50 days had a 50% incidence of sterility). This rose to 70 and 75% sterility in 55 and 75-day -old male pig foetuses. Pregnant goats were irradiated on the thirtieth, fortieth, and fiftieth days of gestation with 300 R. The male offspring were not tested for fertility but there were 32% less sperm, 26% less sperm activity, and 133% increase in abnormal sperm (O'Brien et al., 1966).

A great deal more investigation has been concerned with irradiation induced sterility in the female mouse than in the male mouse. Yet Rugh and Wohlfromm (1964) did expose 10.5 to 12.5-day mice to 100 R but did not observe sterility in the male mice. Although there was some reduction in the number of matings, the litters sired were normal in size. Although Petrosyan and Pereslegin (1962) reported that 300 R administered to neonatal rats sterilized them, Rugh and Wohlfromm (1964) found that 400 R to the neonatal mouse did not permanently sterilize the mice. In fact, they administered 100 R on each day of gestation or 400 R to sexually maturing mice and they concluded that these doses "are not sufficient to seriously affect the reproductivity of male mice over their normal reproductive period". The specific stage of maximal sensitivity for sterilization of male mice embryos or the minimal dose of irradiation necessary to accomplish the sterilization occurs during the latter part of mouse gestation (sixteenth day) (Rugh and Jackson, 1958).

Female

The effects of irradiation on the developing ovary is more fascinating and even less predictable than those reported for the male embryo and neonate. Beaumont (1962) irradiated pregnant rats at either 13.5, 15.5, 17.5, or 19.5 days post-coitus with 100 R and then sacrificed the female offspring at 100 days of age. The population of oocytes was determined. Animals irradiated at the 15.5-day stage with 100 R had the greatest depopulation of oocytes; namely, 241 rather than the 5,025 in control rats. These findings help explain the results of Ershoff and Brat (1960). These investigators reported that 300 R protracted irradiation from the thirteenth to the twentieth day was more effective than one acute dose of 300 R on the eighteenth day. This is understandable, since the eighteenth day of gestation is not the day when the ovary is the most sensitive to irradiation. The course of protracted radiation straddled the sensitive period for the ovary in the rat (15.5 days) as demonstrated by Beaumont (1962). Although sterility was not tested for, there were histologic changes in the gonad. Brown (1964) compared the sterilizing effects of low dose protracted irradiation in the male and female. After 11 generations of rats had received 2 R/day (20 hours/day), there was a decrease in litter size but Brown concluded that the male rat was overall more sensitive to the sterilizing effects of irradiation. This is predominantly due to the very radiosensitive period during the last few days of rat gestation.

The mouse presents a different picture. First of all, the female mouse can be sterilized by a dose of irradiation below 100 R and is, therefore, much more readily sterilized than the females of most other species and the male mouse. Secondly, the mouse ovary has its greatest sensitivity in the neonatal period rather than in utero. Rugh and Wohlfromm (1964a) tested the fertility of mice irradiated with 100 R from the time of conception to the age of 2 months' post-partum. A single exposure of 100 R was given on each day of gestation or to the neonate, 1, 2, or 3-week-old, or the 1 or 2-month-old female mouse. Irradiation with 100 R on any day of mouse gestation from fertilization to the eighteenth day did not result in sterile females, although the litter size of females irradiated on the thirteenth day was smaller (Rugh and Wohlfromm, 1966). An increase in ovarian cyst formation was noted in adult mice irradiated on the twelfth and thirteenth day of gestation. Only 44% of the mice irradiated as new-borns were fertile. One, 2, and 3-week-old mice receiving 100 R were sterile while those irradiated at 1 and 2 months had 16% and 14% fertility. Sterility was not produced by 30 R given to the new-born or 1, 2, or 3-week-old mice. In fact, 30 R to the new-born mouse did not even decrease fertility, but the fertility of 1, 2, or 3-week-old mice was decreased (Rugh and Wohlfromm, 1964a).

The explanation for these findings was demonstrated by Peters (1961), Peters and Levy (1964), Russell and Oakberg (1963), and others. Mice receiving 20 R on the day of birth had 50% of their small oocytes destroyed. On the other hand, the 1, 2, and 3-week-old mouse that received 20 R had 95, 98, and 99% of their small oocytes destroyed, respectively. The exact mechanism of oocyte killing is not understood, but the cells die shortly after irradiation, resulting in partial destruction of the pool supplying future mature ova. Although 50% of the small oocytes are killed in the neonatal mouse, there are 85% of the normal number of oocytes in the ovary at maturity. On the other hand, a 3-week-old mouse that receives 20 R will have only 1% of the normal number of oocytes at maturity. The change in oocyte sensitivity is believed to be due to the synchrony of mouse oocyte development and the transformation of oocytes of the new-born in the early diplotene stage to the highly sensitive late diplotene and pachytene stages in the 1 to 3-week-old mice.

During the sensitive period the oocyte is very sensitive to changes in dose rate. Ten-day-old female mice exposed to 25 R at a dose rate of 0.009 R/min had ten times the number of surviving oocytes than at 2.85 R/min. This indicates that there are repair processes in the oocyte (Russell and Oakberg, 1963). Russell et al. (1959) exposed pregnant mice to 200 R irradiation protracted over the entire period of gestation and noted a slight reduction in adult female fertility.

O'Brien et al. (1966) exposed pregnant goats to 300 R on the thirtieth day of gestation and found that the exposed females had a normal number of oocytes as adults.

Fractionation of the 300 R dose, with exposures at 30, 40, and 50 days, resulted in a decrease in the number of follicles in the ovaries of the surviving goats to 59% of the controls.

Apparently, the rhesus monkey is more resistant to the sterilizing effects of irradiation since the minimal dose to sterilize the monkey foetus was approximately 2,000 R. Although the primary oocytes disappeared within 2 days following 140 to 300 R in the mouse and rat at the primordial stage, the monkey needed 700 R to accomplish the same results (Baker and Beaumont, 1967). The radiation resistance of the monkey oocytes may be due to the asynchronous development of the germ cells.

There is little data on the effect of irradiation in utero on the fertility of the offspring in the human. The large number of survivors in Hiroshima and Nagasaki exposed in utero have not lived long enough to have complete fertility histories. Mondorf and Faber (1968) studied the fertility of 180 females who had been examined fluoroscopically for intussuception during their infancy. They found no difference between the number of children born and the age distribution of births in the controls and the exposed girls. The gonadal exposure dose was estimated to be 1 to 5 R. Tabuchi (1964) reviewed the data of the Atomic Bomb Casualty Commission in Japan and found the menarche was delayed in girls exposed to high doses of irradiation while in utero (1 to 3 months).

It is evident that it is very difficult to generalize about the effects of irradiation in utero during the neonatal period on subsequent sterility. There are marked sex and species differences in the response to irradiation and also marked variations in the response among females.

Induction of malignancy

The embryo and foetus have been considered more sensitive to the effects of irradiation than the adult. This conclusion resulted from observations made on the lethal effects of irradiation. The increased sensitivity is due primarily to the destruction of cells or the disorganization of complicated developmental processes at critical periods of development. At the same time the embryo does have the ability to repair cellular radiation damage and to replace cells that are destroyed. The question then arises, is the embryo or neonate which survives irradiation and appears normal, susceptible to the long-term effects of irradiation such as shortening of life-span or tumour induction? Is the sensitivity of the embryo to these long-term effects greater or less than the sensitivity of the adult organism?

Stewart and her colleagues (1956, 1958) suggested that the human embryo was more sensitive to the leukaemogenic effects of irradiation and more recently they have concluded that other tumours also occur more frequently following diagnostic radiographic procedures performed during pregnancy (primarily pelvimetry). The present estimate is that 1 to 2 rads of in utero irradiation increases the chance of leukaemia developing in the offspring by a factor of 1.5 to 2.0. This increase is considerably greater than the result of 2 R of irradiation to adults. In fact, 2 rads delivered to an adult population would not make a perceptible change in the incidence of leukaemia (Lewis, 1957). Lillienfeld (1966) reviewed the epidemiological considerations of leukaemogenesis. The results of Lillienfeld (1966), McMahon and Hutchinson (1964), Graham et al. (1966), Polhemus and Koch (1959), Yamazaki (1966), Ager et al. (1965), and Ford and Patterson (1959) support the thesis that diagnostic irradiation absorbed in utero increases the risk of leukaemia. Six of nine studies reported in Lillienfeld's paper reported an increase in leukaemia risk of 1.3 to 1.8 following diagnostic irradiation in utero. Lillienfeld states: "When one considers the variety of control groups used and the sampling variability, the results are remarkably consistent in showing an excess frequency of leukaemia among children of radiation exposed pregnant mothers."

There are a number of interesting associations with this data that should be pointed out. In Stewart's studies there was an association of a higher incidence of abortion history in the mothers receiving pelvimetry and also the children in the pelvimetry group had a higher incidence of upper respiratory infections. Tabuchi et al. (1967) reported no increase in leukaemia following diagnostic radiographic procedures. In some of the studies that did not report an increased risk of leukaemia, the number of patients was small. Of the 86 human cases exposed in utero at Nagasaki, none developed leukaemia (Burrow et al., 1964). These individuals received considerably higher doses of irradiation than those patients in the previous studies.

It is of interest that Graham et al. (1966) reported an increased risk of leukaemia that was identical, whether the mother received irradiation from diagnostic procedures before conception or after conception. Hoshino et al. (1965) reported no increase in leukaemia in a study of 17,700 children of parents receiving preconception irradiation. The question arises, do the same biases which contribute to the increased risk of leukaemia in the studies of preconception irradiation appear in the in utero irradiation studies? Graham et al. (1966) pointed out that children of mothers with a history of abortion or stillbirth also had children with a higher risk of leukaemia.

At the present time there are investigators who believe that in utero exposure to low dose radiation can increase the risk of leukaemia and other malignancies and other investigators who question this inference. Until the mechanism for leukaemia induction is understood, there will always be questions about this phenomenon.

It has been thought that the work of Bloom et al. (1968) might explain the increased leukaemia risk of patients exposed to irradiation in utero. They examined 38 survivors of irradiation in utero who received more than 100 rads and found a much higher incidence of chromosome rearrangement in the irradiated group. Since many instances of leukaemia are associated with either diseases transmitted genetically or diseases associated with chromosome abnormalities, the work of Bloom et al. seemed important. Fraumeni and Miller (1967) reviewed the diseases associated with leukaemia. These are Down's syndrome, Klinefelter's syndrome, D-trisomy, Bloom's syndrome, Fanconi's syndrome, the congenital agammaglobulinemias, ataxi telangiectasia, and Wiskott-Aldrich syndrome. The problem with this line of investigation is that two laboratories have now reported that human foetuses or young infants exposed to diagnostic radiographic procedures did not have an increased incidence of cells with chromosome abnormalities (Macintyre et al., 1965; Reisman et al., 1967). Thus it appears that we cannot invoke a cytogenetic hypothesis to explain the increased risk of leukaemia from pelvimetry.

It also appears that infants have an increased susceptibility to the leukaemogenic effects of irradiation. Irradiated children under the age of ten in Hiroshima and Nagasaki had six times greater risk of leukaemia than the control population. Children exposed between 10 and 19 years of age had 18 times the risk of leukaemia compared with the control population. Kitabatake (1966a, b) reported 1,197 leukaemic and 581 lymphoma patients and the association of these diseases with diagnostic and therapeutic doses of irradiation. Only about 20% of the patients in this study were children and there was no association between previous diagnostic irradiation and an increased risk of leukaemia. There was a definite increase in the risk of leukaemia following radiation therapy. This was also true for lymphoma, but the risk was not as great. Simpson et al. (1955) reported an increased incidence of leukaemia in children following irradiation of the thymus in infancy. From these data there is no way to determine whether the infant has greater susceptibility to leukaemia than the adult, since there is no disease or radiation therapy protocol that can be compared with the treatment of children with an enlarged thymus. There are not many animal experiments which can be used for comparison. Billings et al. (1966) reported the incidence of tumours in 4-day-old rats following 0, 5, 25, and 125 R. None of the groups had an increase in the incidence of tumours in spite of the fact that the 125 R group had a 10% reduction in life-span. On the other hand, Toth (1968) reviewed experiments dealing with chemical carcinogenesis in the new-born. He reported that in some instances the new-born had a greater susceptibility to chemical carcinogens compared with adults, although other carcinogens were more effective when administered to adult animals.

There is ample evidence to support the hypothesis that therapeutic doses of irradiation of 250 R to 1500 R can induce carcinoma of thyroid (Duffy and Fitzgerald, 1950; Simpson et al., 1955; Polhemus and Koch, 1959; Toyooka et al., 1963; Hagler et al., 1966; Silverman, 1966; Burke et al., 1967; Albright and Allday, 1967). In most instances the carcinoma followed radiation therapy to an enlarged thymus. Other forms of therapy were radiation to the tonsil and lymph nodes (Hagler et al., 1966), radioactive iodine therapy (Burke et al., 1967), and radiation therapy for the treatment of adolescent acne (Albright and Allday, 1967). It has been estimated that the threshold dose for carcinoma of the thyroid in childhood is 180 R and it has been reported that diagnostic irradiation does not increase the incidence of carcinoma of the thyroid (Silverman, 1966). High doses of radiation (1,000 R) to 6 to 7-week-old rats resulted in an increase in thyroid adenomas and a slight increase in carcinoma of the thyroid. No laboratory has determined simultaneously the susceptibility of infant and adult rats to radiation-induced thyroid cancer.

Rugh et al. (1966) irradiated mice with 100 R on each day of gestation and observed the incidence of tumours in the offspring. There was no statistical increase in the incidence of tumours in adult animals from irradiation in utero on any day. Brent and Bolden (1968) irradiated pregnant mice with 30, 60, and 90 R after $\frac{1}{2}$, $7\frac{1}{2}$, $8\frac{1}{2}$, $12\frac{1}{2}$, and $16\frac{1}{2}$ days of gestation. They also did not observe an increase in the incidence of tumours diagnosed grossly.

It appears that high doses of irradiation can produce malignancy in children. There may even be an increased susceptibility to radiation-induced tumourogenesis in children. The increased incidence of cancer in children exposed in utero to diagnostic radiation has to be clarified in view of the fact that higher doses of irradiation to animal embryos and the children exposed in utero at Hiroshima and Nagasaki do not result in a significant increase in the incidence of malignancy. One cannot overstress either the importance of the multiplicity of factors involved or the difficulties in their identification and control. Even laboratory experiments dealing with tumour production can present serious difficulties. For example, Ross and Bras (1965) reported that the incidence of spontaneous tumours varied with the diet and weight of the animals. Heavier animals on high protein diets had a higher incidence of tumours than did the lighter rats on low protein diets. We, therefore, close this section leaving many unanswered and unanswerable questions concerning the relationship between leukaemia and malignancy in children exposed to diagnostic irradiation in utero.

Neuropathological, neurological, and behaviour abnormalities

There are a number of publications that review, in part, this subject and should be noted as excellent source material (Furchtgott, 1963; Hicks, 1958; Hicks and D'Amato, 1966;

Werboff, 1963; Cowen and Geller, 1960).

Probably the most important information available to investigators interested in the effects of irradiation on the brain and behaviour can be derived from reports dealing with irradiated human embryos and foetuses. The reports suggest that children exposed in utero to doses of irradiation above 100 R and during the third to the twelfth week have an increased probability of being microcephalic, mentally retarded, or both (Burrow et al., 1964; Miller, 1956, 1968; Wood, Johnson and Omori, 1967a, b; Yamazaki et al., 1954). There are individual case reports of pregnant women being treated for carcinoma of the cervix who bore microcephalic infants that were mentally retarded. Dekaban (1968) reviewed 26 cases in the literature and contributed a case report of his own; namely, a woman in the third month of pregnancy, who was treated for rheumatoid spondylitis. The infant received 900 R. The child was severely microcephalic, having hypoplasia of the brain and dilated ventricles. The next commonest pathological finding was microcephaly. It was present in the majority of infants irradiated from the second to the twentieth week with high doses of irradiation. Mental retardation was the third most common finding in this group of patients. There are scores of case reports in the literature but they cannot be all individually discussed (Glass, 1944; Murphy, 1929; Geets, 1967). Several representative cases demonstrated the variability of the human foetuses response. Stettner (1921) reported that an infant was born to a mother who received radiation therapy for a uterine myoma during the latter part of the first trimester. Not only did the child have microcephaly and other malformations but there were also general disturbances of co-ordination. Scharer et al. (1968) reported an infant with microcephaly and severe retardation of motor development whose mother was treated with radiation therapy. Another example is of interest because the child is reported to be normal and the other, who was treated for carcinoma of the cervix during the sixth to seventh month of pregnancy, was cured and is living 11 years after the birth of the child (Ronderos, 1961). A 40-year-old woman was treated with X irradiation and radium therapy over a 2-week period. The $6\frac{1}{2}$-month foetus was exposed to 754 R from X rays and 134 R from the radium. The child is now 11 years old and has grown normally and appears mentally normal. It is likely that exposure at this level resulted in some neuronal depletion. Driscoll et al. (1963) described the neuropathological finding in two foetuses, that received between 400 and 500 R, one at 16 weeks and the other at 22 weeks of gestation. Therapeutic abortion was performed following the radiation therapy and there was neuronal depletion in the cerebral cortex and the cerebellum. The histology was not inconsistent with the results of irradiating other mammalian foetuses later in gestation. The survival without neurological sequelae following exposure of a 6-month foetus to 988 R protracted irradiation suggests that repair processes occur in the developing brain. The fact that this irradiation was protracted may be very important in explaining the results in this particular case (Ronderos, 1961).

Irradiation of pregnant animals from the initiation of differentiation to parturition, results in a high incidence of central nervous system malformations. The exposure used by most investigators has ranged between 50 and 400 R with the lower doses being utilized during differentiation and the higher doses during the late foetal periods. Hicks (1958), Hicks and D'Amato (1966), and Cowen and Geller (1960) have worked out in detail the types of malformations that are produced in the offspring of pregnant rats at various stages of gestation and various doses of irradiation. Their contribution was the concept that the central nervous system maintains its radiation sensitivity throughout gestation in the rat. Many investigators were aware that the mammalian foetal brain could be severely malformed by exposure to 50 to 200 R during the early organogenetic period (Russell, 1954; Rugh and Grupp, 1959b, Wilson et al., 1953; Roizin et al., 1962).

The time-table that has been developed by Hicks and D'Amato and Cowen and Geller can be summarized as follows: Animals irradiated on the fifteenth to the sixteenth day of gestation with 200 to 250 R acute irradiation had severe forebrain defects. Those animals that survived the radiation and grew into adulthood exhibited microcephaly, heterotopia, corpus callosum agenesis, and interhaemospheric third ventricle. Following irradiation after the seventeenth day, absence of the corpus callosum was not observed. By the twenty-first day of gestation, the effects on the cortex were still demonstrable but were less severe than after irradiation on the sixteenth or seventeenth day of gestation. Cerebellar malformations appeared after irradiation later in gestation. Maximal depression of cerebellar growth occurred with exposure after day 18 and cerebellar hypoplasia could be observed following irradiation of rats in the immediate post-partum period. The histological pictures associated with these malformations in adult animals are well described by Hicks and D'Amato (1966). It can be stated that besides the gross morphological alterations, there was evidence of neuron depletion and "scrambling" of neuron fibres. The area and extent of neuron depletion depended on the dose and stage of gestation that irradiation was administered.

Dekaban (1969) has made some generalizations about the mouse that are similar to the findings for the rat. He based his conclusions on studies involving the administration of 200 R to pregnant mice at various stages of gestation. He states: "Diencephalon, olfactory system and a part of the limbic system had low sensitivity in the range of irradiation used; the hippocampus and basal ganglia were moderately sensitive between the tenth and twelfth day of gestation. The neopallium and neocortex were the most sensitive structures and severe damage was caused by irradiation between the tenth and thirteenth gestational days, while milder abnormalities occurred after exposure between the fourteenth and sixteenth gestational days."

There appears to be little disagreement concerning the deleterious effect of high doses of irradiation, but there is some difference of opinion concerning the ability of the irradiated embryo to repair some of the damage that is produced by high or low doses of irradiation. Hicks and D'Amato (1963, 1966) and D'Amato and Hicks (1965) reported subtle changes in the histologic development of the brain following 10, 20, 30, 40, or 50 R at various periods of rat gestation. The brains were studied from a few hours after irradiation until some animals were 5 months old. One problem with the study is that some of their experimental and control groups consisted of one animal each, although the authors stated that usually two animals were examined in each stage. These authors reported that 10 to 40 R regularly initiated changes that led to abnormalities of individual neurons and their organization in the cerebral cortex. They considered the threshold exposure dose for these phenomena was 10 R just after birth and below 10 R in late foetal life. "There was persistent retardation of differentiation of all layers of the cortex well into post-natal life after irradiation on the sixteenth or eighteenth day (rat gestation). In addition to cytologic and architectural abnormalities a notable outcome of irradiation of these foetal rats was a paucity of neurons in all the cortical layers, with a compensatory increase of neuropil so that there was little dimunition in cortical volume. The paucity of neurons was attributed to an injury to the source of neurons, the primitive proliferative-migratory cell system. The injury was sublethal and persistent and must have been transmitted through a number of cell generations because whole series of cell migrations to all layers of cortex, extending over a week in the 16-day irradiated animal was altered. The nature of the injury which seemed to make the proliferative-migratory cells 'forget' how many neurons a cortex should have but not what volume the cortex should occupy is unknown. It is suggested that in producing persistent or delayed changes, radiation may have more specific effects than is often supposed."

While Hicks and D'Amato (1963) have been impressed with the sequalae of high and low doses of irradiation to the developing central nervous system, Altman et al. (1968a, b),

Brizzee et al. (1961a, b, 1967) have been interested in the ability of the foetal and new-born rat to repair radiation damage to the central nervous system. Brizzee and co-workers found that fractionation or protraction of the total dose of irradiation could ameliorate markedly the reduction in cortical thickness produced by irradiating the foetal brain. If the dose rate is low enough or the intervals between irradiation long enough, then the repair processes of the cells of the developing nervous system can function quite well. Brizzee et al. (1967) were impressed with these repair processes even in the groups exposed to high doses at high dose rates. They said: "Although the total number of cells in the cortex is drastically reduced by in utero irradiation at the dose and rate levels employed, the surviving cels tend strongly to follow normal growth patterns and establish their normal spatial integrity." Altman et al. (1968b) irradiated 3-day-old rats with 200 R and observed marked depletion of the granule cells of the cerebellum. The necrosis of the external grandular layer was evident by 4 hours. Yet those animals which were allowed to reach adulthood had a cerebellum which was functionally and histologically normal.

The studies of Hicks and co-workers, Altman and co-workers, and Brizzee and co-workers were all performed with different doses of radiation and at different stages of gestation and the neonatal period. These experimental differences alone may explain why the residual changes in the adult organism were different. In any event, the two important aspects of these projects should be stated:

1. The lowest dose of radiation that causes irreparable damage to the central nervous system at the various periods of gestation.

2. The rate and mechanisms of repair of the developing nervous system irradiated at various stages of gestation.

There are several other interesting reports that relate to the status of the nervous system in adult organisms that have been irradiated in utero or during the neonatal period. Vernadakis et al. (1966) reported that pregnant rats exposed to 100 R on the fourteenth day of gestation resulted in a delay in neuromuscular development, as measured by response to electro-shock. Bonavita et al. (1965) reported that irradiation of the new-born rat with 300 R accelerated the maturation of the lactate dehydrogenase isoenzyme patterns of the developing brain. DeVellis et al. (1967) irradiated 2-day-old rats and found that the total protein content of the brain and the activity of a number of enzymes was depressed. Rugh (1963) exposed rats on the ninth day of pregnancy to 100 R. Those animals which survived the effects of irradiation until 24 weeks of age had electroencephalogram (EEG) patterns which were the same as the controls. Mice that had severe brain abnormalities had abnormal EEG patterns from birth and were destined to die.

Furchtgott (1963) mentioned in his review that there had been a marked increase in the number of publications dealing with the alterations in behaviour of adult animals that had been irradiated in utero. Most investigations have demonstrated that the effect of irradiating a pregnant mammal was due primarily to the direct effect of irradiating the embryo (Neifakh, 1957; Brent, 1960b, 1964; Brent and McLaughlin, 1960; Brent and Bolden, 1967a, b, 1968). In the field of behaviour, the question arose as to whether an indirect effect might be more plausible and so a number of investigations have been carried out to determine whether irradiation of only the mother could contribute to behavioural changes in the offspring.

Brizzee et al. (1961b) demonstrated that irradiation of the mother with 100, 200, or 300 R did not affect the ability of the offspring to function in a water maze. Meier and Foshee (1962) used a Lashley III maze to test animals that had been irradiated in utero or that came from litters whose mothers had been irradiated. They were convinced that irradiation of the mother was more detrimental than irradiation of the foetus. The problem with these experiments was that the shielding and radiation techniques were very primitive. Levinson (1962) suggested that to resolve the dilemma more investigations are needed in this area.

Animals that have been irradiated in utero manifest certain obvious clinical manifestations as adults. Sikov et al. (1960) exposed rats on the tenth day of pregnancy to 20 or 100 R and on the fifteenth day to 50 or 185 R. The offspring of the 185 R, 15-day group, exhibited diminution of the grasp and righting reflex at birth, progressive hind limb ataxia, loss of ability to hop, nystagmus and circling. Some females had myoclonic jerks in response to sensory stimuli. Some males had priapism at 3 months of age. Pobisch (1960) observed ataxia and trembling in the offspring of irradiated pregnant rabbits. Petrosyan and Pereslegin (1962) observed ataxia in adult rats irradiated during the new-born period with 300 R.

The offspring of rats exposed early and late in gestation to 100 and 600 R had difficulty in learning (Levinson, 1952; Brizzee et al. (1961b).

Tests for locomotor function of the offspring of irradiated pregnant rats demonstated diminished function. Werboff et al. (1961b) irradiated pregnant rats on the fifth, tenth, fifteenth, and twentieth day of gestation and the group demonstrating the greatest reduction in motor activity as adults was the group exposed to 100 R on the fifteenth day. It was surprising that Werboff and colleagues reported that 5-day pregnant animals that were irradiated also delivered offspring that had depressed motor activity since differentiation had not begun at the time of the irradiation. Lipton (1966) irradiated pregnant animals on the seventeenth day of pregnancy and 1 and 3-day-old rats with 200 R. All three groups had locomotor deficits. Lipton also correlated these neurological findings with neuropathological studies on these animals. Although the animals irradiated on the seventeenth day of gestation had cytoarchitectural anomalies of the cerebrum, the cerebellar architecture was not as disarranged as in the animals irradiated at 1 and 3 days of age. Furchtgott et al. (1968) irradiated 16-day pregnant rats with 100 or 200 R and noted that the offspring that received 200 R had increased locomotor activity but that this decreased as the animals grew older. Furchtgott et al. interpreted these results to mean that the irradiated rats exhibited fearfulness when exposed to novel situations, but with increased exposure they tend to approximate the performance of unexposed animals.

It has been reported that 150 R administered to pregnant rats between the seventeenth and twenty-second day results in a decrease in mating activity (Hupp et al., 1960). Furchtgott and Kimbrell (1967) reported that 200 R administered to rats on the sixteenth day of pregnancy caused depression of olfactory sensation in the progeny in adults. Tacker and Furchtgott (1963) found that rat foetuses receiving 200 R had a diminished ability to adjust to food deprivation cycles. Sharp (1968) reported that the critical flicker frequency was increased in adult rats that had been irradiated on the sixteenth gestational day. These same animals were similar to controls when tested for the acquisition, retention, and extinction of a conditioned emotional response (Sharp, 1965).

The susceptibility to audiogenic seizures in irradiated and control offspring was tested by several groups. Werboff et al. (1961a) found that adult rats that had been irradiated on the fifth and tenth day of gestation had a decreased susceptibility to audiogenic seizures while adult rats irradiated on the fifteenth and twentieth day of gestation had an increased susceptibility to audiogenic seizures. Furthermore, the relationships were independent of dosage. Cooke et al. (1964) administered 2 R/day for the first 10 days of rat gestation for a total exposure dose of 20 R. They found that the female offspring had an increased susceptibility to audiogenic seizures. The authors suggest that audiogenic seizures may serve as an indicator of low level radiation damage. There are obvious inconsistencies in both these experiments dealing with audiogenic seizures.

Brown (1964) reported that eleven generations of rats had received 2 R/day chronic ^{60}Co gamma irradiation without manifesting behavioural effects as measured by response to gravity, balance, reaction time, and endurance.

Stahl (1963) has reviewed the work of scientists in the U.S.S.R. in this field and summarizes the many experiments utilizing 200 R at various foetal stages. "When the Pavlovian terminology is converted into more conventional modern concepts, one sees that it compares fairly closely with parameters such as emotionality and anxiety level in test animals and it is these same parameters which have often shown deviations in U.S. work on antenatal effects. The published Soviet results are therefore very similar in their implications to the large amount of U.S. work on the same subject." The only work from the Soviet Union that is difficult to accept is the work of Piontkovskii (1958, 1961). He irradiated pregnant rats with 1 R/day for the 20 days of rat gestation. The irradiated offspring exhibited an increase in early motor activity and adapted to test chambers more slowly. The results of this experiment are just as difficult to explain as the results reported by Cooke et al. (1964) since the same low dose rate was used.

Hicks and his co-workers (Hicks and D'Amato, 1966) reviewed their own work which combines histopathological knowledge of the irradiated offspring and behavioural testing. They reported that adult rats irradiated with 200 R on the thirteenth, fifteenth, seventeenth, or nineteenth day of gestation were able to discriminate visual patterns as well as the controls. Rats with small cerebral hemispheres and scrambled cerebral cortices (200 R, seventeenth day) learned to press a bar in response to signals as well as control rats, but did not have the motivation of the control rats when time was limited.

As long as there is little attempt to correlate pathological neuroanatomical findings with behavioural or functional changes, there is only a small chance that this line of investigation will reveal any startling new concepts. Hicks refers to the combination of neuropathology and functional studies as functional teratology. It is the combination of these two disciplines that will aid in the understanding of the development and adult function of the brain.

Eye defects

Rugh et al. (1964a) conducted a very complete study in the mouse embryo dealing with the production of cataracts following in utero irradiation. Although 10 R, at any stage of gestation, did not increase the incidence of cataracts, 100 R, at most stages, increased the incidence of cataracts, with a peak incidence of 60% following the administration of 100 R to mouse ova before the first cleavage. The lack of stage specificity of this effect led Rugh to infer that response was not a direct effect on the embryo. Human embryos and children exposed to much higher doses of irradiation had a lower incidence of cataracts than reported in the experiments with mice by Rugh et al. (1964a). Miller (1968) reported no radiation cataracts in the in utero survivors in Hiroshima and Nagasaki. Dekaban (1968) analysed 27 cases of human embryos that had been exposed to therapeutic doses of irradiation ($<$ 400 R), and noted only two surviving infants with cataracts. Furthermore, one child irradiated during the first 2 weeks of gestation exhibited no malformations.

Cataracts have been produced in rats that were irradiated in the new-born period with 300 R (Petrosyan and Pereslegin, 1962), and in some instances microphathalmia was produced. Griem et al. (1967) reported no increase in the incidence of eye anomalies in human infants exposed to diagnostic irradiation in utero. Jacobsen and Mellemgaard (1965, 1968) reported 11 cases of eye abnormalities in 184 patients either exposed in utero or born to parents who were exposed to diagnostic radiation prior to conception. There were seven different eye abnormalities, but no cataracts. It seems unlikely that the radiation is responsible for these eye malformations but these studies should be continued in order to be certain of the data and also to clarify the aetiological factor or factors.

Longevity

There is at present no body of data dealing with in utero irradiation of human embryos that can be used to determine whether the human embryo and foetus are more sensitive to the life-shortening effects of irradiation than is the adolescent or adult human being. A previous section of this paper did present information which supported the concept that the human embryo was more sensitive to the carcinogenic effects of irradiation. Although there are some qualifications for this, there is no evidence from animal studies that the irradiated animal embryo is more sensitive to the tumourgenic effects of irradiation. Tumour induction is only one contributing factor to shortening of life and, therefore, the controversy over whether the embryo has or has not an increased susceptibility to radiation-induced tumours will answer only part of the question dealing with longevity.

The planning and execution of animal experiments concerned with the life-shortening effects of in utero irradiation should observe the following precautions:

1. The dose of radiation should not be teratogenic.

2. The litter size should not be altered by the in utero irradiation.

3. A minimal number of procedures should be performed on animals in a longevity study.

There are few longevity studies dealing with the irradiated embryo that have considered these pitfalls. In 1961 Brent and Bolden reported that 100 R administered to 9-day-old rat embryos shortened their adult life considerably, but many of these adult rats had obvious congenital malformations. A study just completed in our own laboratory indicates that irradiat irradiation of embryonic mice at five periods of gestation does not reduce life expectancy in the surviving embryos when the embryos were exposed to 30, 60, or 90 R (Brent and Bolden, 1968). It is obvious that more experiments are also needed in this area.

Summary

1. The present understanding of the acute effects of embryonic irradiation can be summarized as follows:

    a. Very few or no congenital malformations are produced by irradiation during the pre-implantation period. Even with exposures to 100 R to 200 R at the time of fertilization, a very low incidence of non-dysjunction appears in the live offspring.

b. The peak incidence of gross malformations will be produced by irradiation during the organogenetic period, although cellular tissue and organ hypoplasia can be produced by irradiation throughout the embryonic foetal and neonatal period, if the dose is high enough.

c. Growth retardation at term results from irradiation of the implanted embryo and exposure throughout the remainder of gestation. Thus, although the growth of the surviving embryo exposed during pre-implantation is not retarded, the implanted embryo shows retardation of growth before it is susceptible to the malforming effects of irradiation.

d. The pre-natal death rate is highest following irradiation in the pre-implantation period and gradually will lower to adult sensitivity in the foetal stages.

e. The neonatal death-rate is highest in the surviving embryos irradiated during the organogenetic period.

f. Effects of exposure to low level X irradiation (50 to 100 R) are seen irrespective of the stage of gestation; death during the pre-implantation period, malformations during the organogenetic period, and cell deletions during the foetal periods. Although lower doses of irradiation have produced effects, the thresholds have not been determined.

2. The effects of exposure of the embryo to 10 to 25 R have been reviewed. There are many questions concerning the significance, incidence, and persistence of the effects observed at these doses, as well as the validity of applying them to the human situation. Intimately related to low level effects are the magnitude of the recuperative powers of the embryo at different doses of irradiation and various stages of gestation. It is obvious that further research is necessary in these areas.

3. Discrepancies in the results of X irradiating the pre-implanted mouse and rat embryo were discussed. Exencephalia and whole-litter resorptions have been reported to occur in the mouse but rarely in the rat.

4. The pathological findings in adult organisms irradiated in utero have been reviewed.

a. Retardation of growth produced by irradiation in utero is not only seen at term but also persists into the post-partum period. The resistance to growth retardation exhibited by the pre-implanted embryo at term persists into adulthood. The retardation of growth produced by irradiation in the pregnant mammal is primarily produced by irradiation of the embryo. There is ample data from human exposures and animal experiments to indicate that growth retardation persists into adulthood. Animal experiments indicate that all embryos exposed to 100 R or more after implantation will exhibit some degree of growth retardation. Although the embryos in the early organogenetic period exhibit the most intra-uterine growth retardation at term, the early foetus exhibits the largest degree of permanent growth retardation. This may be due to the fact that the younger embryo can repair more completely some of the radiation-induced deficits. The threshold dose for radiation-induced growth retardation is below 100 R but the figure will vary with stage of gestation and variations in the dose rate.

b. Investigations dealing with radiation-induced sterility have been directed along two avenues. Some investigators have been primarily interested in the histological picture of the gonads following irradiation while others were interested in the functional capacity of an organism to sire or deliver offspring. In many instances it is impossible to predict fertility from histological examination.

There are marked differences between the intra-uterine and extra-uterine sensitivity of the male and female to radiation-induced sterility. In the mouse the male is more sensitive to the effects of irradiation in utero and the female is more sensitive in the neonatal period. There are also species differences in the minimal sterilizing dose and the optimal stage for sterilization of females. This is primarily due to the nature of the development of ova. In those species in which the ova develop synchronously and have the bulk of the developing oocytes at the same sensitive stage of development, low doses of radiation can eliminate a very high percentage of the future ova. This is an area where generalizations are not applicable. Sterilization following irradiation is dependent on many factors; the sex of the organism, the species, the stage of development at the time of irradiation, the dose, and the dose rate.

c. There is no question that high doses of irradiation administered to man or experimental animals are carcinogenic. The question discussed in this paper, however, is whether the embryo and neonate are more susceptible to the leukaemogenic or tumourogenic effects of irradiation than is the adult organism. Many studies have reported an increase in leukaemia and other tumours in human offspring that received as little as 2 rads in utero. These findings are discussed along with appropriate animal studies and the reports from the Atomic Bomb Casualty Commission. There are many epidemiological and aetiological questions that are still unanswered.

d. There is ample data to indicate that therapeutic doses of irradiation can produce microcephaly and mental retardation in human offspring irradiated in utero. Reproducible central nervous system defects can be produced throughout the foetal period in experimental animals. The type of malformation is determined by the stage of gestation at the time of the irradiation. The results following lower doses of irradiation (10 to 40 R) is yet to be clarified. There is no question that neuropathological changes are produced by low doses of irradiation, but the significance and permanency of these lesions is yet to be determined.

The central nervous system offers an excellent system to study repair processes following irradiation. There is ample indication that the foetal nervous system has significant repair processes.

The literature dealing with behavioural changes in adult organisms that have been irradiated in utero was reviewed. There is controversial and inexplicable information and yet there appears to be ample evidence that in utero irradiation alters animal behaviour. There has been little attempt to correlate the neuropathological with the behavioural changes.

This field of study offers great potential since it is possible to study behaviour in a large group of animals with similar neuropathology since the radiation-induced abnormalities are reproducible.

e. Radiation-induced cataracts and other eye defects have been reported following in utero irradiation. Inconsistencies in the human and animal data are reported.

f. One of the best measures of the long-term effects of irradiation is the reduction in life-span of the irradiated animals. There are no such studies with irradiated humans and the only adequately performed studies indicate that the surviving mammalian embryo is less susceptible to the life-shortening effect of irradiation than is the adult organism.

References

Ager, E., Schuman, L., Wallace, H., Rosenfield, A., and Gullen, W. An epidemiological study of childhood leukemia. J. chron. dis., 18, 113-132, 1965.

Albright, E.C., and Allday, R.W. Thyroid carcinoma after radiation therapy for adolescent acne vulgaris. J. Am. med. Ass., 199, 280-281, 1967.

Altman, J., Anderson, W., and Wright, K. Gross morphological consequences of irradiation of the cerebellum in infant rats with repeated doses of low-level X-ray. Exp. Neurol., 21, 69-91, 1968a.

Altman, J., Anderson, W., and Wright, K. Reconstitution of the external granular layer of the cerebellar cortex in infant rats after low-level X-irradiation. Anat. Rec., 163, 453-472, 1968b.

Baker, T.G., and Beaumont, H.M. Radiosensitivity of oogonia and oocytes in the foetal and neonatal monkey. Nature, Lond., 214, 981-983, 1967.

Beaumont, H. Effect of irradiation during foetal life on the subsequent structure and secretory activity of the gonads. J. Endocr., 24, 325-339, 1962.

Billings, M., Yamazaki, J., Bennett, L., and Lamson, B. Late effects of low dose whole body X-irradiation of four-day-old rats. Pediatrics, 38, 1047-1056, 1966.

Bloom, A.D., Neriishi, S., and Archer, P.G. Cytogenetics of the in-utero exposed of Hiroshima and Nagasaki. Lancet, 2, 10-12, 1968.

Bonavita, V., Amore, G., Avellone, S., and Guarneri, R. Lactate dehydrogenase isoenzymes in the nervous tissue. V. The effect of X-rays on the enzyme of the developing and adult rat brain. J. Neurochem., 12, 37-43, 1965.

Brent, R.L. The effect of irradiation on the mammalian fetus. Clin. Obstet. Gynecol., 3, 928-950, 1960a.

Brent, R.L. The indirect effect of irradiation on embryonic development. II. Irradiation of the placenta. Am. J. Dis. Child., 100, 103-108, 1960b.

Brent, R.L. The modification of the teratogenic and lethal effects of irradiation to the mammalian fetus. In: Effects of Ionizing Radiation on the Reproductive System, edited by W.D. Carlson and F.X. Gassner, Pergamon Press, New York, 1964.

Brent, R.L. The long term effects of embryonic and fetal irradiation. Pediatric Res., 2, 291-292, 1968 (Abstract).

Brent, R.L., and Bolden, B.T. The long-term effects of low dosage embryonic irradiation. Radiat. Res., 14, 453-454, 1961.

Brent, R.L., and Bolden, B.T. The indirect effect of irradiation on embryonic development. III. The contribution of ovarian irradiation, uterine irradiation, oviduct irradiation and zygote irradiation to fetal mortality and growth retardation in the rat. Radiat. Res., 30, 759-773, 1967a.

Brent, R.L., and Bolden, B.T. The indirect effect of irradiation on embryonic development. IV. The lethal effects of maternal irradiation on the first day of gestation in the rat. Proc. Soc. exp. Biol. Med., 125, 709-712, 1967b.

Brent, R.L., and Bolden, B.T. Indirect effect of X-irradiation on embryonic development: V. Utilization of high doses of maternal irradiation on the first day of gestation. Radiat. Res., 36, 563-570, 1968.

Brent, R.L., and McLaughlin, M.M. The indirect effect of irradiation on embryonic development. I. Irradiation of the mother while shielding the embryonic site. Am. J. Dis. Child., 100, 94-102, 1960.

Brizzee, K.R., Jacobs, L.A., and Bench, C.J. Histologic effect of total-body X-irradiation in various dose fractionation patterns on fetal cerebral hemisphere. Radiat. Res., 31, 415-429, 1967.

Brizzee, K., Jacobs, L., and Kharetchko, X. Effects of total-body X-irradiation in utero on early postnatal changes in neuron volumetric relationships and packing density in cerebral cortex. Radiat. Res., 14, 96-103, 1961a.

Brizzee, K., Jacobs, L., Kharetchko, X., and Sharp, J. Quantitative histologic and behavioral studies on effects of fetal X-irradiation in developing cerebral cortex of white rats. In: Response of the Nervous System to Ionizing Radiation, Academic Press, Inc., New York, 1961b.

Brown, S. Effects of continuous low intensity radiation on successive generations of the albino rat. Genetics, 50, 1101-1113, 1964.

Burke, G., Levinson, M.J., and Zitman, I.H. Thyroid carcinoma ten years after sodium iodide I^{131} treatment. J. Am. med. Ass., 199, 247-251, 1967.

Burrow, G., Hamilton, H., and Hrubec, Z. Study of adolescents exposed in utero to the atomic bomb, Nagasaki, Japan. J. Am. med. Ass., 192, 357-364, 1965.

Burrow, G., Hamilton, H., Hrubec, Z., Amamoto, K., Matsunaga, F., and Brill, A.

Study of adolescents exposed *in utero* to the atomic bomb, Nagasaki, Japan. I. General aspects: clinical laboratory data. *Yale J. Biol. Med.*, *36*, 430-444, 1964.

Chang, M.C., and Hunt, D.M. Effects of *in vitro* radiocobalt irradiation of rabbit ova on subsequent development *in vivo* with special reference to the irradiation of maternal organism. *Anat. Rec.*, *137*, 511-519, 1960.

Conard, R., and Hicking, A. Medical findings in Marshallese people exposed to fallout radiation. *J. Am. med. Ass.*, *192*, 457-459, 1965.

Cooke, J., Brown, S., and Krise, G. Prenatal chronic gamma irradiation and audiogenic seizures in rats. *Expl. Neurol.*, *9*, 243-248, 1964.

Coppenger, C.J., and Brown, S.O. Postnatal manifestations in albino rats continuously irradiated during prenatal development. *Texas Rep. Biol. Med.*, *23*, 45-55, 1965.

Coppenger, C.J., and Brown, S.O. The gross manifestations of continuous gamma irradiation on the prenatal rat. *Radiat. Res.*, *31*, 230-242, 1967.

Cowen, D., and Geller, L.M. Long-term pathological effects of prenatal X-irradiation on the central nervous system of the rat. *J. Neuropathol. Exp. Neurol.*, *19*, 488-527, 1960.

D'Amato, C.J., and Hicks, S.P. Effects of low levels of ionizing radiation on the developing cerebral cortex of the rat. *Neurology*, *15*, 1104-1116, 1965.

Dekaban, A. Abnormalities in children exposed to X-radiation during various stages of gestation: Tentative timetable of radiation injury to the human fetus, Part 1. *J. nucl. Med.*, *9*, 471-477, 1968.

Dekaban, A. Effects of X-radiation on mouse fetus during gestation: Emphasis on distribution of cerebral lesions, Part 2. *J. nucl. Med.*, *10*, 68-77, 1969.

DeVellis, J., Schjeide, A., and Clemente, C. Protein synthesis and enzymic patterns in the developing brain following X-irradiation of newborn rats. *J. Neurochem.*, *14*, 499-511, 1967.

Driscoll, S., Hicks, S., Copenhaver, E., and Easterday, C. Acute radiation injury in two human fetuses. *Archs. Path.*, *76*, 113-119, 1963.

Duffy, B.J., Jr., and Fitzgerald, P.J. Thyroid cancer in childhood and adolescence: Report 28 cases. *Cancer, N.Y.*, *3*, 1018, 1950.

Erickson, B., Murphree, R., and Andrews, J. Effects of prenatal gamma irradiation on the germ cells of the male pig. *Radiat. Res.*, *20*, 640-648, 1963.

Ershoff, B., and Brat, V. Comparative effects of pre-natal gamma radiation and X-irradiation on the reproductive system of the rat. *Am. J. Physiol.*, *198*, 1119-1122, 1960.

Ershoff, B., Steers, C., and Kruger, L. Effects of radioprotective agents on foot deformities and gait defects in the prenatally X-irradiated rat. Proc. Soc. exp. Biol. Med., 111, 391-394, 1962.

Ford, D., and Patterson, T. Fetal exposure to diagnostic X-rays and leukemia and other malignant diseases in childhood. J. natn. Cancer Inst., 22, 1093-1104, 1959.

Fraumeni, J.F.. and Miller, R.W. Epidemiology of human leukemia: Recent observations. J. natn. Cancer Inst., 38, 593-605, 1967.

Freedman, L., and Keehn, R. Urinary findings of children who were in utero during the atomic bombings of Hiroshima and Nagasaki. Yale J. Biol. Med., 39, 196-206, 1966.

Furchtgott, E. Behavioral effects of ionizing radiations. Psychol. Bull., 60, 157-200, 1963.

Furchtgott, E., and Kimbrell, G. McA. Olfactory discrimination in prenatally X-irradiated rats. Radiat. Res., 30, 217-220, 1967.

Furchtgott, E., Tacker, R., and Draper, D. Open-field behavior and heart rate in prenatally X-irradiated rats. Teratology, 1, 201-206, 1968.

Geets, W. Influence des radiations ionisantes sur le development du systeme nerveux. Acta Genet. ned. Gemell., 16, 275-309, 1967.

Gentry, J., Parkhurst, E., and Bulin, G. An epidemiological study of congenital malformations in New York State. Am. J. publ. Hlth, 49, 497-513, 1959.

Glass, S.J. Dwarfism associated with microcephalic idiocy and renal rickets. J. clin. Endocr. Metab., 4, 47, 1944.

Graham, S., Levin, M.L., Lilienfeld, A.M., Schuman, L.M., Gibson, R., Dowd, J.E., and Hempleman, L. Preconception, intrauterine and postnatal irradiation as related to leukemia. Natn. Cancer Inst. Monogr., 19, 347-371, 1966.

Greulich, W.W., Crismon, C.S., Turner, M.A., Greulich, M.A., and Okumoto, Y. The physical growth and development of children who survived the atomic bombing of Hiroshima and Nagasaki. J. Pediat., 43, 121, 1953.

Griem, M.D., Meier, P., and Dobben, G.D. Analysis of the morbidity and mortality of children irradiated in fetal life. Radiology, 88, 347-349, 1967.

Hagler, S., Rosenblum, P., and Rosenblum, A. Carcinoma of the thyroid in children and young adults. Iatrogenic relation to previous irradiation. Pediatrics, 38, 77-81, 1966.

Harvey, E.B., and Chang, M.C. Effects of radiocobalt irradiation of pregnant hamsters on the development of embryos. J. cell. comp. Physiol., 59, 293-305, 1962.

Havlena, J.M., Werboff, J., and Sikov, M.R. X-irradiation of the 36-hour rat embryo: Neonatal mortality and post-natal activity, learning and seizure susceptibility. Radiat. Res., 22, 193, 1964 (Abstract 74).

Hicks, S.P. Effects of ionizing radiation on the adult and embryonic nervous system. In: Metabolic and Toxic Diseases of the Nervous System, Vol. 32, Proceedings of the Association for Research in Nervous and Mental Disease, Williams and Wilkins, Baltimore, pp. 439-462, 1953.

Hicks, S.P. Radiation as an experimental tool in mammalian developmental neurology. Physiol. Rev., 38, 337-356, 1958.

Hicks, S.P., and D'Amato, C.J. Low dose radiation of developing brain. Science, N.Y., 141, 903-905, 1963.

Hicks, S.P., and D'Amato, C.J. Effects of ionizing radiation on mammalian development. In: Advances in Teratology, edited by D.H.M. Woollam, Logos Press, London, pp. 196-243, 1966.

Hicks, S.P., D'Amato, C.J., and Lowe, M.L. The development of the mammalian nervous system. I. Malformations of the brain, especially the cerebral cortex, induced in rats by radiation. J. comp. Neurol., 113, 435-469, 1959.

Hoshino, T., Itoga, T., and Kato, H. Leukemia in the offspring of parents exposed to the atomic bomb at Hiroshima and Nagasaki. Presented at Japanese Association of Hematology, 28-30 March, 1965.

Hupp, E., Pace, H., Furchtgott, E., and Murphree, R. Effect of fetal irradiation on mating activity in male rats. Psychol. Rep., 7, 289-294, 1960.

Ivanitskii, A.M. Electroencephalographic analysis of certain individual sequelae of antenatal ionizing irradiation of animals. Patol. Fiziol. eksp. Terap., 3, 21-26, 1959 (in Russian).

Jacobsen, L., and Mellemgaard, L. A retrospective study of the possible teratogenic effects of diagnostic pelvic X-irradiation. Proc. XIth International Congress Radiol. Excerpta Medica Internat. Congress, Series No. 105, pp. 1372-1375, 1965.

Jacobsen, L., and Mellemgaard, L. Anomalies of the eyes in descendants of women irradiated with small X-ray doses during age of fertility. Acta ophthal., 46, 352-354, 1968.

Kitabatake, T. Retrospective survey on medical irradiation and leukemogenesis in Japan. Tohoku J. exp. Med., 90, 25-34, 1966a.

Kitabatake, T. Relationship between medical irradiation and development of malignant lymphoma: A retrospective survey. Nippon Acta radiol., 26, 891-893, 1966b (in Japanese).

Leonard, A., Imbaud, F., and Maisin, J. Testicular injury in rats irradiated during infancy. Br. J. Radiol., 37, 764-768, 1964.

Levinson, B. Effects of neonatal irradiation on learning. J. comp. Physiol. Psychol., 45, 140-145, 1952.

Levinson, B. Effects of neonatal irradiation on learning in rats. J. comp. Physiol. Psychol., 52, 53-55, 1959.

Levinson, B. Comment on Meier's "Prenatal anoxia and irradiation: Maternal-fetal relations. Psychol. Rep. 10, 173-174, 1962.

Levy, B., Rugh, R., Lunin, L., Chilton, N., and Moss, M. The effect of a single subacute X-ray exposure to the fetus on skeletal growth: A quantitative study. J. Morphol., 93, 561-571, 1953.

Lewis, E.B. Leukemia and ionizing radiation. Science, N.Y., 125, 965-972, 1957.

Lilienfeld, A.M. Epidemiological studies of the leukemogenic effects of radiation. Yale J. Biol. Med., 39, 143-164, 1966.

Lipton, M. Locomotor behavior and neuromorphologic anomalies in prenatally and postnatally irradiated rats. Radiat. Res., 28, 822-829, 1966.

McMahon, B., and Hutchinson, G.B. Prenatal X-ray and childhood: A review. Acta Un. int. Cancr., 20, 1172-1174, 1964.

MacIntyre, M., Stenchever, M., Wolf, B., and Hempel, J. Effect of maternal antepartum exposure to X-rays on leukocyte chromosomes of newborn infants. Obstet. Gynec., N.Y., 25, 650-656, 1965.

Meier, G.W., and Foshee, D.P. Indirect foetal irradiation effects in the development of behavior. In: Effects of Ionizing Radiation on the Nervous System, International Atomic Energy Agency, Vienna, pp. 245-259, 1962.

Meyer, M., Diamond, E., and Merz, T. Sex ratio of children born to mothers who had been exposed to X-rays in utero. The Johns Hopkins med. J., 123, 123-127, 1968.

Miller, R.W. Delayed effects occurring within the first decade after exposure of young individuals to the Hiroshima atomic bomb. Pediatrics, 18, 1-18, 1956.

Miller, R.W. Effects of ionizing radiation from the atomic bomb on Japanese children. Supplement to Pediatrics, 41, 257-264, 1968.

Mondorf, L., and Faber, M. The influence of radiation on human fertility. J. Reprod. Fert., 15, 165-169, 1968.

Murphy, D.P. The outcome of 625 pregnancies in women subjected to pelvic radium or roentgen irradiation. Am. J. Obstet. Gynec., 18, 179-187, 1929.

Murphy, W.T., and Berens, D.L. Late sequelae following cancericidal irradiation in children, a report of 3 cases. Radiology, 58, 35-42, 1952.

Murphree, R., and Pace, H. The effects of prenatal radiation on postnatal development in rats. Radiat. Res., 12, 495-504, 1960.

Nair, V. An ontogenetic study of the effects of exposure to X-irradiation on the pharmacology of barbiturates. Chicago med. Sch. Q., 28, 9-25, 1969.

Neifakh, A.A. Role of the maternal organism in the irradiation illness of fetal mice. Dokl. Akad. Nauk., Biol. Sci. Sect., 116, 821-824, 1957.

Nichols, C., Lindsay, S., Sheline, G., and Chaikoff, I. Induction of neoplasms in rat thyroid glands by X-irradiation of a single lobe. Archs. Path., 80, 177-183, 1965.

O'Brien, J.P. Vertebrate radiobiology: Embryology. A. Rev. nucl. Sci., 6, 423-453, 1956.

O'Brien, C.A., Hupp, E.W., Sorensen, A.M., and Brown, S.O. Effects of prenatal gamma radiation on the reproductive physiology of the Spanish goat. Am. J. vet. Res., 27, 711-721, 1966.

Peters, H. Radiation sensitivity of oocytes at different stages of development in the immature mouse. Radiat. Res., 15, 582-593, 1961.

Peters, H., and Levy, E. Effect of irradiation in infancy on the mouse ovary. A quantitative study of oocyte sensitivity. J. Reprod. Fert., 7, 37-45, 1964.

Petrosyan, S., and Pereslegin, I. Acute radiation sickness of newborn rats and its remote consequences. Meditsinskaya Radiologiya, 5, 38-45, 1962 (in Russian).

Piontkovskii, I.A. Certain properties of the higher nervous activity in adult animals irradiated prenatally by ionizing radiations; the problem of the effect of ionizing irradiation on offspring. Biull. Eksp. Biol. Med., 46, 77-80, 1958 (in Russian).

Piontkovskii, I.A. Some peculiarities of higher nervous activity in adult animals subjected to irradiation in utero, Part III. Biull. Eksp. Biol. Med., 51, 27-31, 1961 (in Russian).

Plummer, G. Anomalies occurring in children exposed in utero to the atomic bomb in Hiroshima. Pediatrics, 10, 687-692, 1952.

Pobisch, R. Die einwirkung der Röntgenstrahlen auf den Kaninchenembryo mit besonderer Berücksichtigung der postnatalen Entwicklung. Radioligia austriaca, 11, 19-82, 1960.

Polhemus, D., and Koch, R. Leukemia and medical irradiation. Pediatrics, 23, 453-461, 1959.

Reisman, L.E., Jacobson, A., Davis, L., Kasahara, S., and Kelly, S. Effects of diagnostic X-rays on chromosomes in infants. A preliminary report. Radiology, 89, 75-80, 1967.

Reynolds, E.L. Growth and development of Hiroshima children exposed to the atomic bomb. Three year study (1951-1953). Atomic Bomb Casualty Commission. Technical Report, 20-59, 1954.

Roizin, L., Rugh, R., and Kaufman, M.A. Neuropathologic investigations of the X-irradiated embryo rat brain. J. Neuropath. exp. Neurol., 21, 219-243, 1962.

Ronderos, A. Fetal tolerance to radiation. Radiology, 76, 454-456, 1961.

Ross, M.H., and Bras, G. Tumor incidence patterns and nutrition in the rat. J. Nutr., 87, 245-260, 1965.

Rugh, R. Vertebrate radiobiology: Embryology. A. Rev. nucl. Sci., 3, 271-302, 1953.

Rugh, R. Vertebrate radiobiology: Embryology. A. Rev. nucl. Sci., 9, 493-522, 1959.

Rugh, R. Neurological sequelae to low-level X-irradiation of the developing embryo. In: Effects of Ionizing Radiation on the Nervous System, edited by T.J. Haley and R.S. Snider, International Atomic Energy Agency, Vienna, pp. 202-224, 1962.

Rugh, R. Ionizing radiations and the mammalian embryo. Acta Radiol., 1, 101-113, 1963.

Rugh, R. Effect of ionizing radiations, including radioisotopes, on the placenta and embryo. Birth Defects, Orig. Article Ser., 1, 64-73, 1965.

Rugh, R. Normal incidence of brain hernia in the mouse. Science, N.Y., 163, 407, 1969.

Rugh, R., Caveness, W., Duhamel, L., and Schwarz, G. Structural and functional (electroencephalographic) changes in the postnatal mammalian brain resulting from X-irradiation of the embryo. Milit. Med., 128, 392-408, 1963.

Rugh, R., Duhamel, L., Chandler, A., and Varma, A. Cataract development after embryonic and fetal X-irradiation. Radiat. Res., 22, 519-534, 1964a.

Rugh, R., Duhamel, L., Osborne, A.W., and Varma, A. Persistent stunting following X-irradiation of the fetus. Am. J. Anat., 115, 185-197, 1964b.

Rugh, R., Duhamel, L., and Skaredoff, L. Relation of embryonic and fetal X-irradiation to life time average weights and tumor incidence in mice. Proc. Soc. exp. Biol. Med., 121, 714-718, 1966.

Rugh, R., and Grupp, E. The radiosensitivity of the embryonic nervous system. Bull. Sloane Hosp. Women, 5, 49-52, 1959a.

Rugh, R., and Grupp, E. Exencephalia following X-irradiation of the preimplantation mammalian embryo. J. Neuropath. exp. Neurol., 18, 468-481, 1959b.

Rugh, R., and Grupp, E. Fractionated X-irradiation of the mammalian embryo and congenital anomalies. Am. J. Roentg., 84, 125-144, 1960.

Rugh, R., and Grupp, E. Neuropathological effects of low level X-irradiation of the mammalian embryo. Milit. Med., 126, 647-664, 1961.

Rugh, R., and Jackson, S. Effect of fetal X-irradiation upon the subsequent fertility of the offspring. J. exp. Zool., 138, 209-221, 1958.

Rugh, R., and Somogyi, C. Hematological recovery of mouse following fetal X-irradiation. Biol. Bull., 134, 320-324, 1968.

Rugh, R., and Wohlfromm, M. X-irradiation sterilization of the premature female mouse. Atompraxis, 10, 511-518, 1964a.

Rugh, R., and Wohlfromm, M. Can X-irradiation prior to sexual maturity affect the fertility of the male mammal (mouse)? Atompraxis, 10, 33-42, 1964b.

Rugh, R., and Wohlfromm, M. Prenatal X-irradiation and postnatal mortality. Radiat. Res., 26, 493-506, 1965.

Rugh, R., and Wohlfromm, M. Resistance of the prenatal female mouse to X-ray sterilization. Fert. Steril., 17, 396-410, 1966.

Rugh, R., Wohlfromm, M., and Varme, A. Low dose X-ray effects on the precleavage mammalian zygote. Radiat. Res., 37, 401-414. 1969.

Russell, L.B. The Effects of Radiation on Mammalian Prenatal Development. Radiation Biology; Part II. edited by A. Hollaender, McGraw-Hill, New York, 1954.

Russell, L.B. Effects of low doses of X-rays on embryonic development in the mouse. Proc. Soc. exp. Biol. Med., 95, 174-178, 1957.

Russell, L.B. Ciba Foundation Symposium on Preimplanted Stages of Pregnancy, edited by G.E.W. Wolstenholme, J. & A. Churchill, Ltd., London, p. 217, 1965.

Russell, L.B., Badgett, S.K., and Saylors, C.L. Comparison of the effects of acute, continuous, and fractionated irradiation during embryonic development: A special supplement to International Journal of Radiation Biology. Immediate and Low Level Effects of Ionizing Radiation, Conference held in Venice, edited by A.A. Buzzati-Traverso, Taylor and Francis, London, pp. 343-359, 1959.

Russell, L.B., and Montgomery, C.S. Radiation-sensitivity differences within cell-division cycles during mouse cleavage. Int. J. Radiat. Biol., 10, 151-164, 1966.

Russell, W.L., and Oakberg, E.F. The cellular basis and aetiology of the late effects of irradiation on fertility in female mice. In: Cellular Basis and Aetiology of Late Somatic Effects of Ionizing Radiation, edited by R.J.C. Harris, Academic Press, New York, pp. 224-232, 1963.

Russell, L.B., and Saylors, C.L. The relative sensitivity of various germ-cell stages of the mouse to radiation-induced non-dysjunction, chromosome losses and deficiencies. Reprinted from Sobels: Repair from Genetic Radiation, Pergamon Press, New York, pp. 313-342, 1963.

Russell, L.B., and Russell, W.L. An analysis of the changing radiation response of the developing mouse embryo. J. cell. comp. Physiol., 43, 103-149, 1954.

Sato, H. Chromosomes of irradiated embryos. Lancet, 1, 551, 1966.

Scharer, K., Muhlethaler, J., Stettler, M., and Bosch, H. Chronic radiation nephritis after exposure in utero. Helv. paediat. Acta, 23, 489-508, 1968.

Schwarz, G. Radiation hazards to the human fetus in present-day society. Bull. N.Y.

Acad. Med., 44, 388-399, 1968.

Segall, A., MacMahon, B., and Hannigan, M. Congenital malformations and background radiation in northern New England. J. chron. Dis., 17, 915-932, 1964.

Sharp, J. The effects of prenatal X-irradiation on acquisition, retention, and extinction of a conditioned emotional response. Radiat. Res., 24, 154-157, 1965.

Sharp, J. Critical flicker frequency in albino rats following prenatal X-irradiation. Radiat. Res., 33, 22-29, 1968.

Sikov, M., Meyer, J., Resta, C., and Lofstrom, J. Neurological disorders produced by prenatal X-irradiation of the rat. Radiat. Res., 12, 472, 1960 (abstract 151).

Sikov, M.R., and Noonan, T.R. Anomalous development induced in the embryonic rat by the maternal administration of radiophosphorus. Am. J. Anat., 103, 137-162, 1958.

Silverman, F.N. Thyroid carcinoma and X-irradiation. Therapeutic radiation versus diagnostic roentgenology. Pediatrics, 38, 943-945, 1966.

Simpson, C.L., Hemplemann, L., and Fuller, L. Neoplasia in children treated with X-ray in infancy for thymic enlargement. Radiology, 64, 840-845, 1955.

Skreb, N., Bijelic, N., and Lukovic, G. Weight of rat embryos after X-ray irradiation. Experientia, 19, 1-4, 1963.

Stahl, W. Recent Soviet work on antenatal effects of radiation and a discussion of future implications of general work in this field. In: Proceedings of the Symposium on Prenatal Behavior, held in Washington, D.C., 5-7 October, Division of Biology and Medicine, U.S. Atomic Energy Commission, Conference Report 631008, p. 37, 1963.

Stettner, E. Ein weiterer Fall einer Schädingung einer menschlichen Frucht durch Röntgen Bestrahlung. Jb. Kinderheilk. phys. Erzieh., 95, 43-51, 1921.

Stewart, J., Webb, D., Giles, D., and Hewitt, D. Malignant disease in childhood and diagnostic irradiation in utero. Lancet, 2, 447, 1956.

Stewart, J., Webb, D., and Hewitt, D. A survey of childhood malignancies. Br. Med. J., 1, 1495-1508, 1958.

Sutow, W., Conard, R., and Griffith, K. Growth status of children exposed to fallout radiation on Marshall Islands. Pediatrics, 36, 721-731, 1965.

Svigris, A. Sensitivity of hemopoietic organs of pregnant animals and their fetuses to ionizing radiations. Akush. Ginek., 34(5), 11-17, 1958 (in Russian).

Tabuchi, A. Fetal disorders due to ionizing radiation. Hiroshima J. Med. Sci., 13, 125-173, 1964.

Tabuchi, A., Nakagawa, S., Hirai, T., Sato, H., Hori, I., Matsuda, M., Yano, K.,

Shimada, K., and Nakao, Y. Fetal hazards due to X-ray diagnosis during pregnancy. Hiroshima J. med. Sci., 16, 49-66, 1967.

Tacker, R., and Furchtgott, E. Adjustment to food deprivation cycles as a function of age and prenatal X-irradiation. J. genet. Psychol., 102, 257-260, 1963.

Toth, B. A critical review of experiments in chemical carcinogenesis using newborn animals. Cancer Res., 28, 727-738, 1968.

Toyooka, E.T., Pifer, J.W., and Hempelmann, H.H. Neoplasms in children treated with X-rays for thymic enlargement. III. Clinical description of cases. J. natn. Cancer Inst., 31, 1379-1405, 1963.

Toyooka, E.T., Pifer, J.W., Crump, S.L., Dutton, A.M., and Hempelmann, L.H. Neoplasma in children treated with X-rays for thymic enlargement. II. Tumor incidence as a function of radiation factors. J. natn. Cancer Inst., 31, 1357-1377, 1963.

Vernadakis, A., Curry, J.H., Maletta, G.J., Irvine, G., and Timiras, P.A. Convulsive responses in prenatally irradiated rats. Expl. Neurol., 16, 57-64, 1966.

Vorisek, P. Einfluss der kontinuierlichen intrauterinen Bestrahlung auf die perinatale Mortalität der Frucht. Strahlentherapie, 127, 112-120, 1965.

Wechkin, S., Elder, R., Jr., and Furchtgott, E. Motor performance in the rat as a function of age and prenatal X-irradiation. J. comp. Physiol. Psychol., 54, 658-659, 1961.

Werboff, J., Broeder, J., Havlena, J., and Sikov, M. Effects of prenatal X-ray irradiation on audiogenic seizures in the rat. Expl. Neurol., 4, 189-196, 1961a.

Werboff, J., Goodman, I., Havlena, J., and Sikov, M. Effects of prenatal X-irradiation on motor performance in the rat. Am. J. Physiol., 201, 703-706, 1961b.

Werboff, J. Prenatal irradiation effects on CNS development and postnatal behavior. Conference Proceedings; Conference held in Washington, D.C. on 4-6 October, under the sponsorship of the American Institute of Biological Sciences under Contract No. AT(49-7) 1287 with the U.S. Atomic Energy Commission, Conference Report 631008, 1963.

Wilson, J.G. Differentiation and reaction to rat embryos to radiation. J. cell. comp. Physiol., 43, 11-37, 1954.

Wilson, J.T., and Karr, J.W. Effects of irradiation on embryonic development. I. X-rays on the tenth day of gestation in the rat. Am. J. Anat., 88, 1-34, 1951.

Wilson, J.G., Jordan, H.C., and Brent, R.L. Effects of irradiation on embryonic development. II. X-rays on the ninth day of gestation in the rat. Am. J. Anat., 92, 153-188, 1953.

Wood, J.W., Johnson, K.G., and Omori, Y. In utero exposure to the Hiroshima atomic bomb. An evaluation of head size and mental retardation: Twenty years later.

Pediatrics, _39_, 385-392, 1967a.

Wood, J., Johnson, K., Omori, Y., Kawamoto, S., and Keehn, R. Mental retardation in children exposed _in utero_ to the atomic bombs in Hiroshima and Nagasaki. _Am. J. publ. Hlth_, _57_, 1381-1390, 1967b.

Wood, J., Keehn, R., Kawamoto, S., and Johnson, K. The growth and development of children exposed in utero to the atomib bombs in Hiroshima and Nagasaki. _Am.J. publ. Hlth_, _57_, 1374-1380, 1967c.

Yamazaki, J.N. A review of the literature on the radiation dosage required to cause manifest central nervous system distrubances from _in utero_ and postnatal exposure. _Pediatrics_, _37_, 877-903, 1966.

Yamazaki, J., Wright, S., and Wright, P. Outcome of pregnancy in women exposed to the atomic bomb in Nagasaki. _Am. J. Dis. Child._, _87_, 448-463, 1954.

DISCUSSION OF CHAPTERS I AND II

Henry I. Kohn, Leader

Dr. Henry Kohn: It is very difficult for me to do much "discussing" at this point. Dr. Brill's paper was complete in itself and requires nothing more to be said about its subject matter. He has provided the dosimetric frame of reference for our conference. Dr. Brent, in effect, discussed his own paper. Some things that I thought of saying as I listened to him, were subsequently said by him, and in a more authoritative way than I could do it.

I think, therefore, that I shall go on to make some general remarks, which should apply to other papers at this conference as well as to the biology presented this morning, in order to provide a baseline from which to consider how to study the biological phenomena that are under discussion. This is going to be very, very simple. I hope that it will not be very, very naive.

The model of the mode of action of radiation that I shall employ is one with two stages (Kohn, 1959):

The first or radiobiologic stage begins with the absorption of ionizing radiation and ends in a fraction of a second or so with the production of what I shall call the initial biologic effect - an effect in a cytologic unit (definable in biologic terms) that "ends" a series of physical and chemical reactions.

In the second or biologic stage, a series of physiologic processes occur that were initiated by the initial effect and that lead to the development of the observed effect, the end-point chosen by the investigator.

In considering the use of this model for the study of the late and subtle effects of radiation, we should keep in mind the requirements of preventive medicine, namely, that effects engendered by low dosage, in the range of one rad, are of primary interest.

Considering the two-stage model, the course of events in the radiobiologic stage must be largely controlled by dose; in fact, their magnitude should be some simple function of dose. What happens in the biologic stage will not only depend on the "size" of the initial biologic effect, but also on the nature of the animal; it will largely be determined by the animal's genome, past history, and present environment. The controlling factors in the two stages, therefore, are very different indeed.

Here at this conference we obviously are dealing extensively with the biologic stage, and to much lesser degree with the radiobiologic stage. This fact has some important consequences, and I am going to list a number of them.

1. When the dose is small, the variance of the biologic stage in the exposed population (due to genetics, history and environment) will tend to blot out the dose-effect relationship inherent in the reaction of the radiobiologic stage.

2. The late and subtle effects of radiation can also be induced by many other agents or

"circumstances". There is nothing uniquely radiobiologic about them; they are ordinary biology.

3. The association of an observed end-point with prior radiation-exposure is no guarantee of a causal relationship, since the biological stage is subject to so many factors. (Dr. Brent noted this in the last part of this talk.)

4. The development of the late-effects seen after irradiation can be studied without using radiation to induce them. Even the initial biologic effect can often (theoretically, perhaps always) be induced by non-radiation agents.

These considerations lead to the proposition that in the low-dose range, studies employing radiation must be joined with studies of other agents or variables of practical and theoretical significance.

Now I realize that this is not a thrilling announcement, but at least it does open up, in a systematic way, the whole question of what is, in fact, the proper design of experiments that deal with the low-dose range. For example, Dr. Brent pointed out that the experimentalist can demonstrate effects with exposures of 10 R. Jacobsen (1968) showed that skeletal effects can be consistently produced by 5 rads when the mouse is irradiated during a sensitive period. Is it of any importance that such studies be extended? Would it make any difference if an experiment with mice demonstrated a somatic effect after 1 rad?

Also, thus far such experiments have dealt largely with the mouse and rat. Would it be advantageous to use another species in which the time course of injury or the structure involved (e.g. placentation) is more like that in man?

I am harping on the question of efficient design. In fact, I raise the question of whether or not one can have further efficient animal experiments.

Finally, I would like to include some additional human data. Dr. Brent mentioned the work of MacMahon and Hutchison, and of Stewart, which implicated low-level foetal exposure as a cause of cancer in infants and children. Three low-level studies are mentioned now, and others, no doubt, will come up in further discussion.

First, Lejeune et al. (1960) reported an increase of segmental heterochromia of the iris in children who had been exposed in utero, but this was not confirmed by Cheeseman and Walby (1963) in a subsequent and larger study. Dr. Griem has worked in this area, and perhaps he will discuss the matter.

Second, Griem, Meyer, and Dobben (1967) studied some 900 children who received 1.5 to 3 rads prior to birth (first trimester, 32; second trimester, 363, and third trimester, 562), and who were controlled by two groups of 813 children born before and 963 born after the exposed group. The children were traced, their histories studied, and if possible they were examined about 15 years after exposure. Status with respect to 14 different conditions was determined. The only positive finding was a 70% increase in a history of haemangioma, which was significant at the 5% level. The incidence of leukaemia was one case in each of the three study groups.

Third, there is the monograph of Nøkkentved (1968) - which incidentally reviews a good deal of the literature. On tracing the 5,734 female patients, aged 15 to 49 years, who received abdominal X-ray examinations at a Danish hospital during a 23-year period, she found that 152 of them had been in the first four months of pregnancy (1 month, 29; 2 months, 56; 3 months, 31; 4 months, 38). The history of the resulting 152 children was reviewed, and when possible the individuals were examined. The doses received are presumed to be in the range 0.5 to 5 rads. The controls comprised a group of 141 siblings. No significant difference between the two groups was observed. Nøkkentved raised the question of the importance of non-radiologic factors in determining morbidity.

In conclusion, I have not offered a great deal of discussion, but some basic questions have been asked and perhaps some of you will provide the answers to them.

Dr. Miller: May I ask Dr. Brent why does he think that experimental animals exhibit so many different congenital malformations following irradiation while the human foetus is limited in manifested types of irradiation-induced malformations.

Dr. Brent: The experimental laboratory animal is irradiated during the susceptible period for the induction of malformations, while the human foetus has been exposed to irradiation on a random basis and, therefore, during "sensitive" and insensitive periods. Secondly, the rodent has a proportionately longer sensitive period making up 30% of rat gestation while only 10% of human gestation falls into this category. A random exposure during rat gestation has a greater probability of occurring during the sensitive period. Finally, the dose can be controlled in laboratory exposures so that the dose is kept below the lethal dose to the rat or mouse embryo but not below the malforming dose. As an example, 100 R absorbed by a 9-day-old rat embryo would result in a 30% probability of death and a 95% probability of malformation if it survived. If the dose is raised to 180 R, all the embryos resorb. Thus, a human embryo exposed to radiation therapy doses of irradiation or a nuclear blast during the sensitive period would more likely be killed than survive, malformed. To sum up the human data, it is not surprising that irradiated human foetuses, if they exhibit anything, exhibit microcephaly. In later stages of gestation their LD/50 is higher and the central nervous system still manifests its sensitivity to irradiation.

Dr. Miller: Situs inversus and exencephaly is compatible with life; why don't we see that in man?

Dr. Brent: The probability of irradiating a human foetus during the sensitive period is low and in order to get these two malformations would necessitate greater than 50 R but less than 200 R irradiation during the sensitive period. Situs inversus is most likely produced during a 24-hour period in rat development which would be equivalent to a three-day period in human development. This is unlikely with either radiation therapy or with a small population of pregnant women exposed in Hiroshima or Nagasaki. Do you have a different explanation for these observations?

Dr. Miller: I have no explanation. You say that we see small heads and mental retardation as the only defect in man because the central nervous system has the greatest range of susceptibility?

Dr. Brent: That is a reasonable explanation for the presence of these malformations, but we would have to invoke my previous hypotheses to explain why the other malformations are not observed commonly in the human. Furthermore, the central nervous system of the rat maintains its radiation sensitivity even after birth. Although it is not a common occurrence, radiation effects on the human infant might still have debilitating consequences.

Dr. Kohn: Would you say that there is some other animal whose time course of development is more like man's and, therefore, would give us a better model for predicting and explaining the effects of irradiating the foetus?

Dr. Brent: The rhesus monkey or some other "high" primate has a longer period of gestation and a placenta that is similar to man's and, therefore, would be a better model for the radiation studies we have discussed. On the other hand, one has to be careful about initiating all these studies in another species. If it is to prove a hypothesis that can not be proven in the rat, then it may be worthwhile, but so frequently experiments are initiated in different species, solely because it is a different species. You referred to Lars Jacobsen's data concerning the malforming effects of low dose irradiation as one reason to look for a species that more closely resembles man. You may be right. My feeling is that we have enough data to know that 2 rads of irradiation cannot produce major congenital malformations. This entire problem of low dosage radiation effects frequently comes into the court room. My own experience has been that the emotional aspects of a questionable radiation induced malformation takes precedence over the scientific information. This is true after the child is born with a malformation or during consideration of a therapeutic abortion for a woman who has been "exposed" to diagnostic irradiation. One must be careful in evaluating these cases that he separates the scientific data that is available and is not swayed by sympathy for a family.

References

Kohn, H.I. The late effects of ionizing radiation: some general problems of experimental design. Radiat. Res., Suppl., 1, 235-242, 1959.

Jacobsen, L. Low dose X irradiation and teratogenesis: A quantitative experimental study, with reference to seasonal influence on dose effects. Acta Path. microbiol. scand., Suppl., 193, 208, 1968.

Lejeune, J., Turpin, R., Rethoré, M.O., and Mayer, M. Resultats d'une premiere enquête sur les effects somatiques de l'irradiation foeto-embryonnaire in utero. Revue fr. Étud. clin. biol., 5, 982-989, 1960.

Cheeseman, E.A., and Walby, A.L. Intrauterine irradiation and iris heterochromia. Ann. hum. Genet., 27, 23-29, 1963.

Griem, M.L., Meier, P., and Dobben, G.D. Analysis of the morbidity and mortality of children in fetal life. Radiology, 88, 347-349, 1967.

Nøkkentved, K. Effect of diagnostic radiation upon the human foetus, Munksgaard, Copenhagen, pp. 222, 1968.

CHAPTER III

EFFECTS OF RADIATION EXPOSURE IN THE THERAPEUTIC RANGE: TRUNCATED DOSES AND DOSE FRACTIONATION

J.F. Fowler

with added comments by
Professor Patricia J. Lindop

Introduction and Scope

The term "truncated doses" does not cover either single doses or continuous irradiation for the duration of life. Truncated doses include continuous irradiation for long periods which are, however, short compared with the life span of the organism studied. Truncated doses also include exposures with intervals, such as might be experienced in intermittent accidental exposure. I wish to deal, however, with relatively high doses, given to only a part of the body, in a regular and limited series of dose fractions. The examples I can give are taken from clinical radiation therapy and from radiobiological experiments aimed at discovering more about radiation injury to normal tissues, since normal tissue tolerance is at present the main limiting factor in the treatment of cancer by radiation.

I shall first present results of animal experiments demonstrating various aspects of the link between "early" and "late" injury to normal tissues in vivo, with reference to proliferating cell renewal systems, and then go on to emphasize the differences and some factors which need further investigation. The role of radiation damage to the vascular system is one such factor. Clinical evidence will be presented later.

My two main points will be that early and late injuries do appear to be related in a quantitative manner in some organs; but that the dose-response curves for late injury in certain tissues are steeper than those for early reactions in the same tissues. This finding suggests that different pathological processes are responsible for "early" and "late" radiation injury, as might be expected. The consequence is that the prediction of a late reaction from observations of an early one in a given case is often possible, but must be done with knowledge that the late reaction may increase more sharply with dose than the early reaction does.

Results from Animal Experiments

Nature of early and late reactions

Myelitis in the spinal cord, ulceration or perforation of the intestines, and fibrosis in lungs will be discussed later. The time sequence of reactions in skin will be discussed first since these have been extensively examined recently in animals. They are relevant to radiation injury to mucosa and connective tissue in addition to skin.

In skin there are three waves of reaction following a large single dose: a transient erythaema appearing after a few hours; then a wave of erythaema beginning at about 10 to 15 days and leading directly to a transient peak of desquamation at 20 to 25 days after appropriate doses; and a third wave of reaction with possible desquamation beginning at 2 to 3 months and persisting for many months. The second and third of these waves were called "early" and "medium-term" reactions in our earlier papers since we were concerned also about "late" reactions after a number of years. These two waves will, however, be called "early" and "late" reactions here. They are exemplified in fig. 1 (Field, 1969) which shows the time course of the skin reaction in rats' feet after a single dose of X rays. An arbitrary system of scoring was used (Fowler et al., 1965).

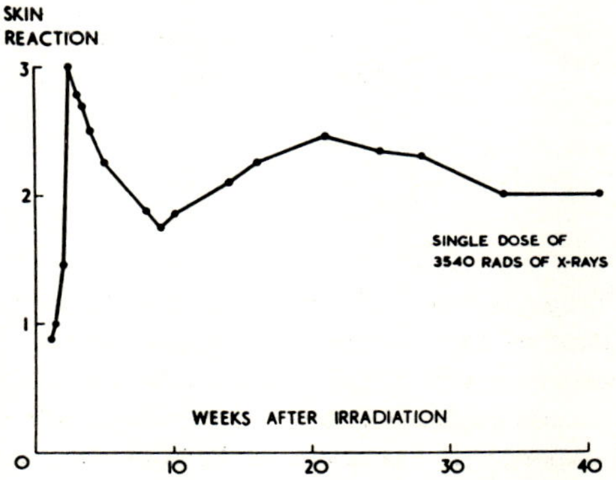

Fig. 1. Skin reaction in rat feet as a function of time after irradiation (Field, 1969).

Figure 2 shows the two waves of reaction observed in pig skin after single and fractionated doses of 8 MV X rays (Fowler, Morgan et al., 1963). The gross appearances of the late and early reactions are usually similar, and the same system of scoring can be

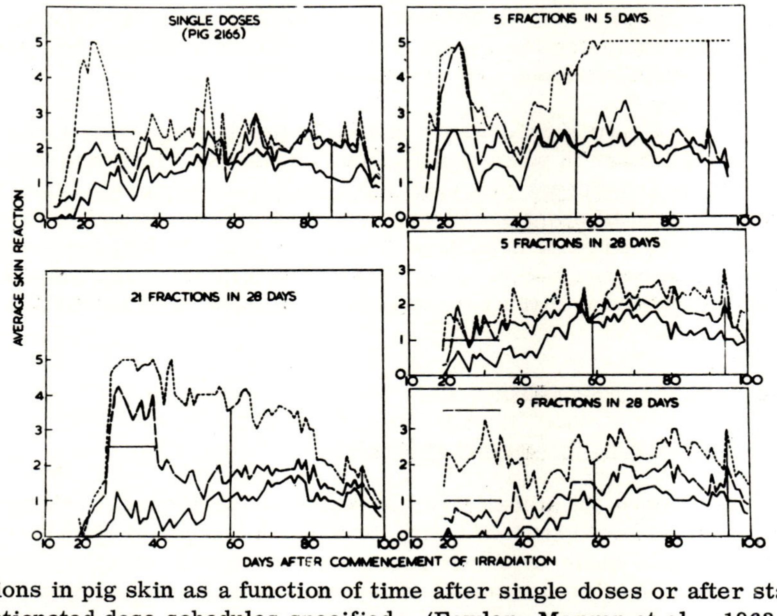

Fig. 2. Reactions in pig skin as a function of time after single doses or after start of the fractionated dose schedules specified. (Fowler, Morgan et al., 1963.)

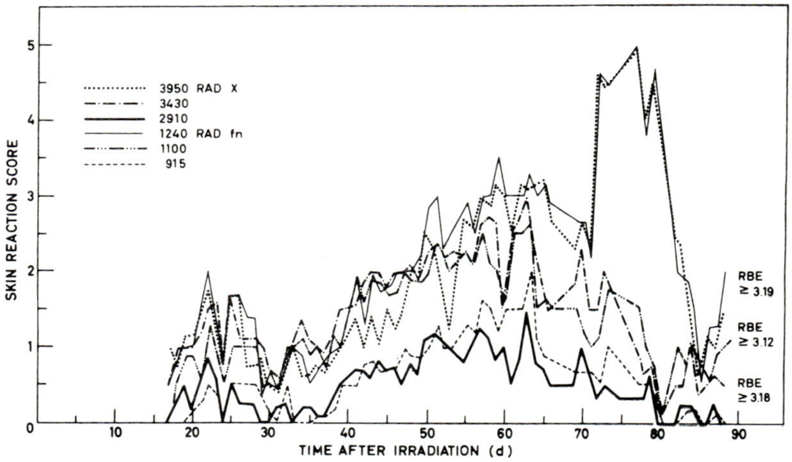

Fig. 2a. Reactions in pig skin as a function of time after start of 6 fractions in 17 days of either X rays or fast neutrons. Here a greater change in "late" reaction than "early" reaction with dose is suggested.

applied to both. The scores are arbitrary and have been used in many experiments: any score over 1.5 involves desquamation. The "early" reactions begin about 15 days after a single dose of 2,000 rads of X rays, and slightly later after the start of fractionated irradiation. The first wave usually subsides after a further 15 days. The second wave rises slowly from 30 or 40 days, and is still subsiding at 100 days.

A main reason for carrying out these experiments in pigs was to investigate the suggestion that very late damage to normal tissues was more severe after fast neutron irradiation than after X irradiation (Stone, 1948). It was found instead that there was no difference in the ratio of "late" (50 to 100 days) skin damage to "early" reaction in pigs as between X rays and fast neutrons (Fowler and Morgan, 1963). A difference of RBE between single and fractionated doses, however, was found which could explain Stone's findings. Some of the pigs have been kept for 7 years; and no more serious long-term effects in skin or subcutaneous tissue have developed in neutron than in X-irradiated fields.

Evidence has been presented previously that the early wave of skin reaction is due to depopulation of the basal layer of the epithelium by irradiation, followed by repopulation (Withers, 1967; Denekamp et al., 1969). The population turnover time of the basal layer (stem) cells is about 5 days in mice and 6 to 7 days in pigs and men (Fowler, 1968). The thickness of the epithelium is 2 or 3 cells equivalent; and the peak desquamation does indeed occur at the time expected from the simple kinetics of this system. Figure 3 illustrates the stem-cell/differentiated-layer relationship for pig or human skin (Fowler, 1968).

After very high doses indeed, such as in accidental over-exposure of the skin, the early wave is indistinguishable from the late wave: desquamation remains present all the time after about 1 to 3 weeks and becomes permanent ulceration.

Time course of injury to blood vessels

Bakowska et al., (1968) have studied the changes taking place in blood vessels in the mouse ear with time after doses of 14 MeV electrons of 1,500 to 4,500 rads. Some changes in permeability were found within hours, but these effects showed no recovery phenomena and

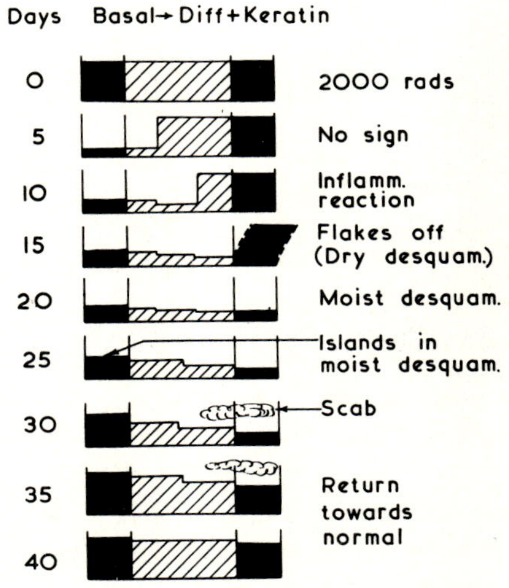

Fig. 3. Schematic diagram of progression of skin reaction with respect to cell population kinetics of basal layer of epithelium (on left of diagram: turnover time about 5 days) and differentiated layer in pig skin or human skin.

their significance is unknown. The relevant effects here were the incidence of tortuosity and segmental arteriolar narrowing which occurred in two peaks, one at 4 to 5 weeks and the other at 12 to 14 weeks after irradiation. These effects did show recovery in split-dose experiments, of about 500 rads as for skin reactions. The timing of these peaks is similar to that of the two peaks of skin reaction, except that the early peak is slightly later than the peak of desquamation.

It is as yet impossible to work out any cause-and-effect relationship, although skin graft experiments are being planned in our laboratory to throw light on this. As stated above, there seems no need to invoke other mechanisms than cell killing in the basal layer to explain the early reactions. It has sometimes been speculated that the second wave of skin reaction might be due to failure of the irradiated vascular system at this time. The suggestion is plausible but not proven. The corollary would be that the cell population turnover time of the vascular endothelium is as long as several months, so that a reduction in cell proliferation would not lead to depletion and hence rupture of blood vessel walls until about this time after irradiation. An alternative hypothesis is that vascular failure is secondary to fibrosis which itself would be a result of an inflammatory reaction to cell killing. This is a subject that would benefit greatly from experimental attention, and surprisingly has received very little to date.

Iso-effect doses in fractionated schedules

Figure 4 shows dose-response curves for the early and late skin reaction following various fractionation schedules (Fowler, Bewley et al., 1965). There are no significant differences in slope, although there is greater variability in the response curves for late reactions.

Figure 5 shows a graph of total dose to produce a given skin reaction in pigs against number of fractions on a double logarithmic scale as used by Strandqvist (1944). As is well known, the total dose required to produce any given level of reaction increases with

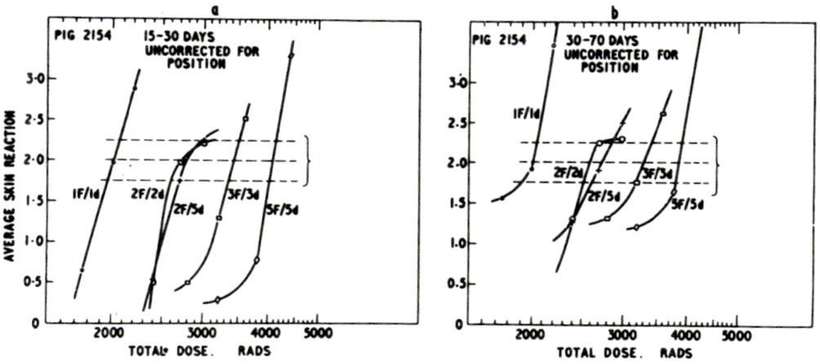

Fig. 4. Average skin reaction plotted against the total dose given, scored over 15-30 days after the start of irradiation (a) and over 30-70 days (b).

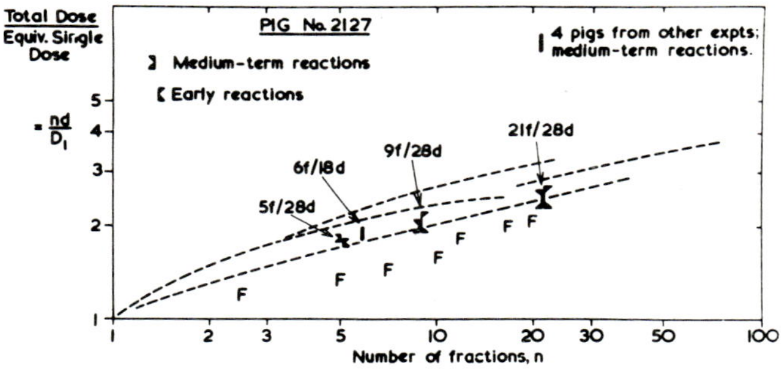

Fig. 5. Ratios of total dose to the single dose required to produce the same skin reaction in pigs. The vertical extent of the "early" and "late" reaction symbols represents the spread of ratios obtained for various degrees of skin reaction between 1.25 and 2.25. The dotted lines and the symbols F are from published clinical observations (Fowler, Morgan et al., 1963).

the number of dose fractions. The early and late reactions are represented by separate symbols. Each symbol represents the ratio of the iso-effect dose to the corresponding single dose. It can be seen that the dose ratios are closely similar for early and late reactions (Fowler, Morgan et al., 1963). This means that for a narrow band of doses and for skin reactions close to tolerance levels, the early reaction observed is a reasonably reliable guide to the degree of the late reaction in the same treated area. Of course, there are statistical variations; and a major difference in that the ratio of doses to produce a given level of reactions, late relative to early, will depend upon the level of reaction, as discussed below.

Ratios of iso-effect doses: oxygen enhancement ratios

Table 1 shows ratios of X-ray doses required to produce the same effect, when the doses are given at three conditions of oxygenation of normal tissues of the mouse leg (Suit and Howard, 1967). Three different biological end-points were studied: the dose required to produce (1) moist desquamation at 21 days in 50% (or in 90%) of animals irradiated; (2) epilation at 40 days in 50% of animals; (3) contraction of the irradiated area from 27.5 mm to 22 mm in 50% of animals. The ratios of doses in the hypoxic to the air-breathing condition,

Table 1

Ratios of doses to produce the same end-point for different conditions of oxygenation during irradiation of mice

Suit and Howard (1967) End-point		Single dose		10 fractions	
		Hypox/Air	Hypox/HPO	Hypox/Air	Hypox/HPO
Desquamation	(DD_{50}	1.2	1.9	1.6	2.5
21 d.	(DD_{90}	1.2	2.1	1.6	2.5
Epilation 40 d.	ED_{50}	1.2	1.9	1.5	2.5
Contraction 27.5 40 d.	22 mm CD_{50}	1.45	2.15	1.57	2.47

and the ratios for hypoxic to high-pressure-oxygen, can be seen in table 1 to be fairly constant for all three biological end-points. The ratios are also the same for eleven dose fractions given at 24-hour intervals as for single doses, in general agreement with the results from pigs quoted in the previous section. These findings suggest that skin desquamation is a reasonable example of normal tissue injury, and that connective tissue damage (e.g. contraction) follows similar oxygenation and fractionation dose ratios as does desquamation.

Ratios for iso-effect doses: fast neutron RBE for early and late skin reaction and for leg deformity in rats

Table 2 shows Field's (1969) values of RBE for neutrons from the M.R.C. Cyclotron at Hammersmith using the rat skin reaction end-point discussed in the section on "Nature of early and late reactions", together with leg deformity at 23 weeks. Here the

Table 2

RBE values for fast neutrons and X irradiation of rat feet

S.B. Field (1969)	Early reaction	Late reaction	Deformity
Single dose	1.69 ± 0.07	1.59 ± 0.13	1.68 ± 0.11
Two fractions	1.93 ± 0.05	2.11 ± 0.07	- -
Five fractions	2.41 ± 0.02	2.38 ± 0.02	2.32 ± 0.02

RBE values did depend upon the number of fractions (as would be expected since there is less prompt repair of intracellular injury after the fast neutrons); but were not significantly different as between late reactions, early reactions, and leg deformity.

Field has also presented a careful comparison of the degree of late skin reaction (mean over 5 to 23 weeks) as a function of the degree of early skin reaction (mean over 7 to 30 days). This comparison is illustrated in fig. 6. A very high correlation is demonstrated between the early and the late reaction, but it should be noted that the correlation is far from being one-for-one. Figure 7 shows a similar correlation plot for leg deformity at 23 weeks against a mean early skin reaction. Again the correlation is extremely good, but the change in deformity is greater than the corresponding change in early skin reaction, from barely perceptible to extremely severe although both scales are of course arbitrary.

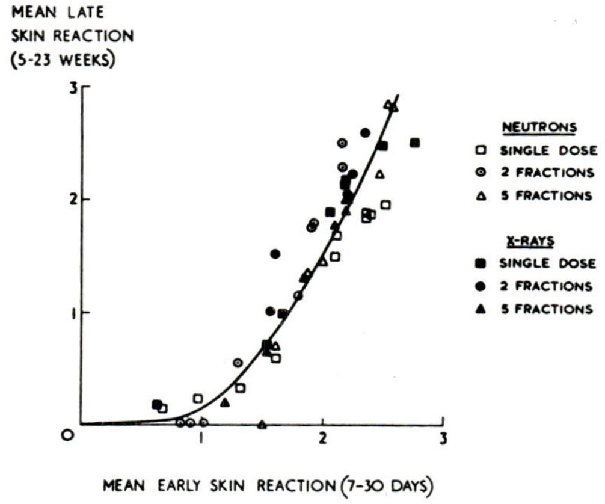

Fig. 6. Late skin reactions in rat feet as a function of early skin reaction after various treatments with X rays or fast neutrons (Field, 1969). The reaction scores are the same for both axes.

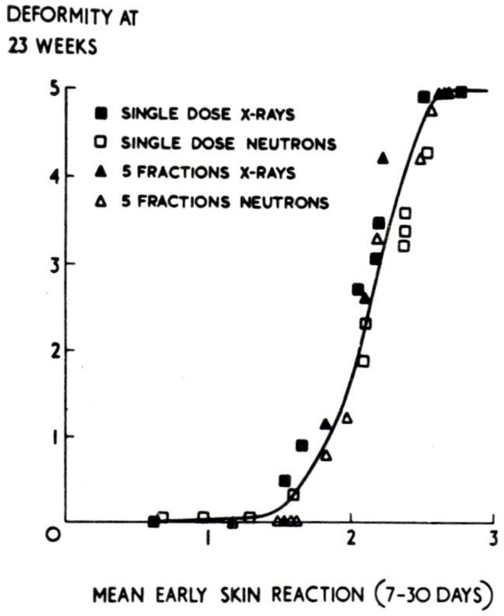

Fig. 7. Deformity of the rat foot as a function of early skin reaction after various treatments (Field, 1969).

Dose-response curves: steeper for "late" than for "early" reactions

Field has summarized the results given in the previous section in fig. 8, which shows early reactions, late reactions, and deformity as a function of dose (for five dose fractions; similar results would be expected for other fractionation schedules, as demonstrated above). This figure shows clearly one of the main points of the present paper: that the increase of late reactions and deformities with dose is much sharper than in the case of early reactions. There is a correlation between early and late reactions — a very good correlation — but the dose ratio varies with degree of injury. It is, therefore, possible to use early injury as a guide to later injury, but with the major caution that the dependence of late injury on dose will be much sharper than for the early reaction.

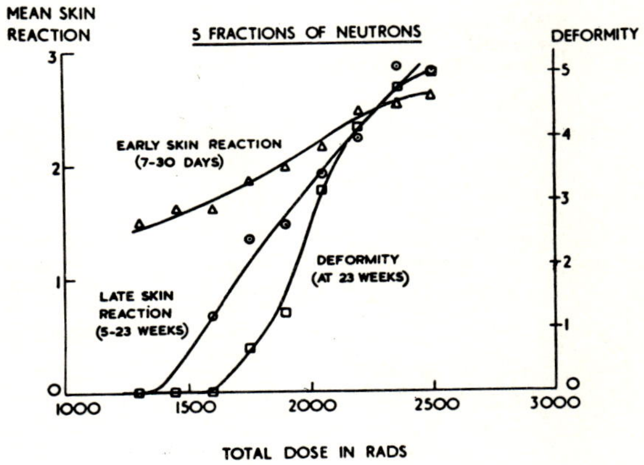

Fig. 8. Dose-response curves for the early and late skin reactions and deformity after irradiation with five fractions of fast neutrons. The scale for scoring deformity has been matched to the crossover point of the other two curves (Field, 1969).

Data from Clinical Observations

Skin reactions

The three waves of skin reaction described above in animals have been well documented in human skin (Miescher, 1924). The time of onset of the second wave, i.e. the "early reaction", after a dose of 1,500 to 2,000 rads of X rays is about 12 to 15 days in pig skin or human skin; the peak desquamation occurs at 20 to 25 days. In the feet of rats or mice the time of onset is 7 to 8 days and the peak desquamation occurs at 17 to 21 days; in mice no third wave of skin reaction (beyond 40 days) has been observed in the skin of feet or of the dorsum. These differences between the time scales of early reactions in human and animal skins are readily explainable in terms of the cell kinetic parameters and thickness of the epithelium.

There is no documented evidence relating late reactions in human patients so definitely to early reactions as in the case of Field's results on rat legs, but there is no reason to suppose that different relationships would apply. In particular, in Stone's patients irradiated with fast neutrons at Berkeley, California in 1937-1942, those patients with very severe late reactions (ulceration of skin or mucosa) had also shown severe early reactions (Stone, 1948; Stone, private communication; Brennan, Field and Phillips, private communication).

Myelitis

Radiation myelitis is a well-known complication of radiotherapy where a high dose was given to the spinal cord. It may appear between a few months and a few years after irradiation, the most likely time of onset being 9 to 12 months. Many mechanisms have been invoked to explain the vulnerability of the neuraxis to radiation damage. These include changes in vascular permeability and focal oedema, primary de-myelinization, inflammatory changes and iso-allergic disturbances, infarction due to vascular damage, or primary radiolytic damage to supporting glial tissues or to neurons. No definite conclusion regarding the pathogenesis of so-called radiation myelitis can be reached. Van den Brenk et al. (1968) pointed out that certain cells (particularly glial cells) are believed to be lost and replaced, so that the C.N.S. should not be regarded simply as a static entity in which the differentiated cell population, once formed, functions till death of the organism occurs. Van den Brenk assumed that the cell-survival model could be applied to radiogenic lesions of the neuraxis. He found, on this basis, that the incidence of myelitis in 239 patients surviving radiotherapy beyond 9 months could be explained as a function of dose by assuming a standard cell survival curve model with D_0 = 130 rads and extrapolation number m = 2 or 4 (fig. 9). These cell survival curve parameters are reasonable. Supporting evidence for a cell depletion mechanism comes from the fact that the latency period in rats is dose dependent (Carsten and Zeman, 1966). The fact that a cell depletion model fits does not prove that C.N.S. cells are involved, of course; the same argument could be used in favour of a reduction in the number of proliferative vascular endothelial cells by irradiation.

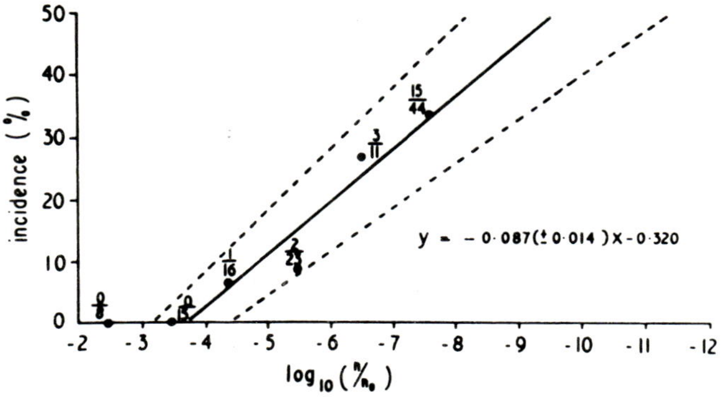

Fig. 9. Incidence of myelitis as a function of dose to spinal cord in terms of calculated cell survival n/n_0, assuming D_0 = 130 rads, m = 2 (Van den Brenk et al., 1968).

A point of interest in Van den Brenk's findings is that the incidence of myelitis is dependent upon the number of fractions given: repair of "intracellular injury" between fractions applies to this type of injury also. Figure 10 illustrates this: a 10% incidence of myelitis would be expected for a single dose of 1,500 rads, or for about 3,200 rads given as 20 fractions. (It should be noted that these doses were to patients treated in the high pressure oxygen tank at 4 atmospheres absolute. A lower incidence would be expected for patients treated in air to the same doses.) The point is that C.N.S. damage is not simply accumulated in proportion to dose; instead, repair or recovery appears to take place in the relevant (but unknown) tissues. This finding is in agreement with earlier but less exact radiotherapeutic results on late brain damage including necrosis and myelopathy (Franke, 1963).

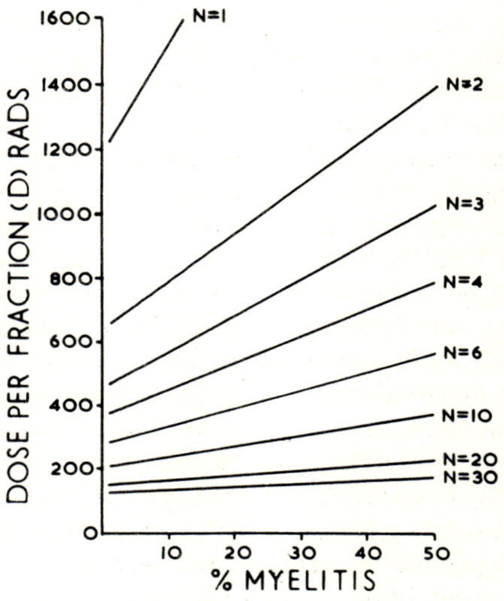

Fig. 10. Calculated risk of cervical myelitis for fractionated 4 MeV irradiation of patients in high pressure oxygen tanks, as a function of dose to spinal cord and number N of dose fractions (Van den Brenk et al., 1968).

Lung fibrosis

The changes in lung following radiation treatment of lung cancer have been reported as being in principle similar to changes caused by radiation in other tissues, where a stage of early reaction to the treatment may be followed by fibrosis (Deeley, 1960). In normal lung tissue there is at first a reaction shown as an increased opacity in lung radiographs, and microscopically as oedema of the tissues with lymphocytic infiltration and exudate into the alveoli. This reaction corresponds to that seen on the mucous membrane in the mouth or in the rectum and to the moist desquamation found in the skin. The reaction may subside as it sometimes does in the other sites mentioned, but with the doses normally given in the treatment of carcinoma the damage to lung tissue is usually too severe for complete resolution to take place and fibrosis occurs.

Deeley (1960) found radiographic evidence of lung shrinkage in all patients with irradiated lungs who survived for 14 months. The time and rate of onset of lung shrinkage in 23 patients treated by 8 MV X rays to a nominal tumour dose of 4,500 rads is shown in fig. 11. The actual doses would be higher by up to 30%, due to the low density of the lung (Svarcer et al., 1965).

Lung shrinkage is shown by movement of the heart, trachea and hilum of the lung, tenting or elevation of the diaphragm, and contraction of the ribs on the affected side as compared with their positions on the radiograph taken before treatment. At the same

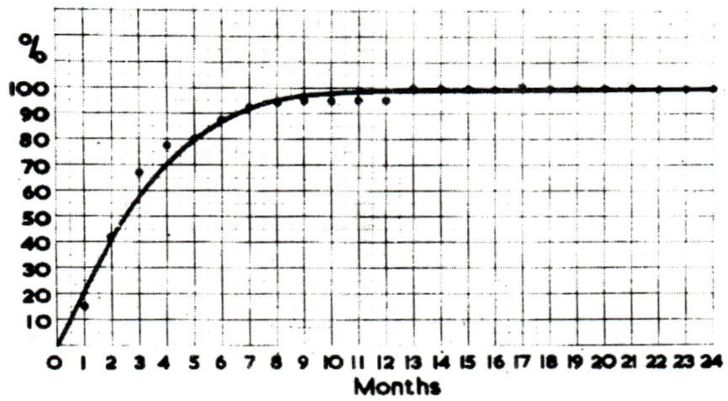

Fig. 11. Percentage of chest radiographs showing any evidence of lung shrinkage for each month up to two years after treatment for Ca bronchus, in 23 patients treated by 8 MV X rays (Deeley, 1960).

time as fibrosis occurs in the irradiated lung, there is often evidence of emphysematous changes in the unirradiated lung. The incidence of fibrosis is higher and occurs earlier in patients given 4,000 rads than in thos given 3,000 rads, both schedules being 20 fractions in 4 weeks (table 3). This long-term damage is so severe that the surviving proportion of patients treated with 4,000 rads is lower than that for 3,000 rads, as shown in table 4 for 51 randomized pairs of patients (Deeley, 1966). The actual doses received by the tumour and the lung could have been greater by up to 30%, as mentioned above. There was no significant difference in the incidence of residual carcinoma within the chest at death (69% in both groups) or in the incidence of distant metastases.

Table 3

Incidence of radiation fibrosis after radiotherapy of lung carcinoma

Deeley (1966)	Tumour dose, 20F/4 weeks	
	3000 rads	4000 rads
0 to 6 months	2/26 (8%)	19/34 (56%)
7 to 13 months	4/15 (27%)	15/19 (79%)
13 to 18 months	4/8 (50%)	7/7 (100%)
19 to 24 months	4/6 (67%)	0

The reason for the poorer prognosis after the higher dose of 4,000 rads appears to be the greater amount of lung fibrosis, which may lead to right-sided heart failure.

Intestinal reactions

Portions of the large and small intestines may come within the field of irradiation during treatment of carcinoma of the cervix uteri or bladder. Two stages of reaction have

Table 4

Proportion of patients surviving after radiotherapy of lung carcinoma

Deeley (1966)	Tumour dose, 20F/4 weeks	
	3000 rads	4000 rads
No. of cases	51	51
6 months	56%	52%
12 months	20%	16%
18 months	14%	0
24 months	6%	0

been described in the intestines. The early reaction may begin at 15 to 17 days after the start of fractionated radiotherapy and persists for about 16 days in the rectum and about 30 days in the small bowel (Deeley, 1969). These time scales are similar to that of the early skin reaction. There is acute inflammatory reaction affecting the mucosa and submucosa, sometimes with bleeding, as seen at other sites where the mucosal membrane is irradiated, for example, the mouth, larynx, and pharynx.

Early reactions may or may not progress into late reactions, which have a more severe prognosis. The picture at the late reaction stage is that of unceration and necrosis of the tissues possibly resulting from fibrosis and reduced blood supply. Surgical repair is hindered by the presence of fibrosis. "Late" rectal symptoms may occur between 1 month and 3 years after irradiation, but the most probable time is within the first year. The tolerance dose depends upon the fractionation, as in skin tolerance doses.

Late reactions in the small bowel may develop as long as 10 to 14 years after treatment. The complications occurring in 16 such cases surveyed by Deeley (1969) included intestinal obstruction, bowel fistulae, persistent diarrhea, pain or bleeding. Fifteen of the 16 patients had had severe early reactions.

It is interesting to correlate the incidence of immediate and late intestinal reactions with the dose given. It is only possible to do this in patients receiving treatment for carcinoma of the bladder, where a uniform dose of radiation has been given throughout the pelvis. Table 5 gives these figures (Deeley, 1969). There is clearly a correlation between the incidence of immediate and late reactions, as noted for rat skin in the section on "Dose-response curves". There is also a much sharper increase of the late reaction with dose than of the increase of the early reaction. This finding too is consistent with the data from rat skin reported above.

Conclusions

A definite correlation has been demonstrated between "early" and "late" reactions

Table 5

Incidence of radiation reactions on small bowel after radiotherapy of carcinoma of bladder

Deeley (1969)	Tumour dose, 20F/4 weeks		
	4000 to 4900 rads	5000 to 5900 rads	Over 6000 rads
No. of patients	179	175	26
Early reactions	4%	5%	15%
Late reactions	0.6%	1.1%	7.7%

in rat skin and in human intestinal mucosa, after irradiation to nearly limiting tolerance levels. In both tissues the late reaction was found to increase much more sharply with dose than the early reaction (fig. 8 and table 5). This observation is in agreement with the response of late and early skin reactions in pigs. There was no difference in the relationship of early to late reactions depending upon dose fractionation. Larger doses were required for both types of damage if many fractions were given. There was also no difference in the relationship of late and early skin reactions in pigs or rats for fast neutron as compared with X irradiation. The latter observations on a small number of pigs have been extended to 7 years after irradiation with no change in the result.

The early reactions discussed here are probably due to cellular depletion of the basal epithelial layer; the processes determining late damage are not known but might include damage to the vascular system and fibrosis.

Acknowledgments

I should like to thank Dr. S.B. Field of the M.R.C. Cyclotron Unit and Dr. T.J. Deeley of the Radiotherapy Department, Hammersmith Hospital, for many stimulating discussions and for permission to quote their results. Thanks are due to the Editors of Radiology for permission to reproduce figs. 1, 6, 7 and 8; of British Journal of Radiology for figs. 4, 5, 9 and 10; and of Clinical Radiology for fig. 11. My own work in this field is supported currently by B.E.C.C.

References

Bakowska, A., Lindop, P.J., and Rotblat, J. Effect of single and divided doses of 14 MeV electrons on blood vessels of the mouse pinna. Br. J. Radiol., 41, 157 (abstract), 1968.

Carsten, A., and Zeman, W. The control of variables in radiopathological studies on mammalian nervous tissue. Int. J. Radiat. Biol., 10, 65, 1966.

Deeley, T.J. The effects of radiation on the lungs in the treatment of carcinoma of the bronchus. Clin. Radiol., 11, 33, 1960.

Deeley, T.J. A clinical trial to compare two different tumour dose levels in the treatment of advanced carcinoma of the bronchus. Clin. Radiol., 17, 299, 1966.

Deeley, T.J. The effects of radiation on the intestines. J. Indian Profess. Med. Assoc.

Denekamp, J., Ball, M.M., and Fowler, J.F. Recovery and repopulation in mouse skin as a function of time after X-irradiation. Radiat. Res., 37, 361, 1969.

Field, S.B. Early and late reactions in skin after irradiation with X-rays or fast neutrons. Radiology, 92, 381, 1969.

Fowler, J.F., and Morgan, R.L. Pretherapeutic experiments with the fast neutron beam from the M.R.C. cyclotron. VIII. General review. Br. J. Radiol.,36, 115, 1963.

Fowler, J.F., Morgan, R.L., Silvester, J.A., Bewley, D.K., and Turner, B.A. Experiments with fractionated X-ray treatment of the skin of pigs. I. Fractionation up to 28 days. Br. J. Radiol., 36, 188, 1963.

Fowler, J.F., Kragt, K., Ellis, R., Lindop, P.J., and Berry, R.J. The effects of divided doses of 15 MeV electrons on the skin response of mice. Int.J. Radiat. Biol., 9, 241, 1965.

Fowler, J.F., Bewley, D.K., Morgan, R.L., and Silvester, J.A. Experiments with fractionated X-irradiation on the skin of pigs. II. Fractionation up to five days. Br. J. Radiol., 38, 278, 1965.

Fowler, J.F. Effect of fractionated irradiation on the skin of pigs and other animals and on tumours in rats. Proc. Symp. on Dose Rate in Mammalian Radiation Biology, Oak Ridge UT-AEC, Paper 21.1 (Conf. 680410; USAEC), 1968.

Franke, H. Der Strahlenempfindlichkeit des menschlichen Rückenmarks. Fortschritte der Medizin, 81 Jg., Nr. 9, 345, 1963.

Miescher, G. Das Rontgenerythema. Strahlentherapie, 16, 333, 1924.

Stone, R.S. Neutron therapy and specific ionization. Am. J. Roentgenol., 59, 771, 1948.

Strandqvist, Magnus. Studien Über Die Kumulative Wirkung Der Röntgenstrahlen Bei Fraktionierung Erfahrungen Aus Dem Radiumhemmet An 280 Haut Und Lippenkarzinomen-Acta Radiologica., Supplementum 55, 1-300, 1944.

Suit, H.D., and Howard, T.C. Normal tissue damage and tumor cure probability for irradiation given under different conditions of oxygenation in hybrid mice. Radiology, 89, 713, 1967.

Svarcer, V., Fowler, J.F., and Deeley, T.J. Exit doses for lung fields measured by lithium fluoride thermoluminescence. Br. J. Radiol., 38, 785, 1965.

Van den Brenk, H.A.S., Richter, W., and Hurley, R.H. Radiosensitivity of the human oxygenated cervical spinal cord based on analysis of 357 cases receiving 4 MeV X-rays in hyperbaric oxygen. Br. J. Radiol., 41, 205, 1968.

Withers, H.R. The dose-survival relationship for irradiation of epithelial cells of mouse skin. Br. J. Radiol., 40, 187, 1967.

Comments by Professor Patricia J. Lindop

In relation to Professor Fowler's suggestions of the relationship between skin damage and vascular changes, we have investigated changes in irradiated blood vessels.

The system which Anna Bakowska is using is local irradiation of one ear-lobe of the mouse. The vessels which are transilluminated are visualized through a stereomicroscope. These are arterioles, venules and capillaries. The extravascular skin response was also studied. The late changes seen are predominantly dilatation of the venules, narrowing in the arterioles, and development of "sausage segments", and dilatation and new growth of the capillaries. We also look at a physiological end-point, the time to full constriction of the arterioles after adrenaline injection.

The reactions seen in these vessels are compared with the skin reaction in the ear scored on an arbitrary scale similar to Professor Fowler's. Figure 1 shows the desquamation reaction with time post-irradiation. The wave forms of these changes are more definite following a single dose with one peak at about 5 weeks, a second peak about 20 weeks, and then a questionable late peak. The dotted line demonstrates the reaction when the dose is fractionated where the subsidiary peaks are not seen.

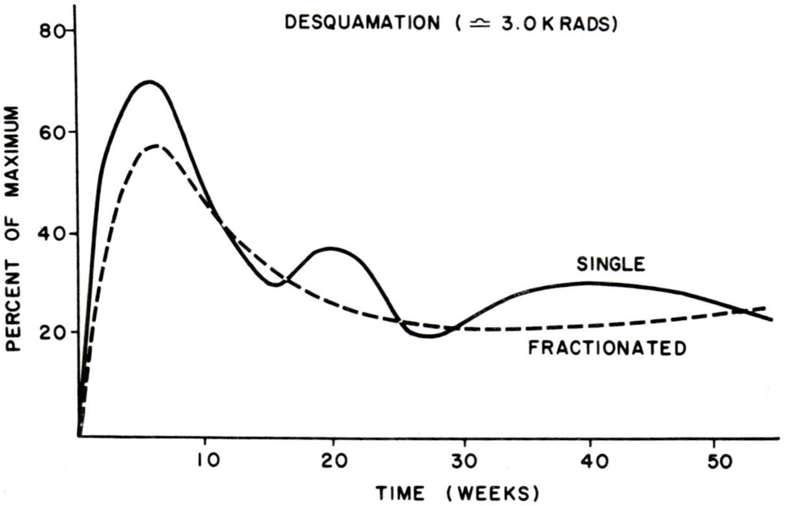

Fig. 1. A comparison of the effect post-irradiation on the skin reaction of the ear-lobe following a single dose of 3 krads — compared with the same total dose, given in two equal fractions — separated by 24 hours. (Bakowska, Anna, Lindop, Patricia J., and Rotblat, J., Br. J. Radiol., 41, 157, 1968.) (With permission.)

Figure 2 (a) shows the reaction of dilatation of the arterioles following single doses of 4.5, 3.0 or 1.5 kilorads. The first peak in this response is within 24 hours, a second peak at about 5 weeks, and then with the highest doses, the dilatation changes to long-term constriction of the arterioles.

There is a similar pattern of response in the venules but no constriction (fig. 2(b)) They remain dilated up to one year post-irradiation.

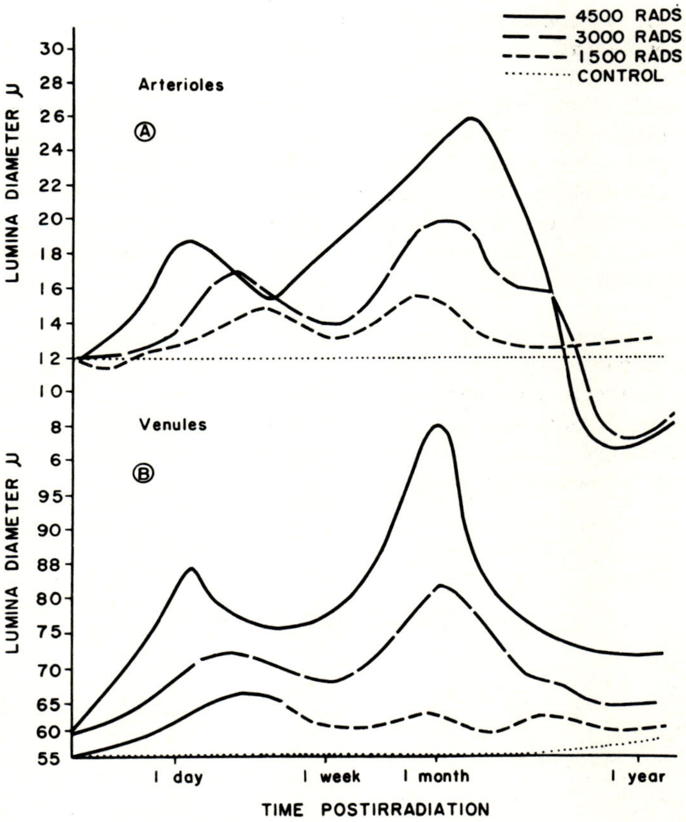

Fig. 2. The response of arterioles and venules at different times after single doses of radiation, observed from 6 hours to 55 weeks post-irradiation. (Bakowska, Anna, 1969, personal communication.)

The arteriolar lumen changed less during 1 to 5 weeks post-irradiation following fractionated doses than with single doses over a range of 1 to 5 kilorads; i.e. an apparent decreased effectiveness of the divided doses. For the late period the divided doses are also less effective using the end point of constriction, and this is more marked than for the early response (fig. 3).

As far as capillary dilatation is concerned, fig. 4 shows that there is a large decrease in effectiveness of divided doses in the early period, but for the late effect, there is, in fact, more persistent dilatation after divided doses than there is after a single dose. In other words, there is a reversal of the sign for the "sparing" effect for the late effect on capillaries.

Figure 5 shows that as far as the physiological end-point is concerned, that is the time from adrenaline administration to constriction of the arteriole, the fractionated dose results in a greater reduction in this time than the single dose, both in the early and

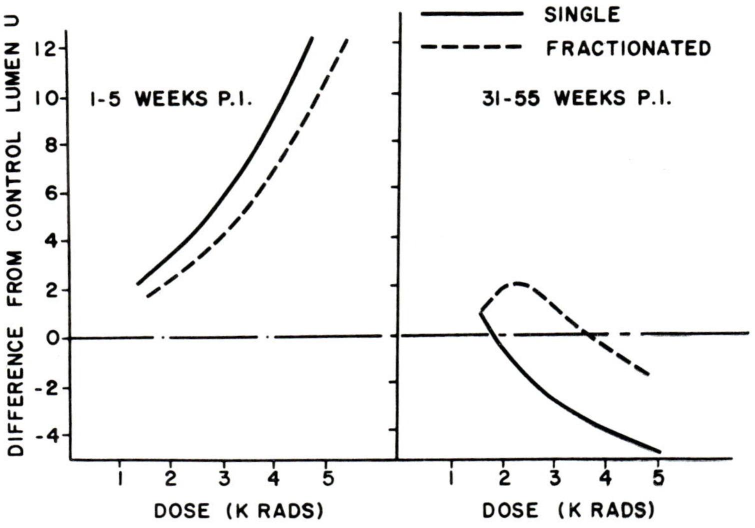

Fig. 3. A comparison of the dose-response curves for changes in arteriolar lumen following single and fractionated doses of radiation, observed at an early (1-5 weeks p.i.) and a late (31-55 weeks p.i.) time period. (Bakowska, Anna, 1969, personal communication.)

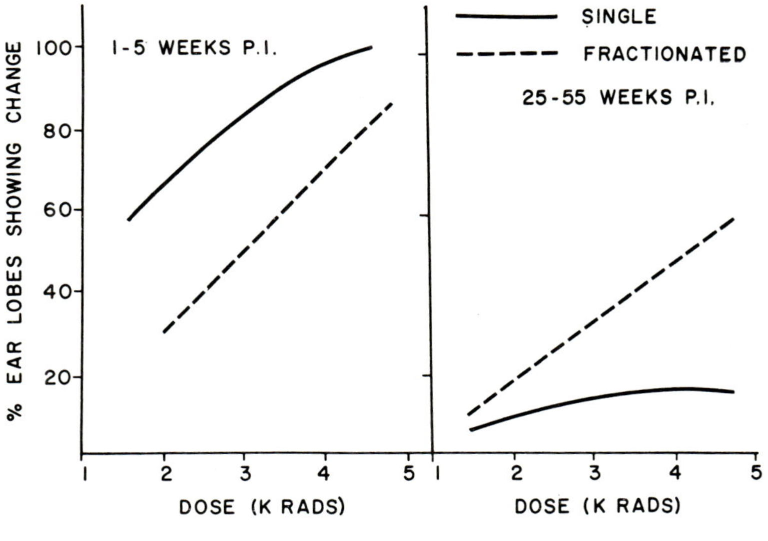

Fig. 4. A comparison of the dose-response curves for capillary dilatation following single and fractionated doses of radiation, observed at an early (1-5 weeks p.i.) and a late (25-55 weeks p.i.) time period. (Bakowska, Anna, 1969, personal communication.)

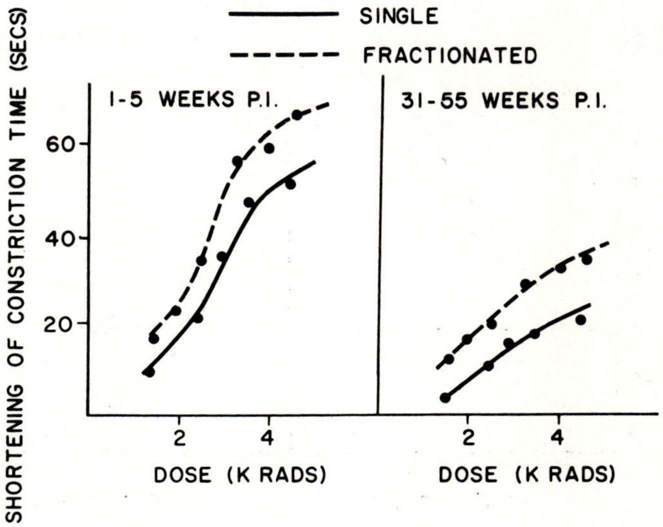

Fig. 5. A comparison of the dose-response curves for shortening of time for arteriolar constriction following adrenaline, after single and fractionated doses, observed in the early (1-5 weeks p.i.) and late (31-55 weeks p.i.) period. (Bakowska, Anna, 1969, personal communication.)

the late period.

Now let us see what is the quantitative difference between the early and late fractionation effects. Table 1 shows the value in rads of the "sparing" effect at the late time period for the different end-points that we have looked at. For constriction of the arterioles, there is a very large "sparing" effect of the order of 1,800 rads. However, for the arteriolar response to adrenaline, there is "negative sparing" of about 1,200 rads. Tortuosity shows about 600 rads and sausage-segments, 200 rads.

There is "sparing" for the effects on the venules. For the capillaries the "sparing" is very large because the fractionated dose curve flattened out, but we can see it as a "negative sparing". For the skin reaction, there is positive sparing of about 500 rads which matches Fowler's sparing effect.

Table 2 shows not only that there is a difference but also there is a much smaller sparing effect for the early time period. In the case of capillary dilatation, fractionated dose results in more marked dilatation at the late periods than with single doses which is just the opposite to that which occurs in the early period.

But for the skin reaction, which is what Professor Fowler was talking about, there is really a good correlation between the sparing effect of 400 rads in the early response with the 500 rads which is shown for the late response.

What we are concerned about is whether you can, in fact, predict late effects in other tissue structures from the early skin reaction, because if any of the late effects depend on vascular changes, there may well not be a comparable response for the early and late effects.

Table 1

A comparison of the "sparing" effect in rads of the fractionated doses, during the long-term observation period

	"Sparing" in rads Time after exposure
End-point	Long-term (23-55 weeks)
Arterioles	
Lumina diameter	+ 1800 (narrowing)
Adrenaline response	- 1200
Tortuosity	+ 600
"Sausage segments"	+ 200
Venules	
Lumina dilatation	+ 500
Tortuosity	+ 1000
Capillaries	
Dilatation	- (very large)
Skin reaction	+ 500

(Bakowska, Anna, 1969, personal communication)

Table 2

A comparison of the "sparing" effect in rads of fractionated doses, during the early observation period

	"Sparing" in rads Time after exposure
End-point	Short-term (1-5 weeks)
Arterioles	
Lumina diameter	+ 300 (dilatation)
Adrenaline response	- 500
Venules	
Lumina diameter	+ 500
Capillaries	
Dilatation	+ 1700
Skin reaction	+ 400

(Bakowska, Anna, 1969, personal communication)

CHAPTER IV

PATHOLOGICAL CHANGES AFTER PROTRACTED EXPOSURE TO LOW DOSE RADIATION *

George W. Casarett

Introduction

This paper is concerned with the late pathologic effects of long-term daily exposure of mature mammals to ionizing radiation at rates of the order of 10 R per day or lower.

Exposure at these rates does not cause acute radiation syndromes in the manner in which they are observed after more intensive exposure. However, substantial accumulation of dose at rates in the upper part of this range may result in depression or depletion of various haemopoietic elements to such an extent as to contribute to the cause of death through mechanisms that also contribute to the causation of death in the acute haemopoietic syndromes; for example, anaemia, leukopaenia, platelet depression, infection and haemorrhage.

In this range of exposure rate, however, the late pathologic effects of extended exposure do not appear to include long-term counterparts to the other acute radiation syndromes, i.e. the central nervous system syndrome and the gastrointestinal or intestinal syndrome.

Although there is advancement in degree of subtle, non-specific degenerative changes in parenchymal and supporting cells and tissues which are similar to changes occurring universally and progressively with increasing time or age in non-irradiated animals (Casarett, 1964), the pathologic effects of extended exposure in this dose-rate range, that apparently are the chief imminent causes or contributors to death, include haemopoietic depressions or disorders, with infection or haemorrhage, and the temporal advancement or induction of neoplasms. Another prominent effect, in organs not vital for survival of the individual, is depletion of gametogenic epithelium.

The haemopoietic, neoplastic and gametogenic effects are the main topics of this paper.

Review of Data

A. Haemopoietic system

Extended low dose radiation exposure in the range of 10 R per day or lower tends

---

* This paper is based on work performed under contract with the U.S. Atomic Energy Commission at the University of Rochester Atomic Energy Project and has been assigned Report No. UR 49-1118.

to depress or deplete various haemopoietic cellular elements at various levels of exposure rate in accordance with the relative radiosensitivity of their progenitors, with respect to effects on cellular viability and reproductive ability. Whether or not the numbers of the various cells in the circulating blood recover to normal after initial depression, or persist at subnormal levels for long periods of time, or decline progressively with increasing time during such exposure, depends much on the capability of the progenitors of the cells to compensate for the repeated or continuous damage done to them. Such compensatory capability may involve an increased rate of cell production in the progenitor cell system and/or increase in radioresistance of cells in this system, whether by selection or acquisition.

In rough, general terms, the persistent decrease in number of a circulating blood cell which is caused by extended low dose radiation exposure, tends to begin earlier, become greater in degree before stabilizing, or become more progressive, the greater the daily dose.

In table 1 the values of lower exposure rates (R or n per day) for extended exposure which have been associated with substantial and persistent depression of blood cell counts in various species, were collected or approximated from data in the various reports discussed below in this section.

In this context, the grouping of species in a rough order of decreasing susceptibility to X or gamma radiation seems to be: for lymphocyte count depression, the guinea-pig, the dog, and the mouse, rat and rabbit; for heterophil (or neutrophil) cell count depression, the guinea-pig and dog, the mouse, and the rat and rabbit; for platelet count depression, the guinea-pig and dog, the mouse and rabbit, and the rat; and for erythrocyte count depression, the guinea-pig, the dog, the mouse, the rat, and the rabbit.

Lorenz et al. (1946, 1947) reported haematologic findings in mice, rabbits, and guinea-pigs exposed daily, in 8 hours each day, 6 days per week, to radium gamma rays at rates of 0.11, 1.1, 2.2, 4.4, or 8.8 R per day for periods in some experiments to more than 3 years. Survival was inversely proportional to dose.

The mice, which accumulated total exposures as high as 5,880 R, showed considerable haemopoietic radioresistance. At 8.8 R/day the mean reductions in erythrocyte, haemoglobin, and platelet values never exceeded 30%, and reduction developed over a period of 79 weeks. Reductions in these parameters were equivocal at 4.4 R/day and did not occur at lower exposure rates. The leukocyte count was reduced at 2.2 R/day or greater, largely as a result of lymphocyte count depression, beginning within the first few weeks and persisting at a fairly constant level thereafter.

There was little evidence of haematologic change in rabbits, despite total exposures as high as 12,000 R. As in mice, the lymphocyte count became depressed within the first few weeks and persisted at a reduced level thereafter for the first 100 weeks. Heterophil leukocyte count increased at all but the lowest exposure level. Erythrocyte and haemoglobin values showed no significant change at any exposure level.

In guinea-pigs the leukocyte count at all exposure levels decreased within a few weeks and the depressions persisted thereafter. The reduction of the leukocyte counts at 0.11 R/day and 1.1 R/day was the result of lymphocyte depression, but at the higher dose rates it was largely the result of neutrophil count depression. The terminal condition was characterized by marked neutropaenia. The erythrocyte counts or haemoglobin values were not depressed significantly at 0.11 R/day or 1.1 R/day. However, with increasing exposure

Table 1

Lower daily radiation exposures associated with substantial and persistent depression of blood cell counts during extended whole-body exposure

Species	Daily exposure (R; n)			
	Lymphocytes	Neutrophils	Platelets	Erythrocytes
Guinea pig	0.11 R;	2.2 R;	2.2 R;	2.2 R; .....
Dog	0.5 R; 0.11 n	3.0 R; 1.7 n	3.0 R; >1.7 n	6.0 R; 1.7 n
Mouse	2.2 R; 1.4 n	4.4 R; 1.4 n	8.8 R; >1.4 n	8.8 R; >1.4 n
Rat	> 1.0 R; 1.7 n	10.0 R; 1.7 n	>10.0 R; >1.7 n	10.0 R; 1.7 n
Rabbit	2.2 R; 1.7 n	>10.0 R; 1.7 n	10.0 R; >1.7 n	>10.0 R; 1.7 n

Symbols:

R - Roentgen, exposure unit for X or gamma radiation.

n - Exposure unit for fast neutrons. See H.H. Rossi, Radiology, 61, 93, 1953.

> - Daily exposure required greater than that indicated.

An approximate value for Kerma can be obtained by multiplying n by 2.5. However, the problems of computing the absorbed dose are great.

rate there was generally an earlier onset and greater degree of anaemia, with severe terminal anaemia developing at the higher exposure rates. Platelet counts did not decline at 0.11 R/day, declined late and slightly at 1.1 R/day, with variable persistence or recovery, and with increasing exposure rate showed greater and more progressive reductions. The majority of the guinea-pigs at 2.2 R/day and 4.4 R/day, and all of them at 8.8 R/day died with anaemia or thrombocytopaenia or both. The size of the daily exposure appeared to be more important than the total exposure in the induction of severe terminal pancytopaenia.

In other experiments to study the patterns of haematologic recovery in guinea-pigs exposed to 8.8 R/day until the erythrocyte count had fallen to slightly less than 3 million per mm^3, Lorenz and his co-workers (Lorenz et al., 1950a, b; Lorenz, 1951) found that the required accumulated exposure ranged from 950 to 1,047 R, and that this anaemia was always associated with leukopaenia and thrombocytopaenia. Three different recovery patterns were observed after cessation of the irradiation. In the first pattern there was continued decrease of erythrocyte count and of haemoglobin and haematocrit values, cessation of platelet decline, rapid recovery of leukocytes (both lymphocytes and neutrophils), and rapid increase of reticulocyte count from normal to supranormal levels, but the animals died within about 9 weeks showing slight to moderate hypoplasia of bone marrow with normal distributions of cellular components. In the second pattern of recovery there were these same changes for the first 9 weeks, and these were followed by several weeks of recovery in which there was partial recovery of leukocytes and persistent increases in reticulocyte count and colour index, but death from recurrent pancytopaenia occurred between the 12th and 24th weeks, in association with normal or hyperplastic cellularity of bone marrow. This suggests a defect in maturation or delivery of cells to the circulating blood. In the third pattern of recovery there was complete recovery from anaemia, beginning about 6 weeks post-exposure, and a rapid recovery of all cellular elements during the next 6 weeks, followed by a more gradual approach over many months toward normal levels. Neutrophil leukocytes showed the most rapid recovery and platelets the longest delay in recovery. Bone marrow cellularity became normal. Recovery of the haemopoietic system was slower after this extended exposure than after single intense exposure.

There was little or no evidence of haemorrhage in these guinea-pigs, even in those which died, despite the rarity of megakaryocytes in the marrow of those which died. The partial recovery of the platelet count in these animals was associated with the presence of megakaryocytes in extramedullary haemopoietic tissue in spleen.

Henshaw et al (1947) observed a marked and uniform reduction of blood leukocyte count, involving both lymphocytes and heterophils, in mice exposed to fast neutrons at the rate of 4.3 n* per day, 6 days per week. Deaths occurred from 8 to 12 weeks after the beginning of exposure. Exposure to 1.15 n per day of fast neutrons, or to 8.6 R per day of pile-produced gamma rays, caused little, if any, haematologic change after 40 to 60 weeks of exposure. Exposure to 0.25 n per day of fast neutrons, or to 8.6 R per day of pile gamma rays, a ratio of 1:35, had the same effect on survival, and for acute lethality the ratio was 1:7.5.

Evans (1948) exposed mice repeatedly to fast neutrons at rates of 0.014, 0.07, 0.14, and 1.4 n per day for periods up to 90 weeks. Mean blood leukocyte counts were lower than controls at all exposure-rate levels, but were substantially depressed, largely due to

---

* The unit n was, at that time, used as an exposure unit for neutrons. See table 1 for further explanation.

lymphocyte count decline, only at the highest exposure rate (1.4 n), with reduction apparent within a month and reaching 50% of control level by the end of exposure at 24 weeks. Erythrocyte, haemoglobin, reticulocyte, or platelet values were not affected.

Ely et al. (1950) reported the pathologic findings in rats, rabbits and dogs given brief daily exposure to cyclotron neutrons, 6 days per week for 1 year, at the rates of 0.012, 0.06, 0.11, or 1.7 n per day. Survivors were sacrificed for pathologic studies after cessation of exposure.

All of the rats at 1.7 n/day died before the end of the irradiation period, but 62 to 68% of the rats in all other groups, including the control group, survived this period. Rats at 0.11 n/day died sooner than those at lower exposure rates. Infectious disease, most frequently pulmonary infections and a paratyphoid infection, although not significantly increased at the three lower exposure rates, was increased to an incidence at 1.7 n/day that was more than twice that in all controls. In fact, in about 40% of the rats at 1.7 n/day, the only lesions to which death could be attributed were infectious diseases. Rats at this exposure level showed hypoplasia of bone marrow, spleen and lymph nodes, marked reduction of blood lymphocyte count, lesser reduction of heterophil leukocyte count, and later a depression of erythrocyte count, but no significant change in platelet and reticulocyte counts. No substantial changes in blood cell counts were observed at the lower exposure levels.

In rabbits, neutron exposure caused significant increase in the mortality during exposure only at the highest exposure rate (1.7 n/day) in which group only 20% survived. The rabbits of this group showed hypoplasia of bone marrow, spleen and lymph nodes, marked reduction of blood lymphocyte count, lesser reduction of neutrophil count, and later depression of erythrocyte count, but no significant change in platelet and reticulocyte counts.

Four of the five dogs at 1.7 n/day died during the 1-year exposure period, but all dogs at the lower exposure levels and in the control group survived this period. At 1.7 n/day all dogs showed haemorrhagic manifestations, the organs most commonly involved being lymph nodes, heart, stomach, small bowel, and kidneys. The bone marrow and spleen were considerably hypoplastic. Peripheral blood cell counts showed marked reduction of lymphocytes, lesser reduction of neutrophils, beginning within 2 weeks, and reduction of erythrocytes beginning after 32 weeks. Lymphocytes were also reduced in dogs at lower dose rates, but neutrophils and erythrocytes were not significantly changed in any group.

Metcalf et al. (1951) reported the pathologic findings in rats, rabbits, and dogs given brief daily exposure to X rays, 6 days per week, at the rates of 0.1, 0.5, 1.0, or 10.0 R/day, with additional groups of dogs at 3.0 and 6.0 R/day. Daily exposure was carried on in rats for 24 months, in dogs at 0.1 to 1.0 R/day for 24 months, in dogs at 3.0 to 10.0 R/day for 19.2 months, and in rabbits for 12 months, after which periods the surviving animals were sacrificed for pathologic studies. Ingram and Mason (1950) reported the haematologic data.

In the rats, mortality during the period of irradiation, which extended over most of the adult life span, increased with increasing daily dose over the whole range of exposure rates. The probable causes of death for the rats that died during this experiment may be assigned to the following diseases in approximately 70% of the cases: pulmonary infection, malignant tumours, chronic nephritis, and Salmonella infection. However, with the exception of certain malignant neoplasms, these diseases were generally not dosage-dependent in absolute incidence, but rather tended to occur earlier and to be more severe at the higher exposure-rate levels. Considerable haemopoietic change in the rats occurred only at

10 R/day and included increased, mild to moderate, hypoplasia of bone marrow, lymph nodes and spleen, and marked depression of blood lymphocyte count.

In rabbits there was no significant increase in mortality during the 1-year exposure period at the three lower exposure rates, but there was such an increase in the 10.0 R/day group, in which 60% died. Causes of death were chiefly infectious diseases. At this exposure rate the rabbits showed moderate hypoplasia of bone marrow, rapid decrease of blood lymphocyte count, which remained depressed thereafter, minimal depression of neutrophil count by 5 weeks, which persisted thereafter, a small and persistent depression of erythrocyte count after 4 months, and a persistent reduction of platelet count after the second month. There was no definite evidence of radiation damage at 1.0 R/day or less.

In dogs there was no significant increase in mortality during the exposure period at the exposure rates below 1.0 R/day, but from 1.0 to 10 R/day there was dosage-dependent increase in incidence of mortality up to 80% at 10 R/day. Focal bowel haemorrhages occurred in 44% of the dogs that died during the 10 R/day exposure, and lymph node haemorrhage, usually severe, also occurred consistently in these dogs. Bone marrow hypoplasia of substantial degree occurred only at 10 R/day and was moderate to marked, including decrease in number of megakaryocytes. Lymph node and splenic lymphoid hypoplasia was more marked at 3 R/day and greater rates than at lower exposure rates. Blood lymphocyte count did not change significantly during the 2 years of exposure at 0.1 R/day, but was decreased substantially at 0.5 R/day and to a greater degree the higher the exposure rate. Depression began abruptly at 3.0 R/day and higher dose levels, becoming marked as early as 1 week and remaining so thereafter. At 0.5 and 1.0 R/day, depressions of lymphocyte count developed more slowly, about the sixth month, and were less marked. Blood neutrophil count was not reduced at 0.1 or 0.5 R/day, was mildly depressed after 1 year at 1.0 and 3.0 R/day, and was moderately depressed as early as 1 month at 6.0 and 10.0 R/day, remaining depressed thereafter. Platelet count was depressed abruptly in all dogs at 3, 6, and 10 R/day within 2 months and showed slowly progressive decline thereafter. Erythrocyte counts and haemoglobin were depressed at 10 R/day, to a marked degree, and to lesser degrees at 6 R/day and 3 R/day. The reticulocyte count was reduced at 3, 6, and 10 R/day to similar degrees in 1 week and remained depressed thereafter.

B. Neoplasms

Henshaw (1944) found an increase in leukaemia in mice after repeated exposures to X rays.

In the study by Lorenz et al. (1947), involving daily (8 hour) gamma ray exposure of mice, guinea-pigs, and rabbits at 0.11 R/day to 8.8 R/day, there was a dose-rate dependent, marked increase in incidence of leukaemia (malignant lymphoma) in the female mice at 4.4 and 8.8 R/day, a greater increase in incidence of ovarian tumours in the female mice, ranging from 60 to 100% from the 0.11 R/day to 8.8 R/day groups as compared with 12% in controls, and a slight increase in incidence of mammary gland tumours and lung tumours in irradiated mice. The incidence of mammary tumours in irradiated female mice was over 20% as compared with 0% in controls. Lorenz et al. (1951) reported that all groups of irradiated female mice, except the 0.11 R/day group, showed an increased incidence of mammary carcinoma ranging from 4 to 14%. Furthermore, in all irradiated groups except the 8.8 R/day group, sarcomas of the mammary gland developed, with incidence ranging from 13 to 25%. Most of the mice having mammary gland tumours also had granulosa-cell tumours of the ovary.

Lorenz et al. (1947) also reported an increase in mammary tumours in guinea-pigs, and an increase in incidence of uterine tumours in rabbits. Uterine carcinomas developed in 11 of 12 rabbits exposed to 1.1 R/day or more, as compared with 2 of 6 non-irradiated controls. These uterine carcinomas appeared within 33 to 50 months in the irradiated rabbits, but not before 57 months in the controls.

In the study by Metcalf et al. (1951), involving brief, daily X-ray exposure of rats (24 months), rabbits (12 months), and dogs (19 to 24 months), at 0.1 R/day to 10 R/day, the incidence of leukaemia in rats increased with increasing exposure rate, from 8% in controls to 35% at 10 R/day.

In the study by Ely et al. (1950), involving brief daily exposure of rats, rabbits, and dogs to cyclotron neutrons, 6 days/week for 1 year, at 0.012 n/day to 1.7 n/day, the incidence of neoplasms in rats at 0.11 n/day (41.6%) was more than three times as great as that in the control group (12.5%), and almost twice that at 1.7 n/day (22.9%). Leukaemia incidence in rats was 0% in controls and in the two lower exposure-rate groups, 4.2% at 0.11 n/day, and 16.6% at 1.7 n/day. Malignant neoplasms other than leukaemia were present in 8% of controls, 14% at 0.012 n/day, 8% at 0.06 n/day, 31% at 0.11 n/day, and only 4% at 1.7 n/day. Benign neoplasms were similar in incidence (2 to 6%) at all exposure levels, perhaps slightly increased at 0.11 n/day. The high death rate and short survival time of rats at the highest exposure rate (1.7 n/day) may have permitted the appearance of leukaemia, with its relatively short induction time, better than cancers with longer induction times. Neoplasms in rabbits were limited to two cases with malignant non-pigmented melanomata that died late in the exposure period at 1.7 n/day.

A comparison of the incidence of rats with neoplasms in the rats exposed to X rays (Metcalf et al., 1951) with that in the rats exposed to neutrons (Ely et al., 1950) reveals certain interesting relations. Owing to the longer duration of exposure in the X-ray experiment, the incidence observed was greater in most exposure groups than in the neutron experiment. In both experiments, however, the differences in total incidence between controls and the two lower experimental groups were not significant. The incidence in the rats exposed to 0.11 n/day was essentially the same as in those exposed to 1 R/day. In the X-ray group the incidence of rats with neoplasms was about the same at the 10 R/day level as it was at the 1 R/day level and much greater than that in rats exposed at 1.7 n/day. Again, the survival time seems to have been an important factor, since the rats at the highest exposure level in the X-ray experiment generally lived longer than those at 1.7 n/day in the neutron experiment. The high incidence of rats with neoplasms at 1.7 n/day was due largely to the larger number of cases with leukaemia, which may have a shorter induction time than other malignancies. Benign mammary tumours, which were increased in incidence in the X-ray experiment, were relatively infrequent in the neutron experiment and showed no increase in any irradiated group. This marked difference in incidence of rats with mammary tumours between these experiments is probably due to the difference in duration of the experiments, 2 years for X rays and 1 year for neutrons, since most tumours of this type occurred during the second year of exposure of the X-ray experiment.

Lesher et al. (1965) exposed mice to duration-of-life ^{60}Co gamma irradiation at daily (10 to 15 hours) dose levels of 5, 12, 24, 32, 43, 49, and 56 R/day. The two lower daily dose levels (5 and 12 R/day) were much more carcinogenic than higher exposure rate levels. Although the incidence of most tumours was increased at 5 and 12 R/day, duration-of-life exposure was less carcinogenic per roentgen of accumulated exposure than single and terminated exposures. There was a reduction in overall tumour frequency at high exposure rates associated with shorter survival times. The incidence and variety of tumours was much higher in the female mice, due largely to their high incidence of lymphoma and of tumours associated with the reproductive system. Lymphoid, pulmonary and mammary tumours appeared earlier in the irradiated mice, while hepatomas, ovarian tumours, and the degenerative diseases, nephrosclerosis and amyloidosis, were not affected. Multiple tumours were common in mice at the lower exposure rates, reaching 50% among the 5 R/day females.

C. Ovarian follicles

There has been relatively little work on effects of extended low dose exposure on ovarian follicles in mature animals, and most of this has been done on mice, a species with relatively sensitive ovaries in terms of single sterilizing doses and susceptibility to induction of ovarian tumours.

Daily gamma irradiation of rabbits with 8.8 R to doses as high as 11,700 R has caused little or no change in ovaries (Eschenbrenner and Miller, 1954).

In experiments with protracted or continuous exposure to gamma radiation (Deringer et al., 1954; Eschenbrenner and Miller, 1954), mice given total exposures of 770 and 880 R at the rate of 8.8 and 4.4 R/day showed some incidence of sterility, and the ovaries showed marked reduction in number of follicles. Some were tumourous. Mice exposed to a total of 550 R at the rate of 4.4 R/day produced litters of reduced size. Throughout these experiments, sterilized females did not recover their fertility, but males did. Daily irradiation caused apparent sterilization of the mouse ovary with 8.8 R/day at 4 months and with 4.4 R/day at 8 months, while with 1.1 R/day there were still some growing follicles at 16 months.

The data from these experiments indicate that the radiation injury to the mouse ovary from chronic exposure is largely accumulative. It is also irreversible in the sense that the stock of follicles or gamete precursors which is being depleted is nonrenewable, in contrast to the male gametogenic system which is a cell renewal system.

D. Spermatogenic epithelium

The order of daily X or gamma-radiation exposure required to cause substantial persistent depression of spermatogenesis during extended low dose exposure seems to be about 0.5 R/day for dogs, and about 2 or 3 R/day for rats, mice and guinea-pigs, and possibly rabbits as well. Larger daily exposures seem to be required to bring the production of sperm down to zero in a relatively short time and to keep it there during exposure.

Figure 1 illustrates the effect of a total, whole-body X-ray exposure of 325 R, given as a single exposure or fractionated into brief daily exposures of 3 R, 5 days/week, on the production of prespermatocytes (i.e. terminal spermatogonia or resting spermatocytes) in the testes of rats (Casarett and Casarett, 1957). Prespermatocytes were counted systematically in tubule cross sections representative of all stages of spermatogenesis in each animal. The counts of prespermatocytes (terminal spermatogonia which have not left the basement-membrane and begun to grow and differentiate as spermatocytes) per tubule cross section were fairly consistent, throughout the study period, with an overall mean of 67.6 ± 0.7.

There was a precipitous decline in the prespermatocyte count in the single exposure group. The minimal count was recorded at day 18 as an average of six

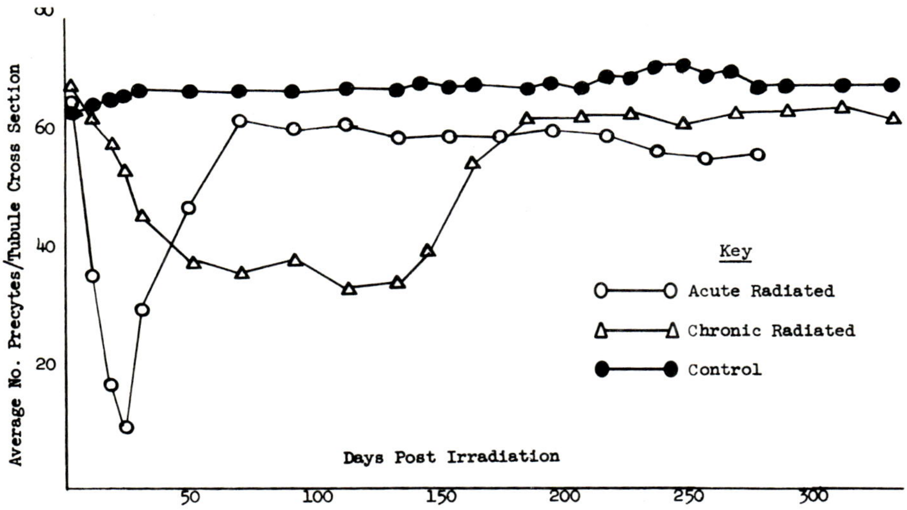

Fig. 1. Prespermatocyte (terminal spermatogonia) counts in testes of rats exposed to 325 R of X rays in a single exposure ("acute radiated") or at the rate of a brief daily exposure of 3 R, 5 days/week ("chronic radiated"). (From Casarett and Casarett, 1957.)

prespermatocytes per tubule cross section. There was rapid recovery thereafter to subnormal levels which persisted. From the 95th to the 284th day (last day of observation) the average of the counts was about 59 per cross section, or 12.6% below the control average, a difference of about 8.5 cells per tubule cross section.

In the fractionated exposure group there was a more gradual depression of the count, the count was depressed to a lesser degree, but the depression was more prolonged. The average count between 53 and 137 days (last day of exposure) was 33.3 ± 4.2. Apparently an equilibrium had been reached between damage and recovery, while extended fractionated exposure was still being carried on. After cessation of daily irradiation at 137 days, there was recovery of the prespermatocyte count, reaching maximal recovery levels by the 169th day which were subnormal and persisted but which were somewhat higher than those for the single exposure group. Thereafter, the average count for the period from 169 days to 337 days was 64.1 ± 1.4, or 5.2% below the mean control count. This difference is statistically significant at the 5% level.

The single exposure seems to have caused about twice as much unrepaired damage as the fractionated exposure, in terms of these cell counts. Although one might argue, on the basis of the areas under these curves, that the fractionated exposure may have been more efficient in maintaining depression of spermatogenic cells, this particular mode of fractionation of this total exposure did not seem to be more effective than the single exposure in terms of unrepaired injury. However, comparison at a total dose level that does not in either mode of administration cause counts of zero, is not necessarily indicative of the relative efficiency of other modes of fractionation of other total doses in causing complete and permanent cessation of spermatogenesis.

In view of the changing radiosensitivity of proliferating spermatogenic cells in various stages of the cell generation cycle, with respect not only to "reproductive death" but also to frank necrosis in post-exposure preparation for or attempts to divide (mitosis-linked necrosis), and in view of the probability that that fraction of the primitive spermatogonia which start each of the cycles in the spermatogenic wave and which have a relatively long interphase, as compared with proliferating spermatogenia in subsequent stages, are relatively radioresistant, it seems likely that there is for each species a highly efficient total dose and mode of fractionation for the causation of complete and permanent cessation of spermatogenesis (Casarett, 1956). This general mode of fractionation would "waste" as little radiation as possible in bringing the production of sperm to zero and in keeping it there, by virtue of continuing to kill the relatively radioresistant spermatogonia which become more sensitive as they enter into regenerative proliferation, and the associated efficient total dose would be the minimal accumulated dose at which regeneration was no longer possible. The inter-related factors which govern the efficiency of the mode of fractionation, in this context, i.e. which reduce "wasted" radiation in killing cells or in allowing regeneration during exposure, are fraction size, dose rate, and inter-fraction interval in relation to the cytokinetics and radiosensitivity changes in the various compartments of the stem cell system.

These are the thoughts that led us to search for a highly efficient mode of fractionation for complete and permanent aspermia in our long-term X-ray (1,000 kVp) experiments on dogs (beagles), which are described below (Casarett, 1950, 1953, 1963; Casarett and Eddy, 1968; Casarett and Hursh, 1956).

In table 2 are given the experimental groups in the life-long irradiation experiment, involving brief (10 minutes), whole-body, X-ray exposure daily, 5 days/week for adult life (beginning 21 months of age) at the rates of 0.0, 0.06, 0.12 or 0.6 R/day and semen analysis biweekly or monthly. In table 3 are given the exposure and survival data for this life-long irradiation experiment. In table 4 are given the experimental groups for limited dose experiments, single or fractionated, whole-body or testicular exposure.

Table 2

Experimental groups in life-long irradiation experiment

Group code	No. of dogs	Intended dosage (R)[a] Daily	Weekly[b]	Yearly[c]
W	20	0.00	0.0	0.0
X	20	0.06	0.3	15.6
Y	10	0.12	0.6	31.2
Z	10	0.60	3.0	156.0

[a]Actual doses about 8% larger than intended doses.
[b]Weekly dose is the addition of the five daily doses per week.
[c]Yearly dose is the addition of the daily doses per year.

In table 5 are given the grand means of absolute sperm counts (total numbers of sperm per ejaculate) in the various exposure groups for various periods in the life-long irradiation experiment to the age of 11 years, i.e. before the rapidly increasing frequency of serious diseases which caused depression of spermatogenesis in increasing numbers of animals in all groups before death. These values reveal the general tendency for the sperm count to decrease with age in the lower dosage groups (0.06 and 0.12 R/day) and control group, without substantial, biologically significant differences among these groups.

Table 3

Life-long irradiation experiment dosage and survival data

Group code	Daily dose (R)	Years exposure	Dose to death (R)	Age at death (yrs)	Ave. death age (yrs)	Median death age
W	0.00	5.4-16.3	0-0	7.1-18.0	12.97	13.14
X	0.06	7.5-15.4	122-257	9.2-17.1	13.76	14.06
Y	0.12	7.3-13.9	243-465	9.0-15.6	13.21	13.78
Z	0.60	6.7-13.2	1088-2198	8.3-14.8	12.33	12.67

Table 4

Limited dose experiments. Single and fractionated

Group code	No. of dogs	Dose rate	Radiation period	Total dose (R)	Part irrad.
S	5	3 R/day[a]	25 weeks	375	W.B.[b]
V-1	5	3 R/day[a]	32 weeks	475	W.B.
V-2	5	3 R/day[a]	42 weeks	635	W.B.
U	4	10 R/min.	30 min.	300	W.B.
T	5	10 R/min.	37 min	375	W.B.
Q	5	64 R/min.	15.6 min.	1000	testes
R	5	70 R/min.	21.4 min.	1500	testes
P	5	70 R/min.	28.6 min.	2000	testes

[a] 3 R in 10 minutes each day (0.3 R/min.), 5 days each week
[b] W.B. is whole-body.

However, there seems to be a consistent trend of somewhat lower values at 0.12 R/day than at the lowest dosage or control levels after 340 weeks of age. Marked reduction of seminal sperm count was caused by irradiation at 0.6 R/day. The absolute sperm counts of these dogs began to decline after 20 to 30 weeks of exposure (60 to 90 R at time of observation) and in 8 of the 10 cases fell to less than 6% of the pre-exposure values within the first year of exposure (150 R). In the other two dogs of this exposure group the absolute sperm count fell only to the 100 or 200 million range (about 20% of pre-exposure values) in the first year of exposure, when their sperm counts became more or less stabilized and remained so for about 5 to 6 years. From the 3rd to the 10th years of exposure all of the dogs at this exposure level became aspermic or almost so.

Table 5

Absolute sperm counts in life-long irradiation experiment to eleven years of age

(grand means in millions[a])

Dosage R/day	Pre-exp. period	Weeks of exposure 0-120	120-190	190-250	250-370	370-420	420-480
0.0	511	518	514	450	400	377	423
0.06	501	570	545	499	460	387	368
0.12	520	517	507	477	375	307	344
0.6	568	493-64[b]	42	46	32	9	5
wks.age	50-90	90-210	210-280	280-340	340-460	460-510	510-570

[a] Excluding dogs which died before 480 weeks of exposure.
[b] Decline of sperm count from 493 to 64 million during period.

A larger daily dose would be required to bring the production of sperm down to zero in much shorter time than that observed at 0.6 R/day. On the basis of previous pathologic studies, a daily exposure of 3 R/day, 5 days/week, was chosen for limited dose fractionation studies in the attempt to find a highly efficient fractionation mode for causing complete and permanent aspermia in dogs. In table 6 is given a general summary of the radiation effects on, and recovery of, seminal sperm count in the limited dose experiments outlined in table 4. In all of these experiments, the beginning of depression of sperm count was observed about 10 weeks after single radiation exposure or after the beginning of fractionated irradiation.

A single, whole-body radiation exposure of 300 R or 375 R (U and T groups) caused a marked depression of sperm count within 3 months, with a maximum depression to nearly zero at about 6 months, followed soon by a recovery trend in which the counts reached almost the pre-exposure ranges in about a year after the maximal depression was observed. In contrast, a total accumulated exposure of 375 R administered whole-body at the rate of 3 R/day, 5 days/week (S group), caused aspermia in all dogs in 6 months, i.e. in the time (25 weeks) that was required for the administration of the total dose; the aspermia persisted in two dogs for about 6 months, in two dogs for about 14 months, and in one dog permanently. Recovery in three of the dogs was only slight and in one case marked but incomplete. Increasing the accumulated whole-body exposure, at this rate of 3 R/day, to 475 R (V-1 group) or to 635 R (V-2) group caused aspermia in all dogs in 6 months and permitted no recovery in any of the dogs thereafter.

Table 6

Reduction and recovery of sperm count in limited dose experiments

Group code	dose rate	Total dose (R)	Part irrad.	Months to aspermia	Months of aspermia	Approx. ave. recovery (%)
S	3 R/day[a]	375	W.B.[b]	6	6 to life	10
V-1	3 R/day[a]	475	W.B.	6	life	0
V-2	3 R/day[a]	635	W.B.	6	life	0
U	10 R/min.	300	W.B.	-[c]	0	90-100
T	10 R/min.	375	W.B.	-[c]	0	90-100
Q	64 R/min.	1000	testes	4	8	75
R	70 R/min.	1500	testes	3	11	50
P	70 R/min.	2000	testes	2	12	10

[a] 3 R/day in 10-minute period each day, 5 days per week.
[b] W.B. indicates whole-body irradiation.
[c] Near-zero counts for brief periods, but aspermia did not occur.

Intense single exposure of testes of dogs with 1000 R, 1500 R, or 2000 R (Q, R, P groups), which would be lethal if delivered to the whole body, caused the development of aspermia within periods of time which were inversely related to the size of the dose, with the duration of aspermia directly related to size of dose, and with the degree of recovery varying inversely with dose size. The recovery of sperm count after these single, high level exposures reached subnormal plateaus 2 to 3 years after exposure.

The marked permanent damage of sperm production by a whole-body exposure of 375 R delivered at the rate of 3 R/day, without the induction of acute illness or death, as compared with the little permanent damage of sperm production caused by a brief single whole-body exposure of 375 R, which caused acute illness, has shown that certain modes of fractionation of dose may be more efficient than intensive exposure in damaging tissue and that male sterility can be a hazard of certain modes of fractionated exposure in the absence of radiation induced acute illness or death.

There were no experiments in which dogs were given localized testicular irradiation at the rate of 3 R/day, and therefore there was no direct test of any possible influence of irradiation of the remainder of the body on the effects on sperm production with this fractionation schedule. However, many experiments, including some of our own (Casarett, 1956; Casarett and Casarett, 1957) have shown that the effects of single exposures of radiation on spermatogenesis are largely the effects of the radiation in the testes, with little or no influence of the irradiation of the rest of the body. If this can be assumed to be true also for fractionation of dose at the rate of 3 R/day in dogs, it would then appear that testicular irradiation at the rate of 3 R/day (15 R/week) is at least four times as effective (or efficient) as a single intensive exposure in causing permanent aspermia in 100% of these dogs, since a single exposure of 2000 R was not sufficient to cause this effect, but a total exposure of 475 R at 3 R/day was sufficient. In any case, this efficiency factor holds for a comparison of the two modes of exposure.

Concluding Comment

The importance of the size of the daily dose to the efficiency of fractionation schedules in damaging sperm production is emphasized by: (1) the failure of whole-body irradiation fractionated at the rates of 0.06 R/day or 0.12 R/day to total accumulated exposures as high as 257 R or 465 R, respectively, to cause any appreciable reduction of sperm count, (2) the long time taken for whole-body irradiation fractionated at the rate of 0.6 R/day (to total exposures of 1,088 R to 2,198 R) to reduce sperm count to zero, after causing early marked reduction of sperm count, and (3) the efficiency of exposures of 375 R to 475 R at the rate of 3 R/day in causing permanent oligospermia or aspermia in comparison with the wasted irradiation involved for these effects in single intensive exposures.

From the data presented on effects of extended low dose exposure on the haemopoietic system, on incidence of neoplasms, and on oogenic epithelium, it is also evident that size of daily dose in fractionated exposure may be of greater importance in many respects than total accumulated exposure, although various specific end-points may be governed considerably by total exposure level. However, in these systems, efficiency factors in terms of minimal daily fraction size and total exposure for production of given degrees of permanent damage have not yet been studied substantially by means of comparisons of effects of single exposures and limited dose fractionated exposures. Such studies in various organs would be of value.

References

Casarett, A.P., and Casarett, G.W. Histological investigations of X-ray effects on spermatogenesis in the rat. U.S. Atomic Energy Commission Document UR-496 (Part I) and UR-497 (Part II), 1957.

Casarett, G.W. Effects of X-rays on spermatogenesis in dogs. U.S. Atomic Energy Commission Document UR-127, 1950.

Casarett, G.W. Effects of daily low doses of X-rays on spermatogenesis in dogs. U.S. Atomic Energy Commission Document UR-292, 1953.

Casarett, G.W. The effects of ionizing radiations from external sources on gametogenesis and fertility in mammals. U.S. Atomic Energy Commission Document UR-441, 1956.

Casarett, G.W. Long-term effects of irradiation on sperm production of dogs. In: Effects of Ionization Radiation in the Reproductive System, edited by W.D.Carlson and F.X. Gassner, Pergamon Press, New York, pp. 137-146, 1963.

Casarett, G.W. Similarities and contrasts between radiation and time pathology. In: Advances in Gerontological Research, Vol. 1, edited by B. Strehler, Academic Press, New York, pp. 109-163, 1964.

Casarett, G.W., and Eddy, H.A. Fractionation of dose in radiation-induced male sterility. In: Proceedings of Symposium on Dose Rate in Mammalian Radiation Biology, edited by D.G. Brown, R.G. Cragle and T.R. Noonan, U.S.A.E.C. Technical Information Division, Washington, D.C., pp. 14.1-14.10, 1968.

Casarett, G.W., and Hursh, J.B. Effects of daily low doses of X-ray on spermatogenesis in dogs. In: Proceedings of First International Conference on Peaceful Uses of Atomic Energy, Vol. 11, Biological Effects of Radiation, United Nations, New York, pp. 184-187, 1956.

Deringer, M.K., Heston, W.E., and Lorenz, E. Effects of long-continued total-body gamma irradiation on mice, guinea pigs, and rabbits. IV. Actions on the breeding behavior of mice. In: Biological Effects of External X- and Gamma Radiation, edited by R.E. Zirkle, McGraw-Hill Book Co., New York, pp. 149-168, 1954.

Ely, J.O., Ross, M.H., Metcalf, R.G., Inda, F.A., Barnett, T.B., and Casarett, G.W. Clinical, pathological, and hematological effects of chronic neutron radiation. USAEC Report UR-92, 1950. Also Chapter 17 in Biological Effects of External Radiation, edited by H.A. Blair, McGraw-Hill Book Co., New York, pp. 419-497, 1954.

Eschenbrenner, A.B., and Miller, E. Effects of long-continued total-body gamma irradiation on mice, guinea pigs, and rabbits. V. Pathological observations. In: Biological Effects of External X- and Gamma Radiation, edited by R.E. Zirkle, McGraw-Hill Book Co., New York, pp. 169-225, 1954.

Evans, T.C. Effects of small daily doses of fast neutrons on mice. Radiology, 50, 811-833, 1948.

Henshaw, P.S. Experimental roentgen injury. IV. Effects of repeated small doses of X-rays on blood picture, tissue morphology, and life span in mice. J. natn. Cancer Inst., 4, 513-522, 1944.

Henshaw, P.S., Riley, E.F., and Stapleton, G.E. The biologic effects of pile radiations. Radiology, 49, 349-360, 1947.

Ingram, M., and Mason, W.B. The effects of chronic exposure to roentgen radiation on the peripheral blood of experimental animals. USAEC Report UR-121, 1950. Also Chapter 11 in Biological Effects of External Radiation, edited by H.A. Blair, McGraw-Hill Book Co., New York, pp. 253-267, 1954.

Lesher, S., Sacher, G.A., Grahn, D., Hamilton, K., and Sallese, A. Survival of mice under duration-of-life exposure to gamma rays. II. Pathologic effects. Radiat. Res., 24, 239-277, 1965.

Lorenz, E. Recovery pattern of the blood picture in guinea pigs following a limited total-body exposure to chronic gamma radiation. J. Chim. Phys., 48, 264-274, 1951.

Lorenz, E., Eschenbrenner, A.B., Heston, W.E., and Uphoff, D. Mammary tumor incidence in female C3Hb mice following long continued gamma irradiation. J. natn. Cancer Inst., 11, 947-965, 1951.

Lorenz, E., Heston, W.E., and Eschenbrenner, A.B. Biological studies in the tolerance range. Radiology, 49, 274-285, 1947.

Lorenz, E., Heston, W.E., Jacobson, L.O., Eschenbrenner, A.B., Shimkin, M.B., Deringer, M.K., Doniger, J., and Schweisthal, R. Effects of long-continued whole body irradiation with gamma rays on mice, guinea pigs, and rabbits. Parts I-IV, USAEC Report MDDC-653, pp. 38-52, 1946.

Lorenz, E., Jacobson, L.O., and Sutton, H. Part I. Survival and blood picture of hybrid guinea pigs exposed to long-continued total-body gamma radiation. USAEC Report ANL-4401, pp. 38-52, 1950a.

Lorenz, E., Jacobson, L.O., Sutton, H., and Schweisthal, R. Part II. Recovery from anemia induced in guinea pigs by a limited exposure to chronic total-body gamma radiation. USAEC Report ANL-4401, pp. 53-71, 1950b.

Metcalf, R.G., Inda, F.A., Barnett, T.B., and Casarett, G.W. Pathology in animals subjected to repeated daily exposure to X-rays. USAEC Report UR-88, 1951. Also Chapter 12 in Biological Effects of External Radiation, edited by H.A. Blair, McGraw-Hill Book Co., New York, pp. 268-338, 1954.

CHAPTER V

BIOLOGICAL EFFECTS OF PROTRACTED LOW DOSE RADIATION EXPOSURE OF MAN AND ANIMALS*

Douglas Grahn

The biological effects of protracted radiation exposure are best evaluated, quantitatively, in terms of the statistics of survival and of the major pathological lesions observed at death of the animal. Although efforts are being made to correlate cellular events with responses of the organism, such comparisons do not yet enjoy the statistical and biological precision necessary for appropriate quantitation. My intent in this discussion is to examine some of the quantitative relations recognized to define or describe the long-term effects of protracted, low dose rate, whole-body ionizing irradiation. I shall very briefly discuss the dose-response data for single doses, briefly fractionated, and terminated exposures to establish a baseline for the discussion of life-shortening effects. The major emphasis, however, will be upon the use of certain lifetable or actuarial statistics and their application to the extensive data of a recently completed study at the Argonne National Laboratory. While this study has involved the talents of many persons, the principal investigators have been D. Grahn, G.A. Sacher and R.J.M. Fry of the Argonne National Laboratory, and Professor John H. Rust of the University of Chicago.

Effects of Single, Fractionated and briefly Protracted Exposures

The life-shortening effects of short-term irradiations have been reviewed recently by Grahn and Sacher (1968), Sacher (1966), and Van Cleave (1968). Single doses of low LET whole-body radiation induce a life-shortening in mice of about 30 days per 100 R; figures of 15% to 35% per $LD_{50/30}$ dose have also been given. Considerable variation in life-shortening can be attributed to genetic, sex, and age factors, in addition to the usual inter-laboratory differences in physical environment. In what appears to have been the only effort to partition this variation into contributing components, Grahn (1959) was able to define the major specific contributions from leukaemia and sex and thus identify a relatively invariant life-shortening parameter common to about six genetically different strains. This was 28 days per 100 R; a primary injury or life-shortening parameter with no implied relation to modes of injury, only its measurement. A 19% reduction at the $LD_{50/30}$ was also shown to be independent of genetic variance. There does not seem to have been any new data that would give reason to modify or adjust these basic parameters.

The life-shortening effects of briefly fractionated doses (dose-free intervals up to about 50 to 100 days for paired doses or total protraction periods of the same duration for multiple fractions) were discussed in detail by Grahn and Sacher (1968), and fig. 1 gives some of their analysis. Briefly, individual dose increments appear to have an additive effect for life-shortening, in most instances. The effect is comparable to that seen for single doses. One might also note here that high LET radiations, such as fission neutrons, have an

* Work performed under the auspices of the U.S. Atomic Energy Commission.

RBE of about three for life-shortening, a value that has been generally observed to describe most short-term end-points.

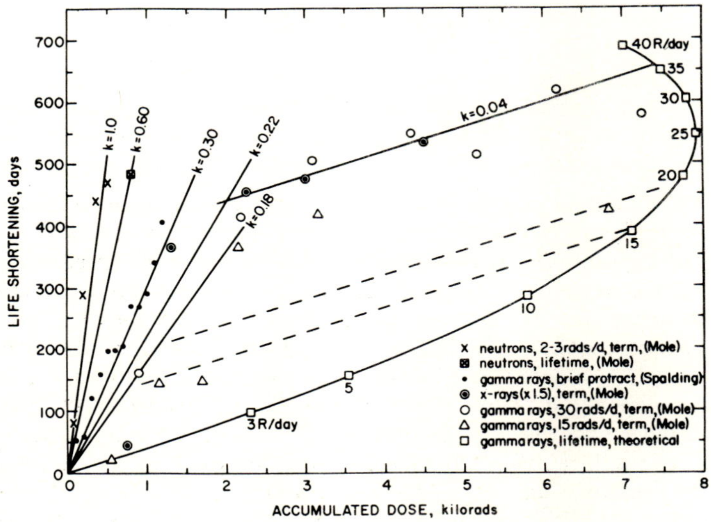

Fig. 1. Life-shortening versus accumulated dose for CBA and RF female mice. See Grahn and Sacher (1968) for specific references to data from Mole and Spalding and for derivation of constants.

Protraction of exposure over periods of 100 days or more, with termination of exposure prior to dying-out of the population, provides a complex array of life-shortening effects. As seen in fig. 1, however, these can be rationalized in relation to the two limiting conditions; single-dose effects and lifetime exposures. There is apparently a daily dose-rate effect as well. A linear relation between log daily dose rate and life-shortening exists for dose-protraction periods of less than 100 days or total doses of less than 1.5 kilorad: days lost/rad = 0.04 + 0.12 log D, where D varies from 1 to 100 R/day. The life-shortening effect at 100 R/day, 0.28 days/R, is assumed to be a maximum effect. It must be appreciated that observed values will run beyond this figure due to superimposed environmental and biological sensitivities.

Beyond total doses of about 1500 rads, the life-shortening constant is observed to drop sharply to a value of about 0.04 days per rad. This is substantially the value derived from low daily dose, duration-of-life exposures. Terminated, protracted exposures of mice that extend beyond 50 to 100 days or 1000 to 1500 rads can therefore bring about a dramatic change in the pattern of injury accumulation from the rapid rise in injury seen at lower total doses. Nevertheless, the late-life injury is apparently accrued additively to that induced at high injury rates in the early period after initiation of exposure (fig. 1). Low daily-dose exposures, at less than 10 R/day for the adult lifetime, produce the minimum injury accumulation from the outset; 0.04 days/rad.

This brief, and somewhat idealized, description of the life-shortening effects of single, briefly fractionated, and terminated exposures is discussed more thoroughly by

Grahn and Sacher (1968). There are some obvious inconsistencies and problems to rationalize, but the described relationships are accessible to experimental validation.

A great deal if information is available on the pathologic sequelae of single and briefly protracted exposures (Furth and Upton, 1953; United Nations Scientific Committee on the Effects of Atomic Radiation, 1964; Upton, 1968; Upton et al., 1963; Van Cleave, 1968). I will not discuss those data here except to note, for reference in a later section, the analysis by Upton et al. (1963) that employed actuarial techniques to evaluate the effects of single doses of gamma and X irradiation on leukaemia, pulmonary tumour, and ovarian tumour death rates. Because it is my major contention from this point on in this discussion that we should analyse and interpret literally all of our toxicity data through lifetable statistics, Upton's data provide one of the few useful comparative analyses for tumour death rates under different patterns of exposure.

Life-shortening Effects and Selected Pathologic Sequelae of Irradiations Protracted over the Lifetime

A great deal has been written on the application of actuarial statistics to the analysis of radiation-induced life-shortening and disease incidence. The most recent complete discussion by Sacher (1966) widely examines their use for single dose effects, lifetime exposures, and the comparison of different species. Probably, the initial application of actuarial methods to radiation toxicity data was given by Brues and Sacher in 1950 (1952). The derivation of the basic method, that of estimating age-specific death rates, has been historically assigned to Gompertz (1825). Concise discussions of the use of these statistics in radiation studies also have been given by Sacher (1956, 1966), Berlin (1960), Jones (1956 a, b), and Mildvan and Strehler (1960).

The basic equation that defines the mortality rate for all causes of death, r, is:

$$r = -\frac{1}{N}\frac{dN}{dt} = r_0 e^{k_0 t} , \qquad (1)$$

where N is the number of animals alive at age, t, r_0 is the intercept, and k_0 is the mortality-rate slope or regression on age. As described by Berlin (1960) and Berlin and DiMaggio (1956), this equation can be used to derive the median survival time, MST, as:

$$MST = \frac{1}{k_0} \ln \left[1 + \frac{0.693\, k_0}{r_0} \right] . \qquad (2)$$

After single doses, the mortality rates are displaced upward but remain essentially parallel to the control population (Berlin, 1960; Sacher, 1956, 1966). The effect of single doses is to displace the intercept upward as an exponential function of dose. Continuous exposure induces a progressive deviation of the mortality rate from the control with increasing age and dose accumulation (Berlin, 1960; Sacher, 1956, 1966). Thus, the effect of protracted exposures is to induce an upward rotation of the death-rate regression, while the intercept, r_0, remains constant. No particular relation between daily dose rate and slope has been suggested heretofore, but data to be presented indicate that this regression is an exponentially increasing function of daily dose.

Age-specific mortality rates for specific causes of death are derived in a slightly different manner. The death rate for a given cause, r_s, is:

$$r_s = \ln \left[1 - \frac{n_i}{N_i}\right]^{-1} \Big/ t_i = r_{s_0} e^{k_s t} , \qquad (3)$$

where n_i is the number of animals dying with specific cause in age interval, i, of t_i days, and in a population of N_i survivors at the beginning, or sometimes middle, of the interval. The definition of N_i is not terribly critical as long as its usage is consistent. In fact, in much of the analysis to be given, an average value of N_i for the interval was used. In terminating populations the rate of change of N for all causes would often be extremely high so that the few animals dying from some specific cause could have their estimated death rate appreciably altered by use of an N for the beginning versus the middle of an interval. The use of average N simply recognizes that the derived rate factor is based upon the average number of mouse days at risk in the interval.

Death rates for populations decremented for specific causes — a procedure we use for the elimination of leukaemia deaths — are based upon values of N corrected for the removed cause by decrementing at the beginning of the interval in which the event occurred.

One important feature to appreciate is the careful use of logarithmic functions, preferably natural logarithms. Some investigators have used simply the log of the percent mortality in the interval; a procedure that impresses an automatic ceiling on the death rate and an artificial flattening of the curve at high rates. It is imperative to use log rates in the manner defined to obtain the best estimate of the instantaneous rates of mortality as if they were derived from an infinitely large population.

Quite recently, a major investigation on the lifetime effects of low daily doses of cobalt 60 γ radiation on mice has been completed at Argonne. While the study has not been fully documented, initial reports on basic survival statistics and death rate analysis have been given (Grahn, 1969; Grahn et al., 1963, 1965; Sacher et al., 1969) and a complete report is in preparation (Grahn et al., 1969). The general experimental conditions are those described for an earlier study reported by Sacher and Grahn (1964). Mice at 100 days of age were placed in a γ radiation facility that automatically irradiated the animals during the night for a period of 7 to 10 hours. The animals were caged in groups of three (except at 0.3 R/day) and irradiated for the duration of life. Both sexes, in equal numbers, of three inbred strains, A/Jax, BALB/c, and C57BL/6, and one hybrid, the BCF_1 (C57BL/6 x BALB/c F_1) were used in the major part of this study. Additional information was obtained on the C57L strain at doses of 12 R/day and above*.

Ten daily-dose levels were employed and are given in table 1 along with the mean after-survival values. From 12 R/day and above, equal sample sizes were used for all genetic groups: 48/sex and strain at 6 R/day, 12 R/day and 24 R/day; 24/sex and strain at 32 R/day, 43 R/day and 56 R/day. At 0 R/day through 6 R/day, a double sample was used for the BCF_1; 168/sex at 0 R/day and 1.3 R/day; 96/sex at 2.6 R/day and 6 R/day. The samples were 84 and 48, respectively, for the three inbred strains.

The dose group at 0.3 R/day was an irregular sample. This exposure condition is behind a bulk lead shield in one corner of the γ radiation facility and does not provide an ideally comparable environment to the balance of the exposure conditions. Caging was also different and involved groups of 12. Originally, only the BCF_1 and BALB/c strains were entered due to space limitation. Sixty mice/sex for the inbred and 120/sex for

---

* These strains are now designated A/JGh, BALB/cJGh, C57BL/6JGh, and C57L/Gh.

Table 1

Mean after-survival and standard errors in days by dose, sex, and strain

Age at start of exposure: 100 days

Strain	Sex	Daily exposure dose, R/day									
		Control	0.3	1.3	2.6	6	12	24	32	43	56
A/Jax	♂	466 ± 16	377 ± 22	433 ± 16	451 ± 19	458 ± 21	388 ± 15	231 ± 8	182 ± 7	111 ± 4	83 ± 4
	♀	538 ± 16	502 ± 21	528 ± 16	533 ± 20	486 ± 19	400 ± 18	228 ± 7	153 ± 8	102 ± 3	59 ± 1
	♂ + ♀	502 ± 12	436 ± 17	480 ± 12	492 ± 14	472 ± 14	394 ± 11	230 ± 5	167 ± 6	106 ± 3	71 ± 3
BALB/c	♂	569 ± 15	520 ± 28	542 ± 20	461 ± 24	526 ± 16	368 ± 14	234 ± 9	166 ± 7	106 ± 3	60 ± 1
	♀	646 ± 14	643 ± 18	592 ± 16	557 ± 17	473 ± 19	395 ± 10	226 ± 7	158 ± 6	99 ± 4	55 ± 1
	♂ + ♀	609 ± 14	583 ± 17	567 ± 13	509 ± 15	499 ± 13	382 ± 9	230 ± 6	162 ± 5	102 ± 3	57 ± 1
C57BL/6	♂	643 ± 19	-	572 ± 20	582 ± 24	576 ± 22	468 ± 14	275 ± 10	209 ± 8	136 ± 4	83 ± 1
	♀	647 ± 22	-	631 ± 16	565 ± 22	581 ± 20	484 ± 14	250 ± 9	179 ± 7	128 ± 3	77 ± 3
	♂ + ♀	645 ± 14	-	602 ± 13	573 ± 16	580 ± 15	476 ± 10	263 ± 7	194 ± 6	132 ± 3	80 ± 2
BCF_1	♂	710 ± 15	762 ± 18	689 ± 13	698 ± 17	599 ± 12	467 ± 17	301 ± 12	207 ± 8	166 ± 5	99 ± 5
	♀	796 ± 14	815 ± 14	722 ± 12	657 ± 15	580 ± 11	448 ± 12	282 ± 12	212 ± 11	160 ± 5	92 ± 3
	♂ + ♀	753 ± 10	788 ± 11	705 ± 9	677 ± 11	590 ± 8	457 ± 10	291 ± 9	210 ± 6	163 ± 3	95 ± 3

the hybrid were used. Late in the study, the A strain was added as space became available, so there is a degree of discontinuity in time between the 0.3 R/day group in the A strain and the balance of the study. Caging and other microenvironmental variables induce a general discontinuity for all animals at this dose. This is emphasized as there are certain inconsistencies in the data at this level that cannot be clearly interpreted.

Control mice were held in a maze corridor to the γ room. Generally, the physical environment was comparable to that in the room itself, but there was more ambient temperature variation and greater contact with the general animal facility environment. Here, too, some mental reservation may be held regarding the most rigorous comparative analysis. At any rate, for the dose groups from 1.3 R/day through 56 R/day, the environment was substantially constant.

Mortality from all causes

The survival data are given in table 1 and fig. 2. In the latter, log MAS (mean after-survival) is plotted against daily dose, and a linear relationship is clearly demonstrated. This was seen earlier by Sacher and Grahn (1964) and has been substantiated in a half-dozen different genetic strains and hybrids (Grahn et al., 1963). The data fit the equation:

$$MAS_D = MAS_0 \, e^{-\beta D}. \qquad (4)$$

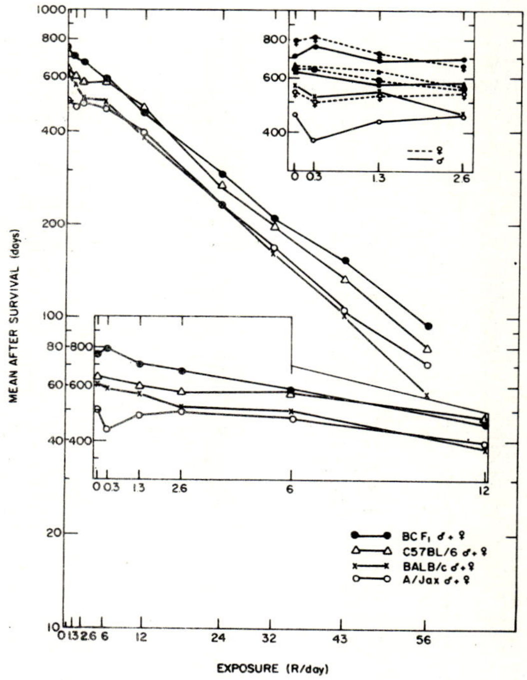

Fig. 2. Logarithm of mean after-survival (MAS) versus daily dose of ^{60}Co γ radiation.

The value of β has only varied between -0.033 and -0.043 for different sexes, strains, and hybrids in nearly two dozen separate estimates over the past 10 to 15 years. The simple average for all strains and sexes is -0.038; that is -3.8% per R per day; -3.8 days per 100 R accumulated; $3.8/MAS_0$ = % lost per R; $(.038)(MAS_0)$ = days lost per R per day.

Because there is no significant genetic variation in this constant, nearly all genetic differences in long-term response are incorporated in the basic differences in life expectancy.

Figure 2 also expands the scale at the lower doses to demonstrate the increase in variation of response. Strain A shows almost no response differential below 6 R/day. Strains BALB/c and C57BL show a steady progression down to 0 R, while the BCF_1 demonstrates a small amount of over-survival at 0.3 R/day. This is statistically significant for the males, but not the females.

The basic age-specific death rates for all causes of death, the two sexes combined, are given in fig. 3 for the four genetic groups. The characteristic fan of mortality-rate slopes is evident in all strains though the A strain reveals an unchanging array for doses 0 R through 6 R/day. The pathological basis for this apparent lack of radiosensitivity is in the susceptibility of this strain to amyloidosis and kidney degeneration (Dunn, 1944).

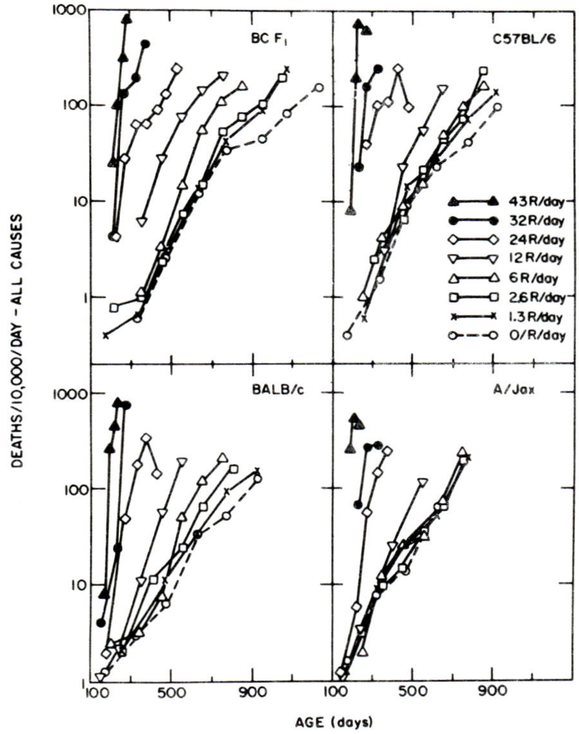

Fig. 3. Age-specific mortality rates for indicated strains and daily doses. Sexes combined; all causes of death.

A careful comparison among the strains indicates that all the A strain low-dose groups and the control have an accelerated mortality rate; the Gompertz slope for the 0 R through 6 R/day groups are all roughly equal to that at 6 R/day for the BALB/c. All radiation injury at doses below 6 R/day in strain A is apparently overwhelmed by the high incidence of degenerative disease. More detailed information on this will be given in a later section, but it should be noted that this suppression of response affects nearly all specific end-points in the A strain at the low doses, although the response at 12 R/day and above is quite typical of the average mouse.

Figure 4 is a more detailed display of the BCF_1 for which more adequate sampling was available. The death-rate curves are nearly all substantially non-linear. This has been discussed by Sacher (1966) and more will be presented in this report when I discuss the matter of risk estimation. It should also be noted here and in fig. 3 that in no case does one find a non-linear relation that is concave upward as described by Neary (1960) for the CBA mouse. The Harwell experience for long-term gamma or neutron irradiation is most peculiar in this regard and is certainly not confirmed by anything we or others have seen.

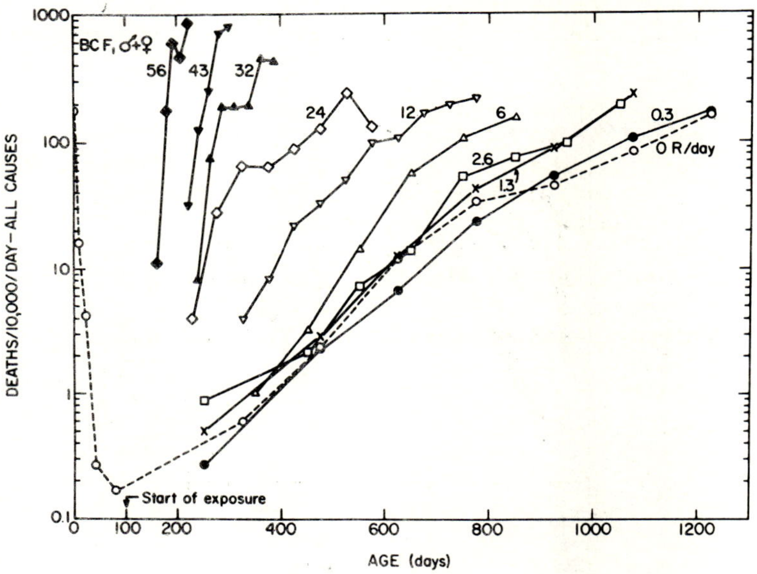

Fig. 4. Age-specific mortality rates for BCF_1 hybrid; sexes combined, all causes of death.

Some of the non-linearity of response can be attributed to leukaemia, which has a phasic non-linear increment of its own. Mortality rates derived from the population decremented for leukaemia mortality are given in fig. 14 and will be discussed in a later section.

The control data are also given for the full neonatal, infant and juvenile period. These data are derived from our breeding records for the first 30 days and from stock cage experience for the period 30 to 100 days. Between 200,000 and 1,000,000 mouse-days of experience are now available for the early part of the life table for this hybrid as well as many of the inbreds. The pre-weaning death rates tend to be about 10-fold higher than those in human experience in the first 30 days, a common feature in littering animals.

Mortality with specific pathology

Autopsies were performed on almost 90% of the mice. Major lesions were grossly defined and tissues from about 25 to 50% were studied by microscopic examination. The percentage examined microscopically was highest in the control and low-dose groups. Since the same degree of detail was not available for all mice, we decided to analyse the data for lesions for which both the information gained from macroscopic and microscopic examination could be used. Our survey concentrated on:

1. Tumours of the reticular tissue, which were subdivided into two groups (a) those with thymic involvement, (b) those with no apparent thumic involvement. This arbitrary subdivision was necessary because data obtained by macroscopic examination alone were used. This subdivision results in an underestimate of tumours of extra thymic origin which occur late in the life-span.

2. Ovarian tumours and cysts.

3. Pulmonary tumours (primary).

4. Hepatomas.

5. Total tumour incidence which also included miscellaneous tumours, including adrenal, skin and connective tissue, mammary gland, haemangiomas.

6. Renal lesions, often detected by cystic degeneration.

The final percent incidence for the major tumour categories is seen in fig. 5.

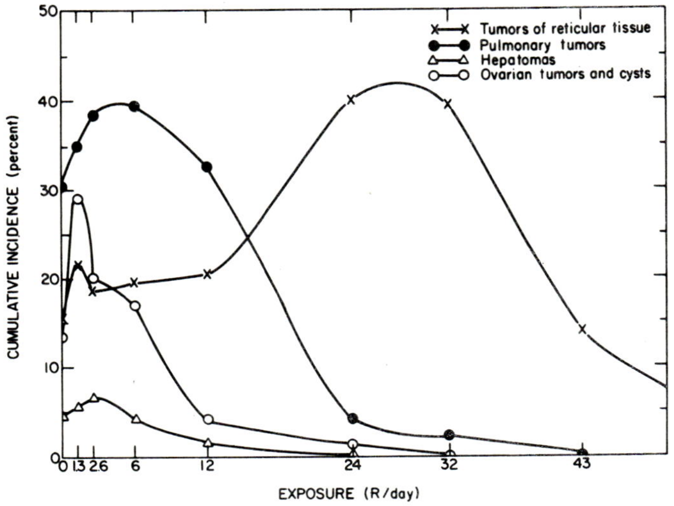

Fig. 5. Final incidence for reticular tissue tumours, hepatomas, and ovarian tumours for strains A/Jax, BALB/c, C57BL/6 and the BCF_1 hybrid combined. Data for pulmonary tumours on A, BALB and BCF_1 only. Sexes combined.

I wish to emphasize the extensive non-linearity manifest so as to <u>discourage</u> the casual reader and experimenter from attempting to draw grand conclusions about dose-response relationships from such simple expressions of data.

All tumours do respond to low dose; the rather extreme response for ovarian tumours at 1.3 R/day is quite significant. The nearly exponential decrease in incidence above 1.3 R/day is apparently a function of two major opposing components — induction by radiation but with little dose-response sensitivity (more of an all-or-none type response; see fig. 10), opposed by progressive life-shortening and truncation of the distribution period of expression.

Pulmonary tumours and hepatomas present a similar picture of a rise at the 2 or 3 lower dose levels, then a steady decline as life-shortening effects predominate. Reticular tissue tumours have a biphasic response; the first rise at 1.3 R/day is significant by a Chi-square test ($P < 0.002$) and generally occurs in both leukaemia subtypes and in both sexes of all four strains. This is followed by a small drop-back and then a steady rise through 12 R/day. Thymic tumours make up only one-fourth to one-third of the total until 12 R/day when these suddenly shift to about 70% and thereafter produce the second phasic response at 24 R and 32 R/day.

<u>Reticular tissue tumours.</u> Figure 6 presents the death-rate data for all strains and sexes combined. At the lowest doses the response is linear and the death rates are generally displaced upward and parallel to the control. This may be a kind of balance

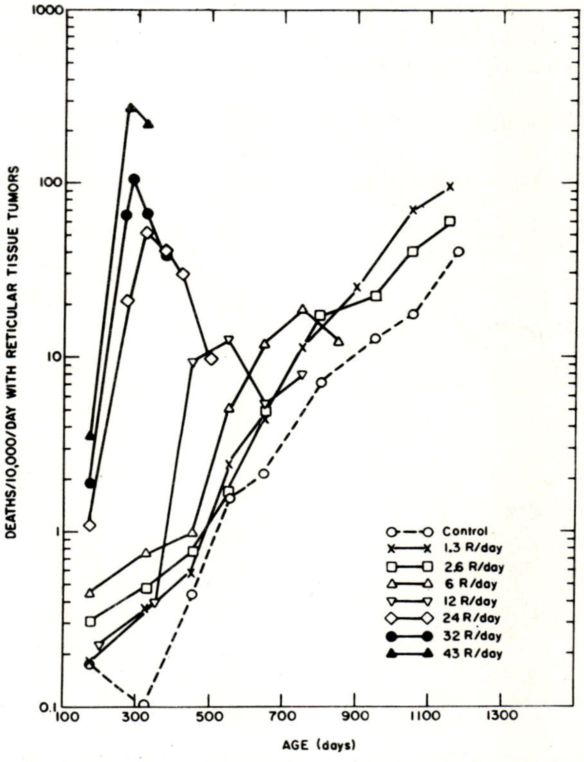

Fig. 6. Age-specific mortality rates for reticular tissue tumours for combined sexes and strains A/Jax, BALB/c, C57BL/6 and BCF_1.

between the early-life thymic tumours and the later increment from those not involving the thymus. At 6 R/day the thymic component is beginning to have its effect and at 12 R/day and above the sharp, but phasic, mortality increment occurs from tumours involving the thymus. At the 6 R, 12 R and 24 R/day levels, there is a definite return to or near the underlying linear trend. The latter is commonly seen after single doses (Brues and Sacher, 1952; United Nations Scientific Committee on the Effects of Atomic Radiation, 1964; Upton et al., 1960, 1963).

The data for each strain are shown in fig. 7 and while the same general pattern is seen in all, there are some exceptions. Data from the BCF_1 are much like those for all strains (this will be generally noted because they make up 40% of the total sample in the pooled data), and the data at 0.3 R show no response above control. The C57BL shows mostly a thymic tumour response component. The opposite is seen in the BALB/c. Here the non-thymic component is predominant in response at 0.3 R through 6 R/day. Although a definite thymic tumour response occurs at the upper dose levels, it is more linear and broadly distributed in time. The A strain shows almost no response at 0 R through 2.6 R/day. A sharp thymic tumour response does ultimately emerge at 12 R/day. As will be noted later, the total reticular tissue tumour response at the four lowest doses is apparently not independent of the pathology defined by degenerative renal lesions.

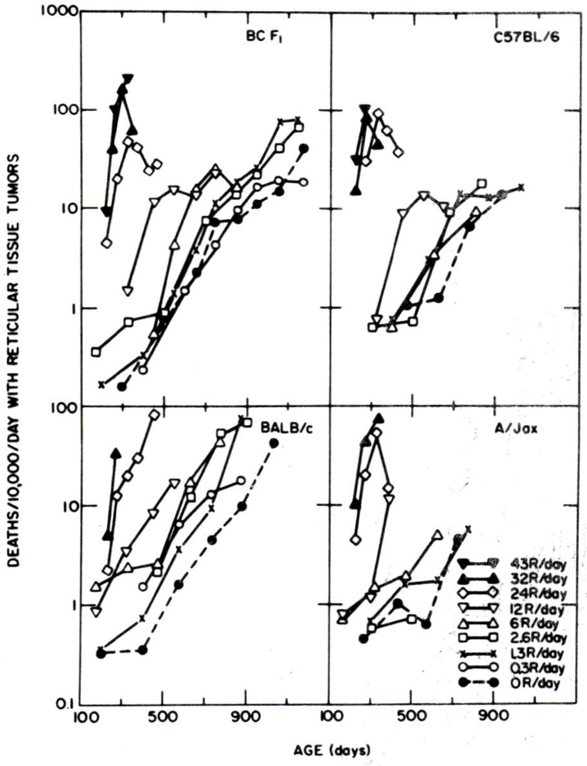

Fig. 7. Age-specific mortality rates for reticular tissue tumours, sexes combined, for indicated strains and doses.

A detailed analysis of the non-thymic tumours in the BCF_1 at the five lower dose levels reveals a family of linearly increasing death-rate slopes (fig. 8). These originate from an apparent common intercept at about 400 days of age. Although 0.3 R/day has no apparent influence on this type of leukaemia, a significant increase in death-rate slope is seen at 1.3 R, 2.6 R and 6 R/day. The only comparable bit of information is Upton's report on non-myeloid, non-thymic tumours of the RF mouse after single doses of X rays (Upton et al., 1963). In that instance, an upward, parallel displacement occurred, which would be expected after single doses in contrast to the present data that show a progressive slope rotation and a common intercept.

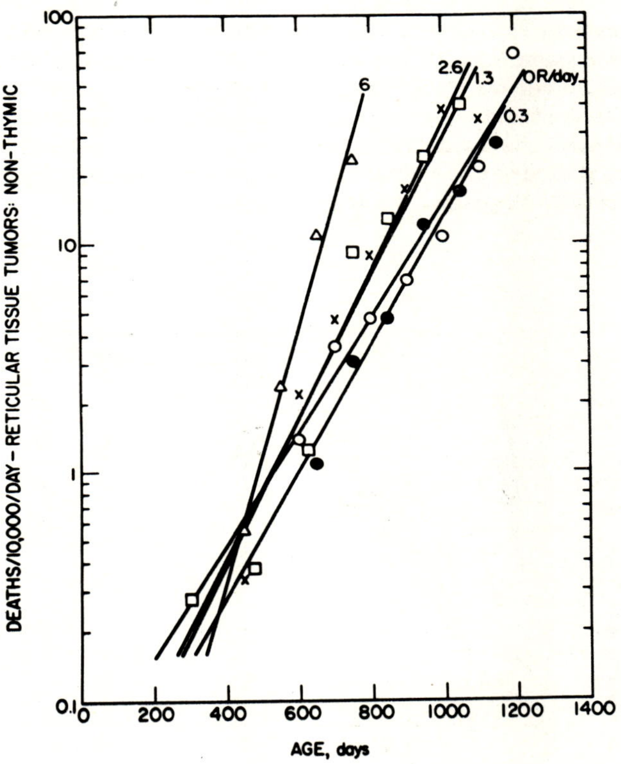

Fig. 8. Age-specific mortality rates for non-thymic reticular tissue tumours in BCF_1, sexes combined. Data fitted by least squares linear regressions; slopes are: 0R: 0.0058 ± 0.0005; 0.3 R: 0.0064 ± 0.0005; 1.3 R: 0.0072 ± 0.0010; 2.6 R: 0.0074 ± 0.0007; 6 R: 0.0127 ± 0.0013.

Pulmonary tumours. The combined data for strains A, BALB/c and BCF_1 are presented in fig. 9. This tumour provides a good array of responses: none at 0.3 R, some progressive divergence of mortality rate at 1.3 R and 2.6 R, and both divergence and displacement at 6 R and 12 R/day. As this array does not lend itself to any preconceived notions of dose response, I will discuss it in greater detail when considering the evaluation of risk.

The three contributing strains are not remarkable. The A strain shows the suppressed response through 6 R/day noted for other end-points. The BALB/c and BCF_1 are individually similar to the combined response. The response in the C57BL/6 was generally below 3 to 5%.

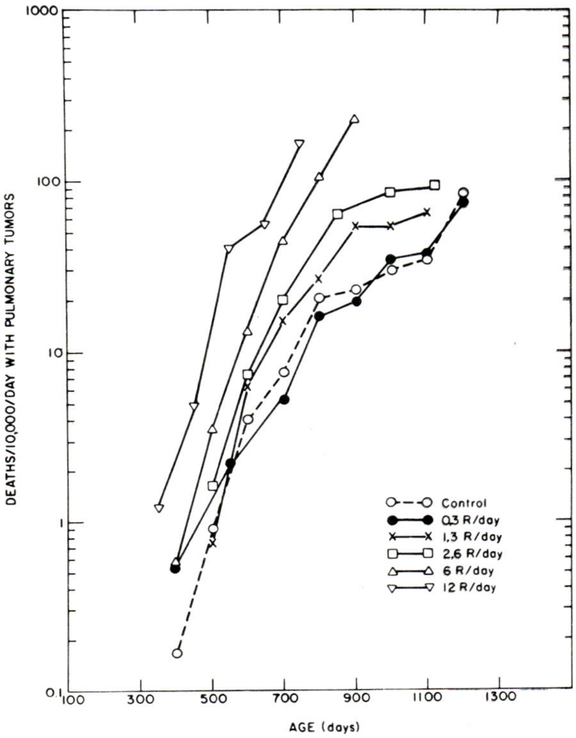

Fig. 9. Age-specific mortality rates for primary pulmonary tumours; sexes and strains combined for A/Jax, BALB/c and BCF_1.

Ovarian tumours and cysts. Figure 10 presents the combined data for the four strains. The characteristic to be noted here is in the similarity of response at 1.3 R, 2.6 R and 6 R/day. The lack of dose responsiveness and minimal divergence through 600 days of age suggests that this tumour requires a long development period and that induction may require a comparatively low threshold of injury to be sustained. Because the female mouse is particularly sensitive to radiation-induced sterility (Rugh and Wolff, 1956), the tumour response may rise rather abruptly to a potential maximum when sterility is induced. Death rates could then be the same for all doses and yields would be a direct function of total time at risk beyond about 500 days of age.

The individual strains show some interesting responses (fig. 11). The incidence in the A strain, again, is suppressed by a degenerative disease mortality while the C57BL shows a tight cluster of death rates at all doses above control. the BALB/c and BCF_1 indicate some minor degree of dose response, though this is still small compared to the basic difference between irradiated and unirradiated. The 0.3 R/day group of the BCF_1 does show an intermediate position but the total dose is only several hundred rads even after two years' exposure. The general conclusions noted from these data confirm many of the observations made on the LAF_1 by Lorenz at doses below 8 R/day (Lorenz et al., 1954).

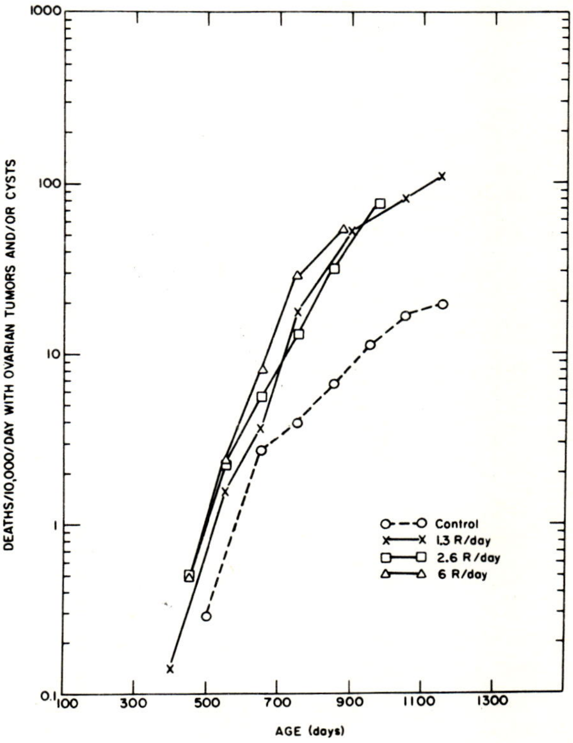

Fig. 10. Age-specific mortality rates for ovarian tumours and cysts; A/Jax, BALB/c, C57BL/6 and BCF_1 combined.

Hepatomas. The data for this tumour are quite meagre, and individual strains never yield more than 14% incidence. The death rates are progressively divergent, linear, and rise from a common intercept of 2×10^{-5} at 500 days of age. To study the dose response of the incidence of hepatomas, the strain of choice is $C3H_f$, which will give yields up to 60% (Grahn and Hamilton, 1964).

Miscellaneous tumours. The incidence of other types of tumours was low. In general, the results on tumour incidence reported here are in substantial agreement with those given by Lorenz et al. (1954) for the LAF_1 exposed daily to doses of 0.11, 1.1, 2.2, 4.4 and 8.8 R/day. Leukaemias, pulmonary tumours, hepatomas and ovarian tumours all demonstrated qualitatively and quantitatively similar levels of response. Unfortunately, earlier studies of our own on the LAF_1 mouse could not fully corroborate those data, as our previous studies did not go below 5 R/day, and it is obvious that much of the valuable tumour information lies at doses below that level. The present data at higher doses are all consistent with our previous reports (Lesher et al., 1957, 1965).

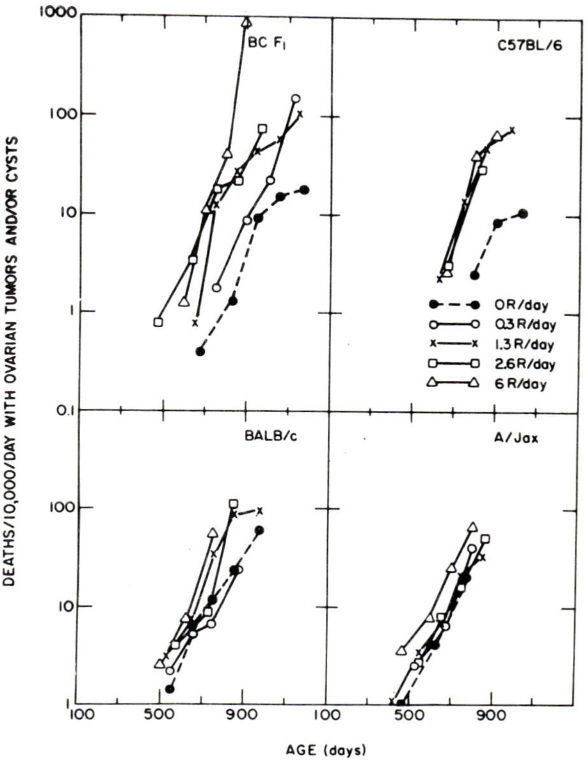

Fig. 11. Age-specific mortality rates for ovarian tumours and cysts for indicated strains and daily dose groups.

Renal lesions. A form of renal disease often grossly characterized by cystic degeneration and microscopically by amyloid infiltration is commonly observed in mice and was a common lesion, particularly, the A and C57BL strains. It reaches a total incidence of 30 to 50% in the A strain, 15 to 35% in C57BL and 5 to 15% in the BCF_1. In the irradiated groups the highest incidence was in strain A, 70% at 0.3 R/day, which accompanied a disproportionately reduced life expectancy (table 1 and fig. 1).

Figure 12 gives a comparative analysis of death rates for the controls of strains A and BCF_1, for all causes, all tumours and renal lesions. The picture presented by strain A is seen at all the doses below 12 R/day with minor exceptions. Deaths from renal lesions overwhelm all other causes and would seem to force the mortality rate upward. At 6 R/day, enough early leukaemia occurs to emerge from the renal lesion background for a few hundred days between 150 and 450 days of age. In a sense, the renal lesions act as a culling force that provides a perfect set of cancer morbidity data. Because the death-rate slope for renal lesions is constant between 0 R and 6 R/day, a redundant series of morbidity data are produced and no information emerges on differential tumour response.

The BCF_1, on the other hand, exhibits no obvious impairment due to the renal lesion. Death rates from all tumours closely follow the death rates from all causes. This is generally seen in the other strains, though the C57BL is somewhat intermediate in its relations between renal lesion and all tumour death rates.

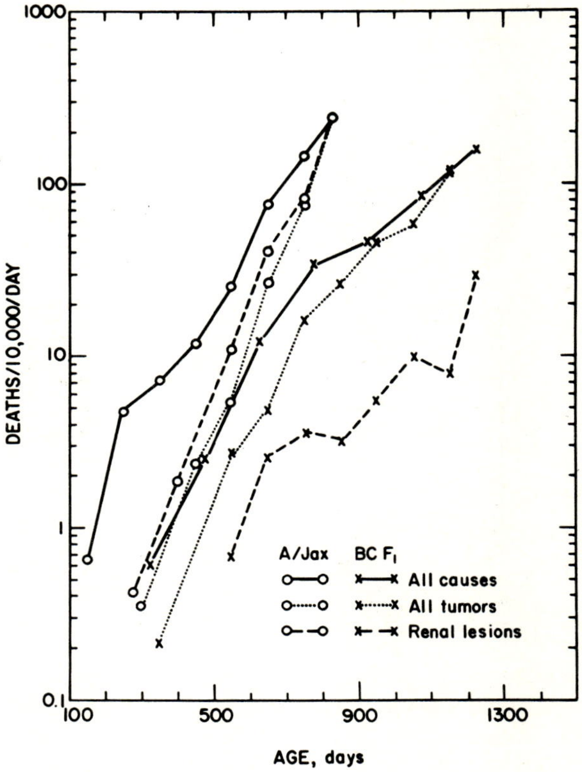

Fig. 12. Age-specific mortality rates for A/Jax and BCF_1 control populations for indicated causes.

The extent of interaction between renal lesions and neoplasia is seen in fig. 13. The final incidence of renal lesions and leukaemias for doses 0 R, 1.3 R, 2.6 R and 6 R/day for the three indicated strains shows an individual and a combined negative correlation between tumour incidence and kidney lesion. It would thus appear that the systemic or basic metabolic events that underly the renal degeneration also act upon reticular tissue tumours. At the four dose groups employed in this relationship, there is no major dose-response for either lesion; the second-degree polynomial that describes the data is thus not an indirect function of radiation level.

Curiously, no particular relation exists between renal lesions and the all-tumour category or ovarian tumours. One is tempted to suggest that this degenerative disease has an auto-immune aetiology that also influences the haematopoietic system.

Estimation of Risk and the Prediction of Low-dose Effects

In the past 30 years, prediction of the late effects of radiation exposure has periodically occupied the time of many individual scientists, sundry committees, individual agencies, or departments of governments around the world. As such, there is really nothing new or untried in this kind of activity, although the emphasis placed upon one or another procedure has varied.

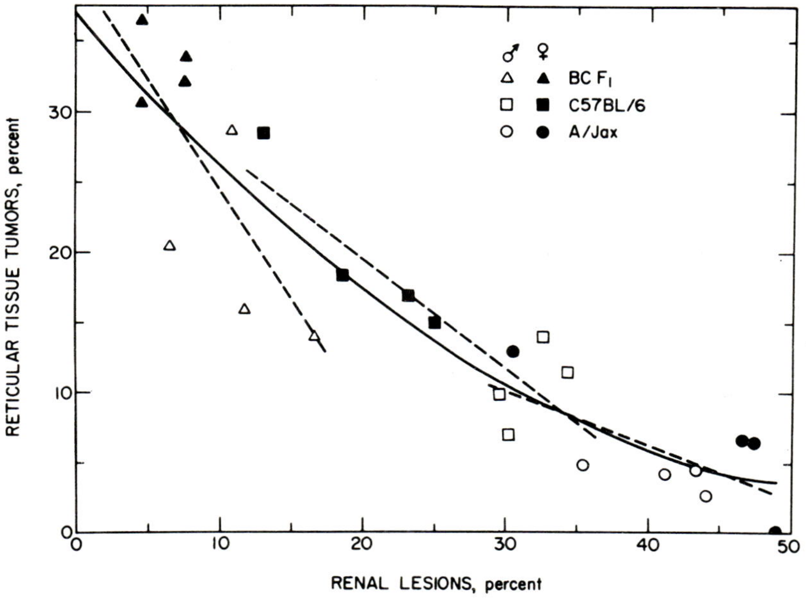

Fig. 13. Final incidence of all reticular tissue tumours versus final incidence of renal lesions for dose groups 0 R, 1.3 R, 2.6 R and 6 R/day. Data fitted by least squares; slopes are A/Jax: -0.384 ± 0.170; C57BL: -0.780 ± 0.177; BCF_1: -1.573 ± 0.556; the combined data were fitted by the equation; $y = a + bx + cx^2$, $a = 36.98 \pm 2.94$, $b = -1.18 \pm 0.27$, $c = 0.010 \pm 0.005$.

Basically, the problem is approached directly by measuring some effect versus dose relationship: the percentage change from control, the elevation of mortality, survival time, tumour incidence, or other effect versus dose. This information is first standardized for a given laboratory animal, usually the mouse, then extrapolated to man through one of several rationales.

One can assume that the percent change per unit dose is constant for all species; a procedure that has been mathematically validated (Sacher, 1956). Another expression of this is to rationalize two species by the ratio of their life expectancies, or some function thereof, such as the age-specific death-rate slope. This is the most widely applied procedure and appears to be biologically most valid. Discussions of this can be found in Brues and Sacher (1952), Sacher (1966), Jones (1956 a, b, 1957), Berlin and DiMaggio (1956), Failla and McClement (1957), Grahn (1962). Nearly all of the past effort at prediction has been concentrated on the life-shortening effects and upon the probability of leukaemia induction (Langham, 1967; United Nations Scientific Committee on the Effects of Atomic Radiation, 1964). Some concern has also developed around thyroid tumours in response to ^{131}I uptake in children (Federal Radiation Council, 1962), bone tumour induction as a function of ^{90}Sr and other bone-seeking radionuclides (Federal Radiation Council, 1964), and pulmonary tumours as a function of uranium mining experience (Federal Radiation Council, 1968).

Prediction activity falls into two nearly separate categories. Life-shortening effects are almost entirely predicted from animal experience, with only minor corroborative efforts drawn from human experience. On the other hand, the prediction of neoplastic disease incidence is almost solely derived from human experience. The reason for the latter does not appear to be due to a lack of animal data — the latter abound. Instead, there seems to be a double bias at work; (1) we appear to innately distrust animal data on specific causes of death as non-human, non-quantitative, diagnostically inaccurate or not comparable; (2) we have neglected the statistics of neoplastic disease incidence in animals and thus we lack the means of comparative analysis. Admittedly, there are scattered efforts to overcome these apparent biases, but if you consider for just a moment the amount of intellectual effort that has been indulged upon the life-shortening prediction problem, then the deficit in such effort on all the specific causes of death should become apparent.

For the prediction of life-shortening effects, the repeatedly proven exponential relationship between log mean after-survival and daily dose rate (equation (4)) is highly dependable for the average mouse. This can be extrapolated to man and other mammalian species by adjusting the slope constant, β, according to the ratio of life expectancies for the compared species, as portrayed by Grahn (1962) and Grahn and Sacher (1968). This procedure for extrapolating to man or other mammals will be re-examined.

Life-shortening Risk Estimates

It was pointed out early in the discussion that any radiation exposure can be expected to modify the life-table of the population. Long-term protracted exposure is expected to effect the life-table as if there had been a series of small single doses, and the ultimate effect is measured by the divergence of the death-rate or Gompertz slope from the control. This, of course, is mathematically straightforward if the death-rate data are strictly linear. Unfortunately, they are not, at least in the mouse. In virtually all the experience in the present series of data as well as that summarized by Sacher (1966), the regression of mortality rate on age is clearly better described by a second-degree polynomial. In order to meet this condition and also handle risk estimation for specific causes of death, for which there is no particular a priori dose-response relation, I have chosen to employ a type of "integrated risk estimation".

The integrated risk over the lifetime of an irradiated population is essentially no more than the sum of all excess mortality experienced by that group over its control. In actuarial analysis with standard mortality tables, the integrated lifetime risk would simply be the ratio of observed number of deaths over the expected number calculated from the control. No statistical standardization procedures are required before dose groups can be compared, as is the requirement for comparison of human populations, because each dose group can be considered a subsample from a common 100-day old base population that was randomly, but proportionately, apportioned by sex, genotype, and dose.

The integrated risk, at the moment, is being calculated for our mouse populations by a computer program that estimates the area under the death-rate curves, in 25-day intervals, from the start of exposure at 100 days of age through the interval where the last animal died. This is being done in considerable detail for only a few conditions now in order to test the procedures and to develop a final program for data management. The conditions we are examining are:

1. BCF_1 - all causes of death, sexes combined, all doses from 0 R to 56 R/day;

2. BCF_1 - all causes less death with reticular tissue tumours, sexes combined, all dose groups;

3. Strains A, BALB/c, BCF_1 combined - pulmonary tumours, sexes combined, doses 0 R to 12 R/day.

Initially, the age-specific death-rate data are fitted by polynomial equations through the fourth degree. These are least-squares estimates using unit weight for all observations. The decision not to employ variable weights for the estimated death rates probably makes little difference in the final steps of this analysis, because the data, at least for all causes, are force-fit through a common 100-day intercept.

The common intercept is chosen from the least-squares estimates at the three or four lowest doses where small deflections in slope have little effect on the intercept. This intercept is then used for re-estimating the mortality-rate regressions so that a choice of equations can be made on the basis of major reductions in the residual error. The use of a common intercept for the analysis of general mortality is biologically valid, since the populations all have a common starting point.

Although we have derived integrated risks for the standard least-squares fitted equations, the results of particular interest are from those data fitted through the common intercepts. We have done this for second-degree polynomials for all causes of death, first- and second-degree equations for the leukaemia decremented population, and a mixture of selected curves describing the pulmonary tumour data. Some of the pertinent results are in tables 2 and 3 for the analysis of the leukaemia decremented population fitted through a common intercept by first-degree equations. The results of this analysis are also portrayed in figs. 14, 15 and 16; fig. 14 is the idealized solution for lifetime protracted exposure. A thorough examination of this idealized population initially will permit a better understanding of the effects of sex, genotype, and the prevalent non-linear components.

Table 2

Linear mortality-rate regression equations for the BCF_1; sexes combined, leukaemia-decremented, constant 100-day intercept (r_0) of 13.5×10^{-6}; $r = 13.5 \times 10^{-6} e^{kt}$

Dose (R/day)	MAS (days)	Mortality-rate slope (k) Prob. of death/mouse day ± S.E. ($\times 10^{-3}$)	$^{k_D}/_{k_0}$
0	752	6.98 ± 0.21	1.000
0.3	781	7.09 ± 0.18	1.016
1.3	686	7.60 ± 0.20	1.090
2.6	678	8.14 ± 0.18	1.166
6	595	9.57 ± 0.21	1.371
12	466	12.78 ± 0.33	1.831
24	340	18.75 ± 0.87	2.687
32	246	29.40 ± 0.64	4.213
43	156	45.72 ± 0.86	6.552
56	96	78.92 ± 4.39	11.309

Table 3

Integrated risk values from 100 days of age expressed as mortality ratios per day or per R; BCF_1 sexes combined, population composition and mortality rate equations as defined*

Dose	Mort. ratio	Days at	Mort. ratio:prob./R		Mort. ratio:prob./day (arith.)		
R/day	ln (prob./day)	risk	ln	arith.	Case 1	2	3
0	0.000	1100	0.000	1.000	1.00	1.00	1.00
0.3	0.061	1100	0.217	1.241	1.06	0.86	0.92
1.3	0.328	1050	0.253	1.287	1.39	1.25	1.42
2.6	0.551	950	0.212	1.236	1.74	1.44	1.54
6	1.101	850	0.184	1.201	3.01	2.37	2.22
12	1.885	650	0.157	1.170	6.58	5.69	6.49
24	2.797	475	0.117	1.124	16.4	16.9	21.7
32	3.363	300	0.105	1.111	28.9	28.5	43.1
43	3.875	200	0.090	1.094	48.2	41.6	48.1
56	5.387	150	0.096	1.101	219.	206.	195.

* Case 1. Leukaemia decremented, constant 100 day intercept, linear equations.

Case 2. Leukaemia decremented, constant 100 day intercept, second-degree equations.

Case 3. All causes of death, constant 100 day intercept, second-degree equations.

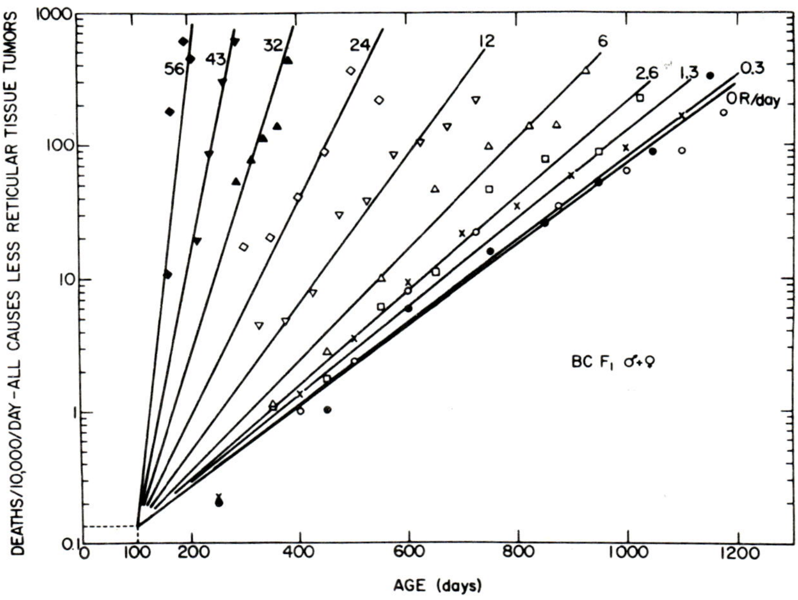

Fig. 14. Age-specific mortality rates for leukaemia decremented populations fitted by first-degree equations forced through common 100-day intercept of 13.5 x 10^{-6}. BCF_1 sexes combined. See table 2.

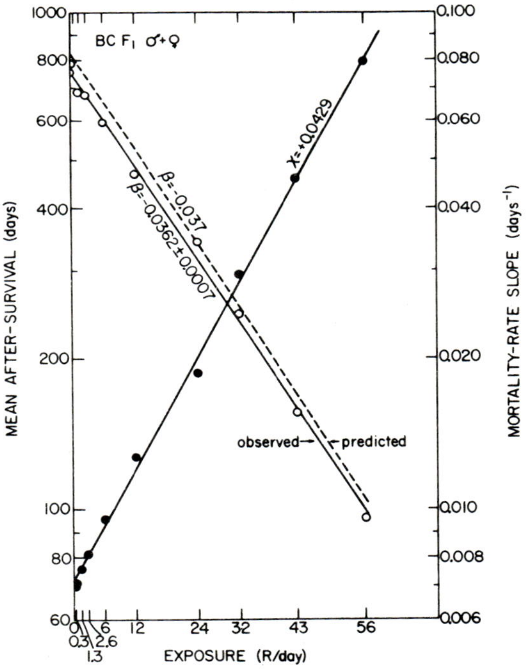

Fig. 15. Log MAS versus daily dose; log mortality-rate slope versus daily dose; BCF_1 sexes combined, leukaemia decremented. See text for equations (4) and (5).

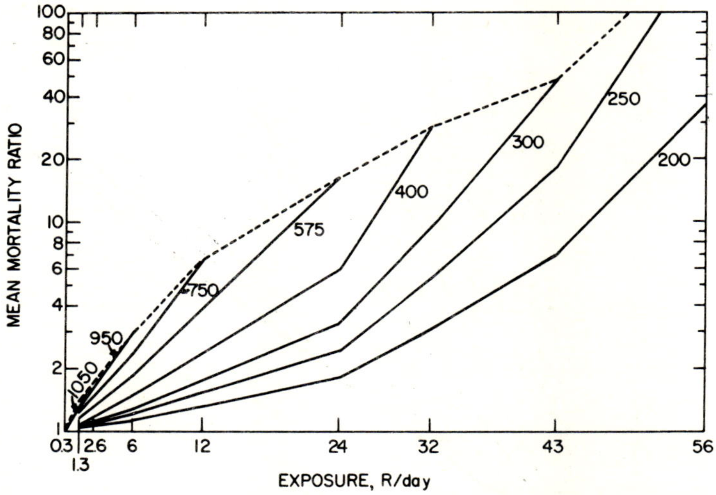

Fig. 16. Mortality ratios for indicated ages (exposure initiated at 100 days of age). Broken line connects final ratios derived from lifetime integrated risks. See table 3.

A most encouraging finding is seen in these data. The Gompertz or death-rate slopes rise exponentially with daily dose rate according to the equation:

$$k_D = k_0 e^{\chi D} \text{ or } k_D = 0.0072e^{0.0429 \pm 0.0016\, D}, \qquad (5)$$

where k_D is the death-rate slope (see fig. 15) and the control slope is 0.0072. Returning to equation (2), which defines MST, a modification to allow for the daily dose rate effect on slope, $k_0 e^{\chi D}$, can be entered to give:

$$MST = \frac{1}{k_0 e^{\chi D}} \ln\left[1 + \frac{0.693\, k_0 e^{\chi D}}{r_0}\right], \qquad (6)$$

which now can be used to re-estimate the relationship given by equation (4) by substituting 0.0429 for χ. The predicted and observed values, as seen in fig. 15, are remarkably parallel.

The existence of an exponential relation between Gompertz slope and daily-dose is predictable from the observation that MAS (or MST) is exponentially decreasing with dose. Starting with the relation:

$$\frac{MAS_D}{MAS_0} = e^{-\beta D}, \qquad (4)$$

and $$MAS_0\ (MST_0) = \frac{1}{k_0} \ln\left[1 + \frac{0.693\, k_0}{r_0}\right], \qquad (2)$$

and $$MAS_D\ (MST_D) = \frac{1}{k_0 e^{\chi D}} \ln\left[1 + \frac{0.693\, k_0 e^{\chi D}}{r_0}\right], \qquad (6)$$

then $e^{-\beta D}$ = the ratio of equation (6) to equation (2)

$$= \frac{1}{e^{\lambda D}} \cdot \frac{\ln\left[1 + \frac{0.693\ k_0 e^{\lambda D}}{r_0}\right]}{\ln\left[1 + \frac{0.693\ k_0}{r_0}\right]}$$

Thus, the value for $e^{-\beta D}$ in equation (4) above is equal to $e^{-\lambda D}$ times a complex term that will be seen to have the value of -0.831.

The area under the death-rate curve, and above the control curve, when divided by the time period at risk, gives a geometric mean mortality-rate ratio or mean difference between slopes in logarithmic transform (table 3). When these values are plotted against daily dose, as in fig. 16, for a series of progressive time intervals from the start of exposure, a family of curves is produced. From 0 R to 24 R/day, a regular and linear increase in risk occurs with dose and time, while the higher three dose levels show an accelerating mortality ratio.

If the final or lifetime mean mortality-rate ratio is divided by the daily dose level, the quotient is equivalent to taking the total area, or integrated lifetime risk, and dividing by the total accumulated dose. Thus, a final risk estimate per roentgen is obtained. This is also given in table 3 and displays a progressive, though not linear, decline with increasing daily dose. This slight but persistent risk increase with decreasing dose and increasing survival time may have two contributing factors. (1) there may be an age:dose interaction that leads to a slight acceleration of injury over long exposure periods or, (2) age itself may promote the more complete expression of low-levels of injury after long time periods of development. This may increase mortality ratios per dose unit accumulated when survival times are 50% or more of the controls. At any rate, the variation across daily dose rates is not great in arithmetic terms; ranging from only about 1.10 to 1.25 per R, and it is opposite to what most persons would have predicted. The predictive value of these risk estimates for conditions other than lifetime exposure will have to be experimentally evaluated.

For more direct prediction, the relations of fig. 17 are offered. Here the mean mortality-rate ratios are plotted against MAS expressed in days and in percent of control. The equations describing the curve in fig. 17 are:

$$MAS_D = 761 - 154 \pm 5\ (X) \qquad (7)$$

$$\%MAS_0 = 100 - 20.2 \pm 0.6\ (X) \qquad (8)$$

In equation (7), if 50% reduction in MAS can be identified by a mortality ratio of 2.303 or, in arithmetic terms, a 10-fold increase in mortality rate, the regression coefficient would be 164. The observed value of 154 ± 5 does not differ significantly from that result (with 7 degrees of freedom). The 50% MAS dose is estimated as 19.4 R/day.

One final prediction equation can be derived from the relation between MAS and the ratio of the mortality-rate slope, k_D, at dose D to the control slope k_0. The ratios, k_D/k_0, and the appropriate MAS_D values form a linear relation on a log-log plot (see fig. 18). The equation is theoretically:

$$MAS_D = MAS_0 \cdot (k_D/k_0)^{-0.831}\ . \qquad (9)$$

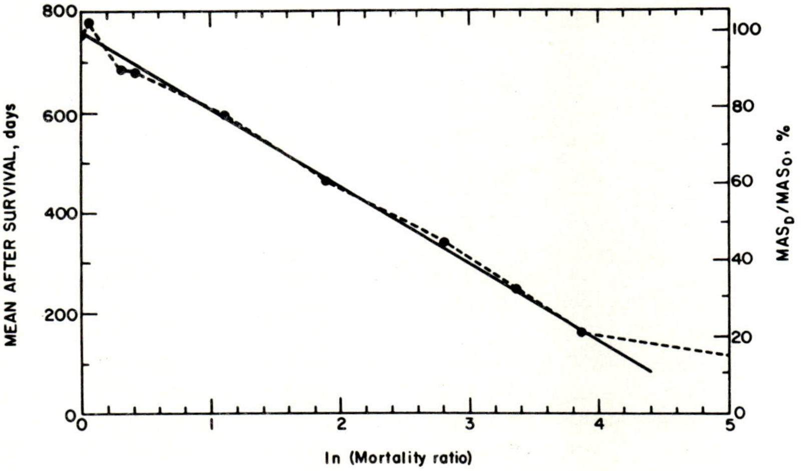

Fig. 17. Regression of MAS in days and as percent of control on mortality ratio in natural logarithms; 0 R - 43 R/day. See text for equations (7) and (8).

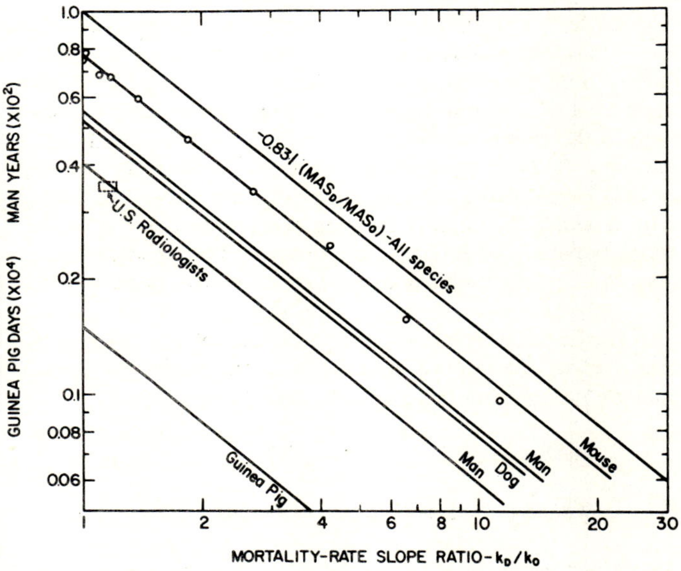

Fig. 18. Log mortality-rate slope ratios versus log MAS for indicated species. Lower line for man based on estimated 40-year after-expectation from 30-35 years for U.S. radiologist controls; upper line for man from Swedish males, 1956-60, with estimated 55-year after-expectation from 20 years. See table 5 for sources of data and text equations (9) and (10).

The least-squares estimated equation is:

$$\ln (MAS_D) = \ln (772) -0.844 \pm 0.014 \ln ({}^{k}D/k_0).$$

The observed slope of -0.844 does not differ significantly from expectation.

This last relationship includes the whole set of dose groups — from 0 R to 56 R/day — thus, it defines the most inclusive prediction equation wherein linearity holds for life expectancies down to only 10% of normal. This is an idealized solution, however, since this is based upon the leukaemia decremented populations fitted by first-degree equations forced through a common intercept.

With equation (9), all the previous relationships between after-survival, daily-dose, mortality ratio, and death-rate slope fall together. The mathematical relationship described by equation (9) has apparently been recognized by epidemiologists, but no reference to it seems available in the literature. The lifetime effects of protracted irradiation may be unique with their progressive expression with age and accumulating dose. At least the expression seems unique in that no comparable mortality experience from other agents appears to have been described for either experimental or human populations. The exponent, -0.831, equals 0.693/-ln (ln 10). This derives from the fact that a 50% reduction in MAS is induced by a 10-fold increase in mortality rate or ratio (equations (7) and (8)).

Equations (4), (5) and (9) can be shuffled around to produce the final result that

$$e^{-\beta D} = \frac{MAS_D}{MAS_0} = \left[\frac{k_D}{k_0}\right]^{-0.831} = \left[e^{\chi D}\right]^{-0.831} ,$$

therefore $\quad -\beta D = -0.831\ \chi D ,$

or $\quad -\beta/\chi = -0.831 = 0.693/-\ln\ (\ln 10). \qquad (10)$

Thus, to establish the life-shortening response of any species under protracted exposure, the value of β or χ must be defined experimentally. Since β is more accessible, and requires only the MAS, the daily-dose duration-of-life exposure regime becomes the method of choice as has been proposed before (Grahn and Sacher, 1968; Sacher and Grahn, 1964).

Interspecific extrapolation requires a means of relating the value of β to some other parameter that characterizes the species under normal conditions. This problem is examined for the mouse-guinea-pig-dog-man relationship in a later section. It will be shown that, in the absence of experimental data, such as in man, an estimate of β or χ can be made by applying a multiple derived by the ratio of control death-rate slopes.

The data of table 3 also present a comparison, in terms of arithmetic mortality ratios, of the three cases mentioned earlier; all causes of death fitted with second-degree polynomials, and the leukaemia decremented populations fitted with either first- or second-degree equations. At the lowest doses, there is no particular consistent difference among the three cases. The second-degree curves are probably more descriptive at least in the sense that for cases 2 and 3 in table 3 the 0.3 R to 0 R ratio is less than 1.0, which matches the observation that MAS at 0.3 R is greater than control MAS.

A comparison of cases 1 and 2 for all doses, does show that the mortality ratios for the second-degree equations are consistently below the ratios from the first-degree equations. Thus, the idealized solution may over-estimate expected mortality by 10 to 20%. If we compare cases 2 and 3 as the most descriptive comparison of the leukaemia decremented population with that for all causes, then a clear measure of the excess mortality due to leukaemia emerges. For doses 12 R, 24 R, 32 R and 43 R/day, a greater mortality ratio for case 3 is seen. This rises from a 15% increase at 12 R to a 50% increase at 32 R, where thymic involvement is about maximum. The increase is about 30% at 24 R/day. A quick look at MAS values in tables 1 and 2 indicates that this excess mortality from leukaemia is also associated with additional life-shortening; MAS is about 50 days shorter at 24 R and 35 days shorter at 32 R (a 17% difference in both cases) for the case for all causes of death.

Although prediction of MAS by slope-ratios (fig. 18) is not directly possible from the second-degree equations, the linear relation between ln (mortality-ratio) and MAS remains as a good prediction equation for doses up to 43 R/day.

Pulmonary Tumour Risk Estimation

The analysis of pulmonary tumour deaths is completely empirical and no common intercept was used. The control data are fitted by a third-degree curve, the 0.3 R, 1.3 R, 2.6 R and 6 R/day data are fitted by second-degree equations and the 12 R/day curve is first-degree. The analysis of integrated risk was taken from 400 days of age (300 days of exposure) to the termination rather than from the 100-day start. Almost no pulmonary tumours appear before 300 days of age even in sample sizes of 300 or more so the early death rates for this cause must be extremely low. If we consider 400 days the time of onset of recognizable risk, then a series of age-risk-dose relations can be derived in addition to the final cumulative risk. The data are in table 4 and figs. 19 and 20. Figure 19 graphically defines the integrated risk estimation procedure for these data and fig. 20 gives some diverse expression of the results.

Table 4

Integrated risk analysis for pulmonary tumours; Strains A/Jax, BALB/c, and BCF_1 and sexes combined

Dose R/day	Days at* risk	Mort. ratio:prob./day ln	Mort. ratio:prob./day arith.	Mort. ratio:prob./R ln	Mort. ratio:prob./R arith.
0	800	0.00	1.00	0	1.00
0.3	800	0.001	1.001	~0	1.00
1.3	700	0.43	1.54	0.334	1.40
2.6	700	0.88	2.41	0.340	1.40
6	500	1.53	4.62	0.255	1.29
12	400	2.59	13.3	0.216	1.24

* Starting at 400 days for all dose groups.

It is clear that the mean mortality-rate ratio rises exponentially with dose at all ages after onset. The final risk for 12 R/day is equivalent to a mortality ratio of about 13.3/1, at 6 R it is about 4.6/1, and 2.4/1 and 1.5/1 at 2.6 R and 1.3 R/day. The final ratio at 0.3 R is only slightly above one, though rough extrapolation from the higher doses suggests the 0.3 R ratio should be about 1.1/1.

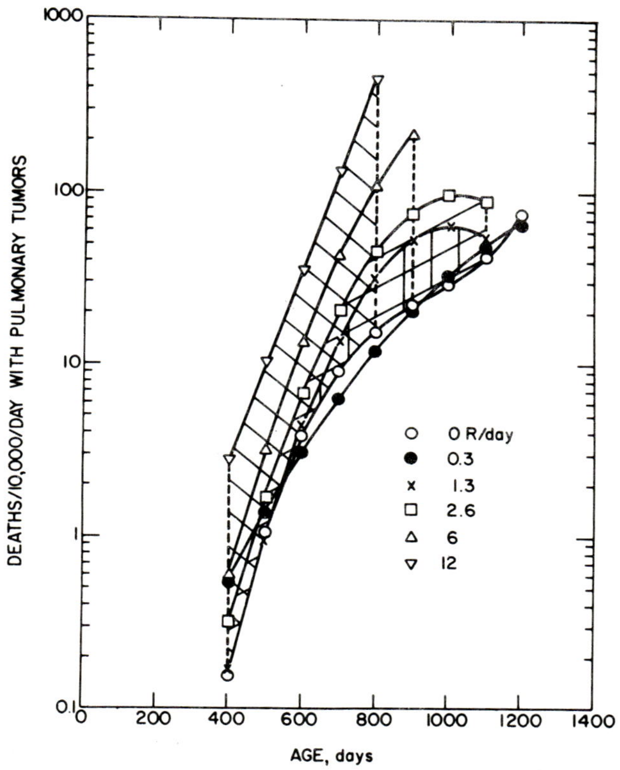

Fig. 19. Age-specific mortality rate data for strains A/Jax, BALB/c, BCF_1 sexes combined, pulmonary tumours, derived equations are third-degree for 0 R, second-degree for 0.3 R, 1.3 R, 2.6 R and 6 R/day, first-degree for 12 R/day. Areas used to estimate integrated risk shown by cross-hatching. See table 4.

The mean ratios divided by their respective daily dose level gives the mortality-ratio per R. As seen in the data for all causes, this ratio tends to decline steadily with increasing dose. Here,too, this could be interpreted to reflect the influence of an age:dose interaction; time permits a continual evolution of injury. For tumour data, this declining ratio can also reflect the effect of the so-called latent period.

The final percentage incidence for pulmonary tumours is also given in fig. 20 to re-emphasize the limited utility of such expressions. The nearly 3-fold increase in average risk between 6 R and 12 R/day is completely lost in the incidence data, as progressive life-shortening truncates the time distribution of tumour events.

Extrapolation between Species

What now can be said regarding other mammalian species and, most important, what about human risk-estimates. Surely, we can all agree that all mammalian species have substantially the same form of actuarial experience. Similarly, the data available on guinea-pigs and dogs under daily irradiation (Casarett and Eddy, 1968; Grahn and Sacher, 1968; Lorenz et al., 1954; Sacher, 1966) would confirm the postulate that MAS is exponentially declining with daily dose and the slope of that function, β, in equation (4), would appear to

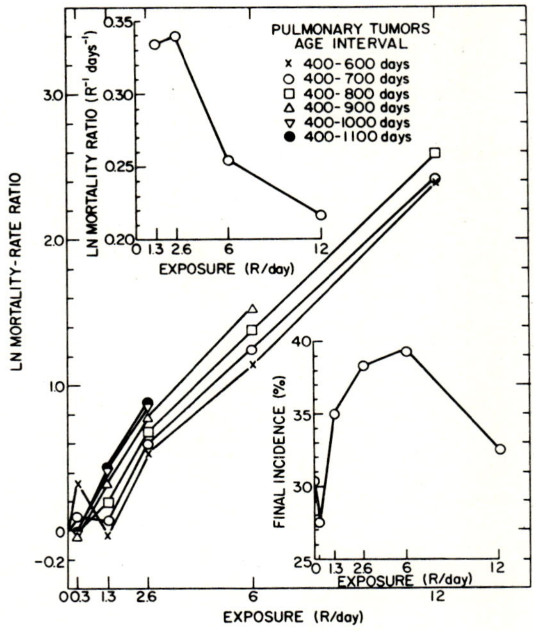

Fig. 20. Mortality ratios versus daily dose for pulmonary tumours at indicated time periods; exposure initiated at 100 days of age. See fig. 19 and table 4.

be an approximate function of life expectancy for these species as compared to the mouse. It would therefore seem reasonable to assume that man should respond in a generally similar manner to that described for the laboratory animals. What would the various constants be in the critical equations (2), (4) and (6) ?

I have compared two selected populations in fig. 21; Swedish males for the period 1956-60 (Larsson, 1965) and the BCF_1 males from the data reported here. Looking first at the death rates for all causes, we see that almost perfect superposition is obtained during the mid-life period for both groups. Early mortality is not strikingly different, but the mouse population drops away from the human population at 70 man years or 700 mouse days. This comparison indicates that although mice have a lower rate of ageing in very late life, the maximum life-span relative to man ($\sim$140 years: 1400 days) may still be in a ratio similar to that seen in mid-life.

The ratio of time scales to equate the two populations is 10 mouse days to 12 man months or one mouse day to 36.5 man days. This is exactly what Jones employed (1957), and is slightly above the 30:1 to 33:1 ratios used by Grahn and others (Grahn, 1962; Grahn and Sacher, 1968) and well above the 20:1 used by Failla (Failla and McClement, 1957). If we assume a common slope for the two species for the mid-life period, this ratio is also the ratio of Gompertz slopes.

The value of k_0 for man in these data is 0.272×10^{-3}/day or 8.28×10^{-3}/month and the death rate at 20 years of age is 25×10^{-6}/month. This predicts an MST of 55 years (53.5 is observed in the life tables (Larsson, 1965)). The ratio of mean after-survivals from

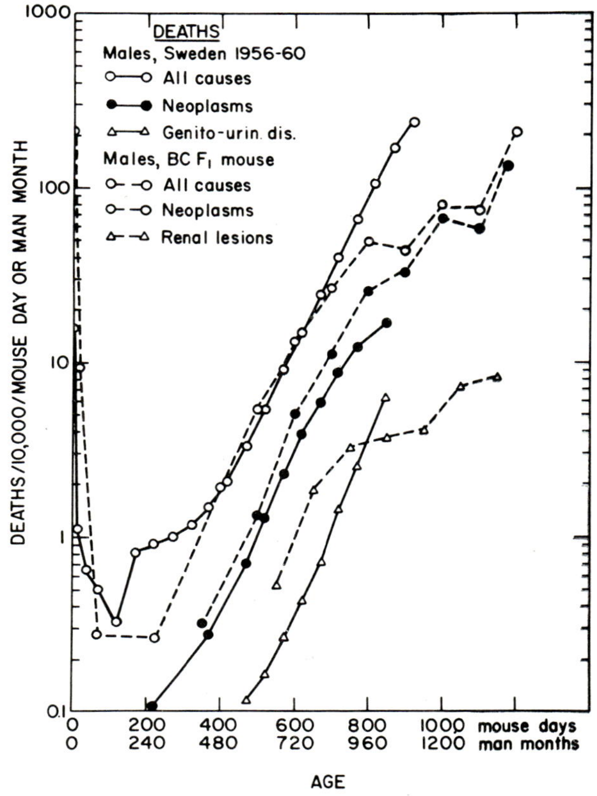

Fig. 21. Age-specific mortality rate for indicated causes for Swedish males (Larsson, 1965) and BCF_1 male controls. See text for details of derivation and comparison.

100 days in the mouse and from 20 years in man is (55 x 365/710) = 28.3. It is 27.5 when compared to the observed expectation of 53.5 years.

Observed values of k_0 for mice are generally below the value of 9.93×10^{-3} that would be estimated by the product (0.272×10^{-3}) (36.5). The BCF_1 combined sex estimate of k_0, from equation (5), is 7.2×10^{-3}/day. The ratio of slopes $7.2 \times 10^{-3}/0.272 \times 10^{-3}$ = 26.5:1. It would seem, therefore, that the man-mouse ratio is somewhere between 25 and 35; a factor of 30 will be assumed as a best estimate for further calculations.

With a ratio of 30, the value of β in equation (4) becomes -1.09 days per R. In equation (2), $k_0 = 8.28 \times 10^{-3}$/mo., $r_0 = 25 \times 10^{-6}$/mo. and MST = 660 months or 55 years. If we accept the ratio of 30 to "humanize" the β-term in (4) and the proof that $e^{-\beta D}$ is a function of $e^{\chi D}$, then the χ-term can be estimated as (30) (0.0429) = 1.287. The death-rate slope for 50% reduction of after-survival would be (8.28×10^{-3}) (2.303) = 19.1×10^{-3}. If $\chi = 1.287$, the daily dose that would induce a 50% reduction of life expectancy in man is 0.831/1.287 = 0.65 R/day. This compares with 19.4 R/day in the mouse.

The man-mouse relation can be explored a bit further by examining the published data on American radiologists (Seltser and Sartwell, 1965; Warren, 1966; Warren and Lombard, 1966). The radiologists, as a group, are apparently the only well-documented source of information on the possible lifetime effects of protracted exposure at or near the tolerance-dose levels. The more recent data on the American group show an average reduction in after-expectation of life of about five years as compared to other classes of medical specialists that did not have a radiation exposure factor in their routine clinical practice (Seltser and Sartwell, 1965). This is relative to deaths in the calendar years 1930-1955; since that time there has been little or no excess mortality (Warren and Lombard, 1966). The exact time of entrance into radiological practice is not clearly defined in these studies but appears to be about 30 years of age. At that age, the cohort would have an after-expectation of about 35 to 45 years, depending upon the "control" employed — general U.S. white males or selected medical specialists. If 40 years is set as the "control" after-expectation, and 35 years is set for radiologists, then the average daily dose can be estimated through the various relations developed in this discussion. This is the lower curve for man in fig. 18.

A five-year reduction in life expectancy, from 40 to 35 years, predicts a ratio of death-rate slopes, (k_D/k_0), of 1.174 in equation (9). This ratio is the value of the term, $e^{\chi D}$, in (5). Since χD will be 0.16 for that term and χ is set at 1.287 for man, the average daily dose to the radiologists would have been about 125 milliroentgens per day, 45 R/year, or between 1350 R and 1575 R accumulated in 30 to 35 years of professional practice. No one really knows what the practising radiologist experienced in the years prior to 1934, when the ICRP set an MPD of 1 R per week for occupational exposure. This was lowered to 0.1 R per day in 1936 by the NCRP, then to 0.3 R/week in the late 1940's, and finally to 0.1 R/week in 1956. Thus, total lifetime doses of as little as 500 R or as much as 2500 R could have been justified by the individual radiologist. Estimates reported by Lewis (1957) are in the range of 100 R to 1000 R. The estimate above, which lies between 1300 R and 1600 R, seems reasonable in relation to changing standards, without assuming either vigorous adherence or careless abuse of those standards.

An additional check is possible from the data given by Seltser and Sartwell (1965). Their death-rate data for radiologists give a slope of 7.6×10^{-3} per month. The slope for other specialists lies between 6.3 and 6.8×10^{-3}, which give ratios between 1.12 and 1.21. These bracket the estimate of 1.174 calculated on the basis of a five-year life-shortening. Curiously, the "control" data for man are quite variable and not easily described by a simple function, even though the death rates are always below the radiologists. The latter group have a uniformly and linearly increasing death-rate.

One last approach is through the mortality ratios for all causes of death. This is about 1.4 for the period 1935-1954 (Seltser and Sartwell, 1965); a value comparable to the mouse experience at 1.3 R/day where a slope ratio of 1.09 pertains. Although this is a little below the lower range of ratios estimated above, it would still predict a daily dose of 70 milliroentgens or a lifetime dose of between 800 R and 1000 R, similar to the range quoted by Lewis (1957).

A quick check of some data on dogs and guinea-pigs offers further support for the relationship of equation (10) and fig. 18 as a substantially dependable prediction equation for life-shortening from protracted irradiation. Data for mouse, guinea-pig, dog, and man are collected in table 5. The values for β (equation (4)) are derived directly from experimental data for mouse, guinea-pig and dog; the human value is 30 times the mouse number. The control Gompertz slopes are from this paper, for the mouse and man, and from Sacher (1966) for man, dog, and guinea-pig. The life expectancies for dog and guinea-pig are estimated from the intercepts of lines fitting the ln MAS versus daily-dose relation.

It is not possible to actually check the fit for dogs in the absence of a mortality-

Table 5

Comparison of mouse, guinea-pig, dog, and man regarding normal life-table and radiation sensitivity parameters

	Normal life expect. (days)	Ratio	Mort. rate slope: k_0 (10^{-3}/day)	Ratio	β (days/R)	Ratio	χ (per R)	Ratio
Mouse	750	1	7.2	1	-0.036	1	0.043	1
G.pig	1,500 (est.)	2	1.6	$^1/_{4.5}$	-0.156	4.3	0.18-0.26	4-6
Dog	5,200 (est.)	7	2.3	$^1/_{3.1}$	-0.195	5.4	0.234	5.4
Man	20,075	27	0.22-0.27	$^1/_{27-33}$	-1.09	30	1.29	30

Source of data: Mouse - this paper; G.pig - Sacher (1966), Lorenz et al. (1954);

Dog - Casarett (1968), Sacher (1966); Man - Sacher (1966), this paper.

rate slope for at least one dose in addition to the control. The ratio of dog:mouse β terms, 5.4, is between those derived from the ratio of life-expectancies or control slopes (table 5). Thus, estimating β or χ by the ratios of 3:1 or 7:1 would give values that would predict the observed life-shortening at 0.6 R/day in the Rochester dogs to have been attributed to a dose between 0.45 and 1.10 R/day.

The guinea-pig data are more erratic. Values of χ can be derived that lie between 0.18 and 0.26; the ratio to the mouse is between 4 and 6. This range matches the ratio of control mortality-rate slopes, but is well above the ratio of life expectancies. In detail, the estimate of χ derived from the Lorenz data at 2.2 R/day is 0.233 for a guinea-pig to mouse ratio of 5.4:1. The ratio of slopes for the Argonne data at 1.8 R/day and control is 1.61:1 to give an χ-term of 0.265, while the life-shortening at that dose yields an χ-term of 0.245. The value of 0.188 is derived from the relation $\beta/\chi = 0.831$. In addition, Sacher's analysis (his fig. 9 in (Sacher, 1966)) gives a guinea-pig to mouse ratio of Gompertz increments per R as 4:1. All of this suggests the guinea-pig is a relatively radiosensitive species in the framework defined by mouse-dog-man.

This radiosensitivity difference does not prevent the guinea-pig from fitting the prediction equations; the question merely recurs — how do we estimate the dose-response relationship for mortality-rate increases in the absence of experimental data. The ratio of control population Gompertz, or death-rate, regressions between the mouse and the species in question seems the most accurate means of establishing an adjustment factor to convert the mouse constants into those for the other species.

Discussion

Although the available data on experimental animals have not been exhaustively presented, it should be noted that the new data confirm much of that previously recorded regarding life-shortening and pathologic effects of duration-of-life irradiation and add significantly to both categories of effect in several ways. Life-shortening prediction equations can be defined more rigorously for reductions that span nearly 90% of the normal life expectancy. The statistical parameters of death-rate or Gompertz slopes, mortality ratios, dose rate, total dose and life expectancy can now be rationally inter-related. The relationship between man and mouse is also clarified by the present data and the experience drawn from American radiologists seem to comfortably comply with expectations derived from the mouse experience. The guinea-pig and dog are also in good general agreement with man to mouse expectations, though control survivals seem underestimated for both guinea-pig and dog while data on death-rates are not complete.

The analysis of tumour incidence is far from complete. The data given here at the lowest doses confirm the original findings of Lorenz et al. (1954), and both confirm and add to those of Lesher et al. (1965). The multiple-risk problem, discussed to some extent by Lesher et al. still remains rather obscure. The antagonistic effect of renal lesions on reticular tissue tumours has not previously been reported, though the LAF_1 mouse used by Lorenz et al. and Lesher et al. did show a high incidence of kidney degeneration in late life (Lesher et al., 1957, 1965; Lorenz et al., 1954).

It may be possible to manage the prediction of human neoplastic responses to radiation in a manner similar to life-shortening effects. Figure 21 clearly indicates that the death-rates from all tumours and from genito-urinary diseases are strikingly comparable for man and mouse and bear a close relation to the death-rates from all causes. Thus, the integrated risk analysis for specific tumours or degenerative diseases in the mouse may offer at least empirical risk estimates for human expectations. This will be examined as we continue the analysis of the mouse data.

A few final general comments might be in order. It should be apparent to many in the field of environmental hazards evaluation that the systems of experimentation and analysis developed for the study of radiation hazards are not only well proven, but are also analytically precise. They can be considered models of experimental methodology that could have direct and immediate applicability to the study of other toxic agents. And in this application, the mouse still stands out as the animal of choice for population-type statistics, good general relationships to man, economy of maintenance, and for its broad spectrum of realistic biological end-points. As methods of risk-estimation become better defined, it may then be possible to predict with considerable accuracy expected responses to environmental hazards in man long before the human experience has developed to the extent it has for radiation hazards. This would enable corrective measures to be instituted on the basis of scientifically justified anticipation, rather than wait for the results of a first retrospective analysis of perturbed rates of morbidity and mortality.

References

Berlin, N.I. An analysis of some radiation effects on mortality, pp. 121-127. In: The Biology of Aging, A Symposium, Edited by B.L. Strehler, AIBS, Washington, D.C., 1960.

Berlin, N.I., and DiMaggio, F.L. A survey of theories and experiments on the shortening of life span by ionizing radiation. Tech. Staff Study Armed Forces Special Weapons Project Report AFSWP-608, 1956.

Brues, A.M., and Sacher, G.A. Analysis of mammalian radiation injury and lethality, pp. 441-465. In: Symposium on Radiobiology, edited by J.J. Nickson, J. Wiley & Sons, New York, 1952.

Casarett, G., and Eddy, H.A. Fractionation of dose in radiation induced male sterility, pp. 14.1-14.10. In: Dose Rate in Mammalian Radiation Biology, edited by D.G. Brown, R.G. Cragle, T.R. Noonan. Div. of Tech. Inform., USAEC Report CONF-680410, 1968.

Dunn, T.B. Relationship of amyloid infiltration and renal disease in mice. J. natn. Cancer Inst., 5, 17-28, 1944.

Failla, G., and McClement, P. The shortening of life by chronic whole-body irradiation. Am. J. Roentg., 78, 946-954, 1957.

Federal Radiation Council. Pathological Effects of Thyroid Irradiation. Federal Radiation Council Report No. 3. Washington, D.C., 1962.

Federal Radiation Council. Implications to man of irradiation by internally deposited Strontium-89, Strontium-90, and Cesium-137. Report of an Advisory Committee, U.S. Nat. Acad. Sci. - Nat. Res. Council, Federal Radiation Council. Washington, D.C., 1964.

Federal Radiation Council. Radiation Exposure of Uranium Miners, Report of an Advisory

Committee. U.S. Nat. Acad. Sci. - Nat. Res. Council, Federal Radiation Council. Washington, D.C., 1968.

Furth, J., and Upton, A.C. Vertebrate radiobiology: Histopathology and carcinogenesis. A. Rev. nucl. Sci., 3, 303-338, 1953.

Gompertz, B. On the nature of the function expressive of the law of human mortality and on a new mode of determining life contingencies. Phil. Trans. R. Soc., 513-585, 1825.

Grahn, D. Genetic control of physiological processes: The genetics of radiation toxicity in animals, pp. 181-200. In: Radioisotopes in the Biosphere, edited by R.C. Caldecott and L.A. Snyder, University of Minnesota, Minneapolis, 1959.

Grahn, D. Late effects in man following exposure to ionizing radiations, pp. 275-290. In: Protection against Radiation Hazards in Space. Div. Tech. Inform., U.S. Atomic Energy Comm. Doc. TID-7652. Dept. Commerce, Washington, D.C., 1962.

Grahn, D. Late effects of external irradiations in animals and the prediction of low-dose effects. In: Biological Implications of the Nuclear Age. Div. of Tech. Inform., USAEC Symposium Series, CONF-690303, 1969.

Grahn, D., and Hamilton, K.F. Influence of sex, environment and radiation factors on life shortening and tumor incidence in $C3H_f$ mice. Rad. Res., 21, 191, 1964.

Grahn, D., and Sacher, G.A. Fractionation and protraction and the late effects of radiation in small mammals, pp. 2.1-2.27. In: Dose Rate in Mammalian Radiation Biology, edited by D.G. Brown, R.G. Cragle and T.R. Noonan. Div. of Tech. Inform. USAEC Report CONF-680410, 1968.

Grahn, D., Sacher, G.A., and Hamilton, K.F. A uniformity of life shortening among genetically different mice under daily gamma radiation. Radiat. Res., 19, 239, 1963.

Grahn, D., Sacher, G.A., and Hamilton, K.F. Survival of mice under daily gamma irradiation: progress report, pp. 18-20. Argonne Nat. Lab., Biol. and Med. Res. Div., Ann. Report ANL-7136, 1965.

Grahn, D., Sacher, G.A., Fry, R.J.M., and Rust, J.H. Lethal and pathological effects of life-time exposure to low daily doses of gamma radiation in inbred and hybrid mice. (in preparation)

Jones, H.B. A special consideration of the aging process, disease and life expectancy. Adv. biol. med. Phys., 4, 281-337, 1956a.

Jones, H.B. Estimation of effect of radiation upon human health and life span. Proc. Hlth. Phys. Soc., 1, 114-126, 1956b.

Jones, H.B. The nature of radioactive fallout and its effects on man, pp.1100-1137. Hearings, Joint Committee on Atomic Energy, Special Subcommittee on Radiation, 85th Congress, Part 2, U.S. Government Printing Office, Washington, D.C., 1957.

Langham, W.H. (Editor) Radiobiological factors in manned space flight. U.S. Nat. Acad. of Sci. - Nat. Res. Council Publ. No. 1487, Washington, D.C., 1967.

Larsson, T. Mortality in Sweden. Acta genet. Statist. med., 15, (Suppl.), 1-143, 1965.

Lesher, S.W., Grahn, D., and Sallese, A. Amyloidosis in mice exposed to daily gamma irradiation. J. natn. Cancer Inst., 19, 1119-1127, 1957.

Lesher, S., Sacher, G.A., Grahn, D., Hamilton, K.F., and Sallese, A. Survival of mice under duration-of-life exposure to gamma rays. II. Pathologic effects. Radiat. Res., 24, 239-277, 1965.

Lewis, E.B. Leukemia and ionizing radiation. Science, N.Y., 125, 965-972, 1957.

Lorenz, E., Jacobson, L.O., Heston, W.E., Shimkin, M., Eschenbrenner, A.B., Deringer, M.K., Doniger, J., and Schweisthal, R. Effects of long-continued total-body gamma irradiation on mice, guinea-pigs and rabbits. III. Effects on life span, weight, blood picture, and carcinogenesis and the role of the intensity of radiation, pp. 24-148. In: Biological Effects of External X and Gamma Radiation, edited by R.E. Zirkle, McGraw-Hill, New York, 1954.

Mildvan, A.S., and Strehler, B.L. A critique of theories of mortality, pp. 216-235. In: The Biology of Aging, A symposium, edited by B.L. Strehler, AIBS, Washington, D.C., 1960.

Neary, G. Aging and radiation. Nature, Lond., 187, 10-18, 1960.

Rugh, R., and Wolff, J. X-irradiation sterilization of the female mouse. Fert. Steril., 7, 546, 1956.

Sacher, G.A. On the statistical nature of mortality, with especial reference to chronic radiation mortality. Radiology, 67, 250-257, 1956.

Sacher, G.A. Problems in the extrapolation of long term effects from animals to man, pp. 3-10. In: Delayed Effects of Whole-Body Radiation, edited by B.B. Watson, J. Hopkins Press, Baltimore, 1960.

Sacher, G.A. The Gompertz transformation in the study of the injury-mortality relationship: application to late radiation effects and ageing, pp. 411-441. In: Radiation and Ageing, edited by P.J. Lindop and G.A. Sacher, Taylor & Francis Ltd., London, 1966.

Sacher, G.A., and Grahn, D. Survival of mice under duration-of-life exposure to gamma rays. I. The dosage-survival relation and the lethality function. J. natn. Cancer Inst., 32, 277-321, 1964.

Sacher, G.A., Grahn, D., Fry, R.J.M., and Rust, J.H. Epidemiological and cellular effects of chronic radiation exposure: A search for relationship. Proc. of the First European Symposium on Late Effects of Radiations, Casaccia, Italy, 22-23 April, 1969.

Seltser, R., and Sartwell, P.E. The influence of occupational exposure to radiation on the mortality of American radiologists and other medical specialists. Am. J. Epidemiol., 81, 2-22, 1965.

United Nations Scientific Committee on the Effects of Atomic Radiation. General Assembly, Nineteenth Session, Suppl. No. 14 (A/5814), New York, 1964.

Upton, A.C. Effects of radiation on man. A. Revue nucl. Sci., 18, 495-528, 1968.

Upton, A.C., Kimball, A.W., Furth, J., Christenberry, K.W., and Benedict, W.H. Some delayed effects of atom-bomb radiations in mice. Cancer Research 20 (8/2): 1-62, 1960.

Upton, A.C., Kastenbaum, M.A., and Conklin, J.W. Age-specific death rates of mice exposed to ionizing radiation and radiomimetic agents, pp. 285-297. In: Cellular Basis and Aetiology of Late Somatic Effects of Ionizing Radiation, edited by R.J.C. Harris, Academic Press, New York, 1963.

Van Cleave, C.D. Late Somatic Effects of Ionizing Radiation. Div. Tech. Inform. U.S. Atomic Energy Comm., Doc. TID-24310, 1968.

Warren, S. The basis for the limit on whole-body exposure-experience of radiologists. Hlth Phys., 12, 737-741, 1966.

Warren, S., and Lombard, O.M. New data on the effects of ionizing radiation on radiologists. Arch. Environ. Hlth, 13, 415-421, 1966.

DISCUSSION OF CHAPTERS III, IV AND V

Dr. Lamerton: One must draw a clear distinction between the late effects of radiation doses in the therapeutic range discussed by Dr. Fowler and the late effects of the smaller or protracted doses of radiation with which Dr. Casarett and Dr. Grahn have mainly been concerned.

The appearance of a late effect of radiation is the manifestation of a deficient or overwhelmed repair system. With doses of the order of one or several thousands of rads, as discussed by Dr. Fowler, only a small proportion of the proliferating cells, 1% or perhaps less, will survive. It is small wonder then that repair processes will not be fully efficient and that late effects, often severe, may occur. However, when dealing with lower levels of cell damage, one would expect the repair and homeostatic mechanisms of the body to be able to cope, if not fully, at least to a large extent. The extent to which repair mechanisms can cope is, of course, the basic problem behind all considerations of radiation hazard, and this is still an area of great ignorance.

I believe this conference to be useful and timely because one of its aims is to attempt to relate the late effects of radiation with those of other environmental agents. And it gives us an opportunity to look anew at two problems which have concerned many people for a long time. The first of these is the quantitative assessment of late effects in man from small doses of radiation, and the second is the mechanism of the production of the various late effects arising from radiation.

I have become despondent about progress in both of these fields. Certainly practical and theoretical radiobiology has had little effect so far on the levels of radiation regarded as permissible. The maximum permissible levels are still based essentially on inspired guesses made a long time ago. Perhaps my despondency has been increased by the part I have had to play recently with two task groups of the International Commission on Radiation Protection, particularly in the most recent one on the spatial distribution of radiation. Our aim was to try to improve the present Recommendations on this matter, and although we recognized that the present system was in many ways inconsistent and illogical, we could not suggest anything else. In fact, we prefaced our report with a quotation from the French which translated says: "If it's simple, it is bound to be wrong. If it's not simple, you can't use it anyhow". Much of our thinking on effects of low radiation doses, so far as man is concerned, seems to oscillate between an unjustified simplicity and an unmanageable complexity.

I am going to be provocative, as I was told to be, and suggest that the two papers by Dr. Grahn and Dr. Casarett in a way represent these two extreme positions.

Dr. Grahn said quite clearly that he was not concerned with the initial pattern of damage or with the mechanisms of the various late effects, but with the actuarial analysis of duration of life under radiation. His paper is, I think, a tour-de-force. It is very elegant indeed, but I have a sort of ambivalence in my mind about it. One half of me is full of admiration for what has been achieved. The other half of me says that the amount of information obtainable must be very limited unless one goes into the biological mechanisms involved. My immediate concern is about the use of life-shortening as a measure of radiation effect, whether it is not too academic a concept, and how far it has real significance in setting dose limits, as compared with the incidence of specific diseases. Also studies on radiation life-shortening can relate only to the response to radiation. Insofar as they do not involve biological mechanisms, they have little relevance to the late effects of other hazardous agents and other forms of initial damage, which is, I feel, a considerable limitation.

If Dr. Grahn's presentation represented the simple approach to the problem, then Dr. Casarett's seemed to demonstrate the complexities.

From his quite encyclopaedic knowledge of radiation effects, he brought together a number of observations which are fascinating in themselves, but which indicated to me how difficult it was to make useful generalizations. He demonstrated, for instance, how very different were the responses of different tissues and different species to protracted or fractionated doses, and also the degree of species specificity in the type of tumour produced.

I have exaggerated the problems, but they exist. As Dr. Kohn said this morning, we have to rethink our approach to the experimental work on the effect of low doses of radiation and I believe that his suggestion was the right one, that we must combine the study of radiation effects with that of other agents and variables. In experimental radiation studies, particularly those concerned with radiation hazard, we may have become too inward-looking and have tended to concentrate our attention on the late effects of a "thing" called radiation instead of on the late effects of a given pattern of cellular damage.

Cellular radiobiology is now at the stage where we can begin to define quantitatively the pattern of cellular damage produced by radiation in terms of effects upon various proliferative and non-proliferative populations. The possibility is now open to modify these effects in quite specific ways and observe what change this has upon the subsequent response of the tissue.

One can modify the pattern by changes in radiation conditions, by changes in LET*, by fractionation, by protraction, and so forth. It is also important, as Dr. Kohn suggested, that we should introduce other noxious agents into the system. We require to know precisely what we are doing to the pattern of cellular change, and the cytotoxic drugs represent one group of such agents which could usefully be used in combination with radiation.

These are vague generalizations, for which I apologize, but I suspect that the demand for "numbers" in radiation effects conflicts with attaining an understanding of the underlying mechanisms. We will have to feel our way to these new approaches, particularly if we want radiation studies in animals and man to have any relevance to the effects of other agents.

The approach I have been discussing is certainly not a new one. In a way, it is very much what Dr. Fowler and Dr. Lindop have done at higher doses of radiation. They had modified the initial pattern of damage by changes in LET and fractionation, and they have noted what had happened to the late effects. I am certain that those who are working on low dose effects of radiation are looking with very envious eyes at this work where the late effects are well defined and occur with high frequency!

---

* Linear energy transfer (LET).

CHAPTER VI

CYTOGENETIC CHANGES AFTER RADIATION EXPOSURE

Michael A. Bender

Chromosomal aberrations are produced soon after exposure to ionizing radiation. They are not, however, ascertainable unless and until the cell containing them enters cell division and they may persist unmodified in interphase cells for many years. At cell division some aberrations are modified and may even be lost for mechanical reasons, but even in rapidly dividing tissues a few aberrations persist and may be seen years after a radiation exposure. In this sense, then, I suppose that chromosomal aberrations qualify as a late effect of radiation. Also, of course, aberrations induced in germ line cells may be transmitted to subsequent generations, causing congenital defects, deaths, or lowered fertility many years after the radiation exposure. Naturally, whether one considers that chromosomal aberrations can ever be considered a subtle effect of radiation depends entirely on one's own point of view.

Mammalian cytogenetics is, of course, a comparatively recent development, and it is perhaps not surprising that relatively little information is now available on radiation-induced chromosomal aberrations in human and other mammalian material. It is important to keep in mind, though, that radiation cytogenetics itself is not a recent development, even though until quite recently it did not include much work on mammalian material. Extrapolations to mammals may be made from the large body of data obtained mainly from work with plant cells. Such extrapolations must be made with caution, and their validity must be checked experimentally. In fact, much of the work that has been done during the relatively brief history of mammalian radiation cytogenetics has consisted of just such demonstrations. These studies have shown that predictions that could have been made from prior work on other organisms were in fact true in mammals, although this has not been generally recognized, especially in reports on human chromosome aberrations. There have, however, been surprises, and the subject is, in my opinion, certainly worth pursuit on its own scientific merit. My purposes here are two-fold: to discuss some of the interesting areas and especially to call attention to some of the points that require further investigation.

Aberration Types

Radiation may be considered to induce chromosomal aberrations by producing breaks in the chromosome's continuity. This may or may not be followed by recombination between various broken ends. Revell (1959) has actually proposed that all aberrations result from recombination, but for our purposes we may consider the various aberration types in terms of the classical "breakage-first" model (Stadler, 1931; Sax, 1938).

There are two major classes of chromosomal aberrations, designated the chromosome and the chromatid types. Chromosome-type aberrations are induced by radiation during the pre-DNA-synthesis portion of the interphase, during which the chromosome behaves as though it were a single thread. Breaks and recombinations occurring at this stage are later replicated when the chromosomes replicate in preparation for a cell division, so that they always involve both chromatids of the chromosome as seen at metaphase. Chromatid-type aberrations, on the other hand, are induced after the chromosomes become effectively two-stranded during the DNA synthesis and post-DNA-synthesis portions of the cell cycle. Whereas an ionizing event may sometimes break both chromatids at the same apparent level (an isochromatid break), in general the individual chromatids are the units of breakage and recombination. Chromatid aberrations (with the exception of isochromatid breaks) seen at metaphase involve only one of the two sister chromatids.

The least complicated type of aberration is the simple break or deletion (fig. 1A). This aberration is seen as a shortened chromosome (or chromatid) plus a fragment that lacks any attachment to the centromere. Such acentric fragments will be either single or paired, depending on whether they are from cells irradiated before or after the chromosomes split.

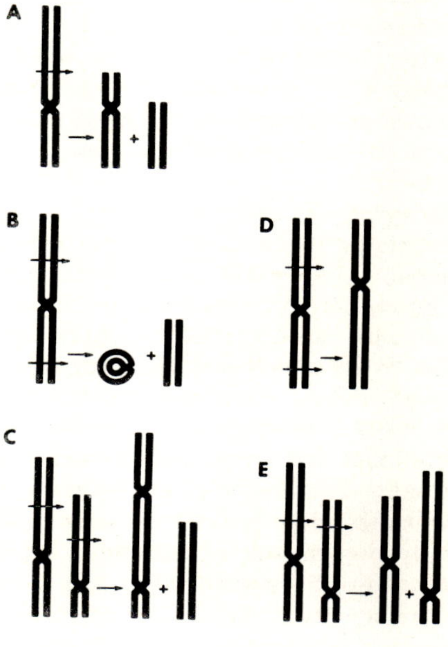

Fig. 1. Schematic diagram illustrating the origin and appearance of various types of chromosome type aberrations. A. Deletion; B. Ring (asymmetrical intrachange); C. Dicentric (asymmetrical interchange); D. Inversion (symmetrical intrachange); E. Translocation (symmetrical interchange).

If several breaks are present in the same cell at the same time, various types of recombination are possible. The breaks do not, however, have to interact; if they do not, the result is simply several deletions. Nor, incidentally, do the recombinations have to be complete; it is possible for some of the broken ends to recombine, but for others not to. But this is a complication we need not bother with here. To take the simplest case, that of two breaks, it is clear that they could be in the same or different chromosomes. In either case, recombination can be symmetrical (i.e. the centric portion of each broken chromosome or the centric ends of a doubly broken chromosome with the acentric portions) or asymmetrical (centric portion recombining with centric portion and acentric with acentric). We thus have four possibilities for two-break aberration types: symmetrical intrachanges (inversions), asymmetrical intrachanges (rings), symmetrical interchanges (translocations), and asymmetrical interchanges (dicentrics). These four types are illustrated in fig. 1 B-E. More complicated aberration types are seen, involving more than just two breaks. For example, tricentric and even tetracentric chromosomes occur, and at least theoretically one can find any of the complex types one might imagine from various types of recombination between multiple breaks. And of course any of the multiple-break aberrations can be of either chromosome or chromatid type, depending on when in the cell cycle the breaks are induced.

The various recombination aberration types are not all equally obvious upon cytological examination. Ring and dicentric chromosomes are easy to ascertain under the microscope because of their novel morphology, but inversions and translocations are frequently impossible to detect by inspection at metaphase because they alter the chromosomes' morphology little, if at all, for example paracentric inversion where both breaks are in the same chromosome arm. Thus, although the symmetrical exchange aberrations are expected to be just as frequent as asymmetrical ones, they are commonly not reported, and scoring is often limited to the deletions, rings, dicentrics, and, provided the dose is large enough that they are seen at all, asymmetrical exchanges involving more than two breaks.

It was certainly no surprise when the earliest observations on irradiated human somatic cells confirmed the expectation that radiation broke their chromosomes, just as it did in the organisms studied previously, and that all the expected aberration types resulted. The surprising thing was that this confirmation came only so recently (Bender, 1957; Puck, 1958; Chu et al., 1961). Subsequently, the expectations have been confirmed in a variety of cells, both in vitro and in vivo, from various tissues of a number of different species of mammals. Naturally, these confirmations come from tissues that normally have high mitotic rates, such as bone marrow, corneal epithelium, and testicular germinal epithelium, or from tissues that can be stimulated to produce many mitoses, such as peripheral lymphocytes and regenerating liver. Similarly, they tend to come either from species of particular interest, such as man, or those in which low chromosome numbers make investigation easier, such as the Chinese hamster and certain marsupials. But there is certainly no reason to believe that radiation does not produce chromosomal aberrations of all the expected types in cells of all tissues of all mammals, including man.

Persistence of Aberrations

Chromosomal damage in the form of aberrations cannot be repaired in the ordinary sense, at least not for more than a few hours after the radiation exposure that induces them. Nevertheless, there are a number of reasons to expect the loss or modification of many types of aberrations at cell division, thus decreasing their frequency in the cell population. This might be thought of as repair of chromosomal damage on the tissue level (though this is not by any means the usual usage of the term "repair").

First, deletions and the asymmetrical-exchange aberrations involve acentric chromosomal fragments. These, lacking any attachment to the cell's spindle apparatus, fail to move to the poles with the centric chromosome at anaphase and most often fail to be included in the daughter nuclei. When this happens, the daughter cell is deficient in the genetic sense, since it lacks a portion of its genome. It is clear that such deficiencies, if they are of appreciable size, are very likely to be lethal to a zygote; however, there seems to be no a priori reason to expect them to be lethal or even particularly detrimental to a somatic cell. Such deficient somatic cells should often survive and even mutliply. This is because many of the functional changes that might prove lethal to a relatively isolated zygote could be compensated for by materials supplied by the normal cells surrounding the somatic cell containing a deletion.

Second, the asymmetrical-exchange aberrations can experience mechanical difficulty in segregation during anaphase, preventing normal separation and possibly eliminating the dividing cell from the population. Dicentric chromosomes or chromatids, for example, can form anaphase bridge structures if the two centromeres are pulled toward opposite poles. Although the ultimate fate of such bridges is not known precisely, they must often result in the elimination of the dicentric chromosome from one or both daughter cells, the formation of polyploid or binucleate giant cells, or the outright killing of the dividing cell. Evidence has been presented that the risk of dicentric loss through bridge formation is about 50% per cell generation in dividing human lymphocytes in culture (Sasaki and Norman, 1967). While this appears to describe the risk for the average dicentric, it is still important to note that some dicentrics may have a very low probability of experiencing the alternate centromere segregation that leads to bridge formation (consider a dicentric with the centromeres quite close together).

Ring chromosomes are also lost through anaphase bridge formation, though the mechanisms is quite different. Any exchange between the two chromatids (sister strand exchange or somatic crossing over) can lead either to interlocking of the two daughter ring chromatids or to the formation of a double-sized ring whose centromeres must segregate, to opposite poles, because they are homologous. Various examples of ring chromosomes seem to have quite different loss risks, some being quite stable and others very unstable. It is clear, however, that rings can be lost at cell division through bridge formation, though some, like some dicentrics, may have a negligible probability of loss at a given division.

Third, even though there is no frequent loss and no consequent partial haploidy, rearrangements of both the symmetrical and the asymmetrical types do change the cells' genome in the position-effect sense. It is thus likely that at least a few such aberrations may have detrimental or even lethal effects even without fragment loss or anaphase bridge formation. Such effects might be manifested during interphase, at cell division, or simply in a lowered "fitness" in the evolutionary sense.

These considerations, mainly from classical cytogenetics, would lead us to expect that acentric fragments would disappear very quickly from rapidly dividing tissues of irradiated mammals, that asymmetrical exchange aberrations would disappear less rapidly, and that symmetrical exchange aberrations would disappear very slowly. Furthermore, one would expect to see many cells with deleted chromosomes, but without the acentric fragments, after one or a few post-irradiation divisions, that would disappear slowly from somatic tissues. Also, one might expect that clones of cells, all with the same aberration, would appear as the aberrant cells multiplied. One would expect such cloning to be most common for cells with symmetrical-exchange aberrations.

Observations that are available on cells from men and other mammals bear out these expectations without exception. Some of the first observations on men, previously irradiated, established that even years after irradiation cells with exchange aberrations were still present (Buckton et al., 1962; Bender and Gooch, 1962). Similar observations have since been made on people irradiated under a wide variety of circumstances, including the Hiroshima and Nagasaki populations exposed during the atomic bombings about twenty years previously (Bloom et al., 1966, 1967). Most of the observations have been made on peripheral lymphocytes induced to divide in short-term tissue culture. Goh (1968), however, reported finding aberrations in direct bone marrow preparations from men irradiated years before in a criticality accident. It is expected, of course, that the residual levels at a given time after irradiation should vary as a function of the rate of cell turnover in different tissues. There is some suggestion of this in Goh's report, as the levels of asymmetrical exchange aberrations seemed to be lower in the bone marrow than in peripheral lymphocyte samples obtained at the same time. However, it seems that the frequencies of these aberrations in peripheral lymphocytes are somewhat erratic in samples taken years after irradiation (Bender and Gooch, 1966); so the differences in Goh's samples may have been fortuitous. In any case, the experiments of Curtis and his collaborators on regenerating mouse liver (see Curtis, 1963) clearly demonstrate the effect of cell replacement rates on residual aberration frequencies in irradiated mammals.

Cloning of aberration-bearing cells (or at least the presence of several cells with what appeared to be the same aberration) has been observed in peripheral lymphocytes from previously irradiated people (Bender and Gooch, 1966; Bloom et al., 1967; Court Brown et al., 1967). In all cases the apparent clones involved symmetrical translocations. Cloning of aberration-bearing bone marrow and lymphoid cells was earlier observed by Ford et al., (1957) in lethally irradiated mice kept alive by isologous, unirradiated bone marrow transplantations. In this case, the clones of irradiated cells were not only able to survive and multiply despite their aberrations, but they were actually able to compete successfully with the unirradiated donor cells as well. In observations of the peripheral lymphocytes of people irradiated years before it was noted early that an occasional cell was present which not only contained an asymmetrical exchange aberration but also the expected acentric fragment (Court Brown et al., 1965). This has been taken as evidence for the existence of long-lived cells that might get into the peripheral circulation without an intervening cell division during the years after irradiation. The frequency of such cells is certainly very low, however. It is not impossible that an occasional acentric fragment may be accidentally included in a daughter-cell nucleus and thus survive a cell division. Also, the acentric fragments observed may have arisen spontaneously as deletions shortly before the cells were sampled and may be quite independent of the exchange aberration. Hence, the evidence for persistence of cells for years without cell division still seems inconclusive.

Several groups have attempted to use the persistence of asymmetrical exchange aberrations in peripheral lymphocytes as a means of measuring the lifespan of the small lymphocyte in humans (Court Brown et al., 1965; Norman et al., 1965, 1966; Buckton, Court Brown and Smith, 1967; Sasaki and Norman, 1967). Unfortunately, the observations of the two groups lead to very different estimates of life-span. Also, the observations of Court Brown's group suggest a two-component curve, which they interpret as evidence for two different cell populations, one with a much longer lifespan than the other. It may well be, though, that the slower component of the curve simply results from those aberrations that have a much lower than average risk of loss at cell division.

It should be noted that the peripheral leukocyte system may have some unique features because of involvement in normal immune mechanisms. Nowell (1965, 1967) has presented evidence that there may be subpopulations of immunologically committed lymphocytes that can "dump" aberration-bearing cells into the peripheral circulation long after the radiation experience that induced the aberrations. Nowell observed that the use of different mitogens in cultures of peripheral lymphocytes from therapeutically irradiated patients yielded different frequencies of asymmetrical exchange aberrations in samples obtained months after irradiation. Such a mechanism may account for the temporal variability in aberration frequencies observed in previously irradiated subjects.

It has been suggested that the peripheral lymphocyte system may be quite different in different species of mammals. Weber and Nowell (1965) subjected Rhesus monkeys, pigs, rabbits, guinea-pigs and rats to partial-body irradiation and then followed aberration yields in peripheral lymphocytes as a function of post-irradiation time. In the monkeys the frequencies of cells with asymmetrical exchange aberrations fell rapidly (apparently during the first two days) following irradiation and then remained essentially constant during the seven months they were observed. In the pigs, the aberration frequencies fell to low levels within 24 hours after irradiation and remained there during the 50 days they were observed. In the rabbits, asymmetrical exchange aberrations were seen only in the culture of one sample obtained an hour after irradiation, and none were observed in samples obtained later. Practically no aberrations were seen in samples from the irradiated guinea-pigs or rats. On the basis of these observations, the authors suggest that the lymphocyte population dynamics show species differences and that perhaps some of the species studied do not have any long-lived subpopulation as postulated for humans. This is, of course, an interesting possibility which has important implications. It seems wise to be somewhat cautious, however, until further data are available. Because the irradiations were of only part of the body (as were the human exposures), the early drop is expected because of dilution and equilibration of the exposed cells with unexposed cells in lymphoid tissues outside the radiation field. This phenomenon has been clearly demonstrated in the case of humans whose peripheral cells were irradiated extracorporeally (Sharpe et al., 1967, 1968). The differences between species may have been caused, at least in part, by the differences in the areas irradiated and in the doses given in Weber and Nowell's experiments.

Aberration Rates and Kinetics

Acute doses of low-LET radiations, such as X or γ rays, induce breaks in chromosomes at random in the exposed cell population. Breaks are distributed at random not only among cells, but also among chromosomes and even along the lengths of chromosomes. This, naturally, dictates the dose-effect kinetics for the various aberration types and, consequently, aberration yields per unit dose. Because most breaks induced by low-LET radiations are induced by separate ionizing events, breaks are statistically independent, or virtually so. Consequently, the yield of single-break aberrations increases as an approximately linear function of the dose. The yield of two-break aberrations, on the other hand, increases as a function of the square of the dose, and the yield of three-break aberrations as the third power of the dose, and so forth. It was, in fact, the observation of such dose-effect kinetics early in the study of chromosomal aberration production by radiation that established the independence of breaks induced by low-LET radiations and led to the "breakage-first" hypothesis.

Naturally, there are various factors that modify the shapes of aberration dose-effect curves somewhat from those expected strictly on the basis of statistical independence of breaks. Thus some fraction of what we score as deletions is actually the result of two separate ionizing events (for example, the fragment resulting from an incomplete asymmetrical exchange), and so the single-break aberration curves typically have some dose-square component. Also, two-break aberration curves tend to saturate at higher doses, probably because the number of chromosomes that can participate in exchanges is limited, so that a given set of data may better fit a function of somewhat less than the square of the dose, especially if high doses are used. Nevertheless, all the experience of classical radiation cytogenetics would lead one to expect that mammalian chromosome aberrations would display the same dose-effect kinetics found earlier in plant material.

Most observations have appeared to confirm these expectations for both chromatid and chromosome type aberrations in human and other mammalian cells (Bender, 1957; Bender and Gooch, 1961, 1962; Chu et al., 1961; Bell and Baker, 1962; Brewen, 1962, 1963; Gooch et al., 1964; Kelly and Brown, 1965; Norman and Sasaki, 1966; Brooks and Lengemann, 1967, 1968; Schmickel, 1967; Brewen and Brock, 1968). Recently, some doubt has arisen over whether the yields of rings and dicentrics in irradiated human peripheral lymphocytes really conform to the dose-square expectation. In a series of papers, Evans (1966, 1967 a, b, c, 1968) has reported that in vitro X-irradiation of human lymphocytes induces rings and dicentrics as a function of only approximately the 1.2 power of the dose. In other words, his dose-effect curve is virtually linear. Not only is such a finding in conflict with all of the observations of classical radiation cytogenetics, but it also conflicts with what was reported by earlier workers with the human lymphocyte system.

Evans has suggested that his kinetics are the "true" ones and that the dose-square kinetics observed by others were an artifact arising from the fact that they fixed their cells after a longer culture period than he did. Norman and Sasaki (1966), however, had actually fixed their cells even earlier than had Evans, and they found a strict dose-square dependence. Evans later suggested that the reason for the discrepancy between his data and those of other workers lay in his use of a special modification of the culture techniques used by others. Recently, though, we tested this idea by repeating Evans' experiments as precisely as possible, using his own culture technique (Bender and Barcinski, 1969), and we still got dose-square kinetics. And K.E. Buckton (personal communication) has also recently attempted to duplicate Evans' results, but again without success.

Similarly (quite possibly because of Evans' results), Buckton, Langlands and Smith have recently interpreted data, obtained from patients irradiated as palliation for advanced cancer, as evidence for a significantly less-than-dose-square relationship for rings and dicentrics induced in the lymphocyte system in vivo (Buckton, Langlands and Smith, 1967; Langlands et al., 1968). Unfortunately, however, their data points show considerable scatter and give little statistical justification for rejecting the dose-square hypothesis. Furthermore, it seems that the treatments their patients received were not uniformly distributed through their bodies and that this might have distorted the expected relationship between the two doses they used. It appears, then, that although Evans' reports have caused much controversy, there is really little reason to doubt the generality of the dose-square relationship, even for human lymphocytes.

One of the main practical reasons for studying chromosomal aberration production in mammalian cells is, of course, to obtain estimates of human radiosensitivity. It thus becomes important to know not only the shapes of the dose-effect curves but also their slopes, or what are known as the coefficients of aberration production. Clearly it is difficult to obtain such information directly on humans because of the lack of suitable irradiated subjects. The peripheral lymphocyte system has been used many times to make determinations of aberration yields in irradiated people. However, the lymphocyte system is sufficiently complicated that, to yield meaningful information, the subjects' irradiations must be acute, single, homogeneous, whole-body exposures, and the blood samples must be obtained promptly. These conditions have rarely been met. Of course, determinations of aberration coefficients could be made directly in solid tissues such as bone marrow, thus avoiding some of the requirements imposed by the peripheral lymphocyte system (though incidentally introducing other complications), but to my knowledge this has not yet been done. Two alternative approaches have been used.

First, one can make precise determinations with cells irradiated and allowed to enter cell division in vitro. This, however, always raises the question of possible in vivo-in vitro differences in response. Peripheral lymphocytes irradiated as freshly-drawn whole blood samples would seem to be the closest approach possible to working with cells in vivo, and this, indeed, is one reason so many experiments have been done with this sytem. Unfortunately, it has turned out that this system is much more complicated than was originally thought (Heddle et al., 1967; Bender and Brewen, 1969), and different laboratories have obtained somewhat different absolute values for the coefficients of aberration production. Under standardized conditions in a particular laboratory, however, the values are quite reproducible. A few very limited tests of the in vivo-in vitro question have thus been possible with the lymphocyte system. Sasaki et al. (1963) compared dicentric yields in two patients who had received acute, whole-body exposures with the yields predicted from their in vitro irradiations. The yield from neither patient was significantly different from the in vitro value, and furthermore the mean from the two patients was very close to the predicted value.

In later observations our group had the opportunity to compare the yields of aberrations in lymphocyte samples from men exposed in several radiation accidents with the yields predicted from coefficients of aberration production derived from in vitro experiments (Bender and Gooch, 1966; Bender, 1969). Although the doses the men received were low and the aberration yield consequently not very high, and in spite of complicating factors such as the fact that some of the men had been exposed to a mixture of γ rays and neutrons, the agreement between the observed and the predicted values was quite reasonable.

Sharpe et al. (1967, 1968) recently made another comparison that tends to give one confidence in the validity of in vitro-in vivo extrapolations. They compared the prompt dicentric yields in lymphocytes of two patients receiving extracorporeal irradiation of their blood with the yields predicted by determinations on cells from blood irradiated as isolated samples in vitro. Although in one case the yield from the extracorporeal irradiation appeared somewhat low, in the other case the agreement between the extracorporeal and the in vitro samples was very good.

A second, more indirect approach to the problem of estimating human chromosomal radiosensitivity is to use other mammals as surrogates in irradiation experiments. In this way, actual in vivo experiments can be done, but naturally the question of possible inter-species differences in radiosensitivity is raised. This question can, though, be attacked experimentally, if only indirectly. Some predictions from classical radiation cytogenetics are pertinent to such inter-species comparisons. The yields of various classes of aberrations are expected to vary from species to species as a function of differences in karyotype even if primary breakage rates, repair rates, and recombination probabilities are the same. If, for example, the total effective chromosome length in a diploid cell is different in two species, we should expect fewer breaks in the species with the lower total, simply because there is less chromosome length to be "hit". Also, even if the total length is the same, the chromosome number should have an effect on the number of interchange aberrations that result. To carry this to a ridiculous extreme, just consider the case of a species with only one chromosome! Similarly, one would anticipate that the centromere positions of the chromosomes would affect the yields of inter-arm intrachanges. One would expect, for example, that centric ring formation would be very unlikely in a species that had all acrocentric or telocentric chromosomes, such as the mouse.

In an early attempt to test the validity of inter-species extrapolations, we measured aberration yields in irradiated diploid spider monkey and human-kidney tissue cultures (Bender, 1957, 1960). Although in such a tissue culture system one is working mainly with chromatid-type aberrations and, thus, variations in yield with small changes in time between irradiation and fixation of the cells (stage sensitivity effect) are a real problem, the human and the monkey cells gave almost exactly the same aberration yields. As a further portion of a sort of "round-robin" validation of extrapolations from monkeys irradiated in vivo to human chromosomal radiosensitivity, we also irradiated the legs of spider monkeys and determined chromatid aberration frequencies in femoral bone marrow cells. The aberration yields are somewhat lower than those from the kidney cultures, but this was almost certainly due to the difficulty of selecting comparable post-irradiation sampling times (in terms of cell cycle time, not clock time) for the two test systems; in any case, these limited experiments failed to demonstrate any very large in vivo-in vitro or inter-species differences.

When the peripheral lymphocyte technique became available, we made the same inter-species comparison for this system (M.A. Bender and P.E. Eide, unpublished data). Only a limited number of samples were tested, but the agreement between the aberration yields in the blood from the two species irradiated in vitro was fairly good, although, as might be expected from the difference in chromosome number (the spider monkey has only 34 chromosomes), the dicentric yields in the monkey samples tended to be somewhat lower than those in the human samples. Again, in a limited attempt to test the validity of the in vivo-in vitro extrapolation, we also exposed some monkeys to whole-body γ irradiation and then determined aberration frequencies in peripheral lymphocyte samples. Although only a few animals were done, the agreement between the in vivo- and the in vitro-irradiated samples was reasonably good.

A.F. McFee (personal communication) is carrying out an in vivo-in vitro comparison with the peripheral lymphocytes of pigs, which have a diploid chromosome number of 38. The animals were given whole-body irradiation with γ rays and the aberration yields compared with those from simultaneously irradiated whole blood samples from the same animals. Although the data are not yet complete, there does not appear to be any significant difference between the yields of either single- or multiple-break aberrations obtained in vivo and in vitro. Preliminary calculations give a coefficient of deletion production of about 1×10^{-3} per cell per rad, very close to that observed in our laboratory under comparable conditions (Bender and Barcinski, 1969; Bender and Brewen, 1969). However, the coefficient of ring and dicentric production in the pig appears to be much lower than that for humans. A rough calculation from McFee's data yields an estimate of only 1.6×10^{-6} per cell per rad^2, whereas comparable estimates for human cells range from about 6 to about 12×10^{-6} per cell per rad^2 (Gooch et al., 1964; Norman and Sasaki, 1966; Bender and Barcinski, 1969; Bender and Brewen, 1969).

Brewen and Brock (1968) recently reported data on chromosome aberration frequencies in in vitro-irradiated peripheral lymphocytes from yet another species, *Wallabia bicolor*. This animal has the rather low diploid chromosome numbers of 10 and 11 (there is an X, Y_1, Y_2 sex-determining mechanism). In contrast to the situation in human and apparently monkey and pig lymphocytes, where terminal deletions display only moderately non-linear dose-effect kinetics, terminal deletions in the wallaby were found to display virtually dose-square kinetics. This makes comparisons difficult. Yet the species are certainly not too different in sensitivity, as shown by comparable yields resulting from doses of 150-300 rads. The coefficient of ring and dicentric production, however, is clearly much lower in the wallaby. Brewen and Brock obtained a best-fit value of about 2.9×10^{-6} per cell per rad^2 which, while higher than that from McFee's data for the pig, is no more than half the lowest estimates for humans.

We can only speculate on the reasons for this inter-species difference. As already mentioned, one expects chromosome number, and probably also the relative proportions of acrocentric, submetacentric, and metacentric chromosomes in the karyotype to influence two-break aberration yields. It seems possible that this may account for the differences, but it is also possible that there is some basic difference in, for example, the probability of recombination in different species of mammals.

Another question that arises in making such comparisons is whether there are differences in chromosomal radiosensitivity between different tissues within the same animal. I have already mentioned our very limited data on spider-monkey bone marrow and peripheral lymphocytes. Only one such comparison has been attempted in man. De Grouchy (de Grouchy, Vallee and Lamy, 1963; de Grouchy, Vallee, Nava and Lamy, 1963) has made a comparison between chromosomal aberration yields in human bone marrow cells and peripheral lymphocytes, both irradiated in vitro. He found that the yields were slightly higher in the bone marrow cells, but the difference, if real, is at best small.

Chromatid type aberration frequencies have been measured in a number of different tissues of the Chinese hamster following in vivo irradiation. We measured aberration frequencies in the bone marrow (Bender and Gooch, 1961) and found coefficients of deletion (chromatid and isochromatid) production of about 5×10^{-3} per cell per rad two hours after irradiation and about 2×10^{-3} per cell per rad six hours after irradiation. Very few exchange aberrations were seen, and no meaningful coefficient can be calculated.

Brewen (1962, 1963) measured chromatid aberration frequencies in the corneal epithelium of the Chinese hamster. At a dose rate comparable to that used in our bone marrow experiments and fixing the cells after six hours, he found a coefficient of about 1.7×10^{-3} per cell per R for deletions. Rather few exchanges were induced, and calculation of a coefficient of exchange production is probably not very meaningful. These results are certainly not very different from the bone marrow results.

Brooks and Lengemann (1967, 1968) have recently made more extensive comparisons between chromatid aberration rates in bone marrow and in spermatogonia of γ-irradiated Chinese hamsters. In experiments with cells fixed six hours after irradiation, they obtained coefficients of deletion production of 1.5×10^{-3} per cell per R for bone marrow and 4.1×10^{-3} per cell per R for spermatogonia. The bone marrow value is the same as we obtained for hamster bone marrow at this fixation time, but the spermatogonial value is clearly much higher. In more extensive time-series experiments Brooks and Lengemann confirmed this difference in sensitivity and concluded that the breakage rate in the spermatogonia must be at least twice that found in the bone marrow. Their data on chromatid exchanges also support this idea. Exchanges were not frequent in bone marrow cells, in agreement with our bone marrow data and Brewen's corneal epithelium data, but, in contrast, the frequencies were fairly high in the spermatogonia, yielding a coefficient of about 1.6×10^{-5} per cell per R^2.

So far I have only considered the case of acute exposures to low-LET radiation. Data from classical radiation cytogenetic studies allow us to predict that a change to high-LET radiation or a change from acute single exposures to fractionated or low dose rate exposures would affect aberration yields. The approximately dose-square kinetics we have discussed for two-break aberrations are predicted because the breaks caused by low-LET radiation are usually the result of separate ionizing events. With high-LET radiation such as fission neutrons or α particles, however, one does not expect the breaks to be statistically independent because the particles lose energy very rapidly and a cell, if it is "hit" at all, is quite likely to sustain many chromosomal breaks. We thus expect multiple break aberration yields resulting from irradiation with these particles to be a function of the first, rather than higher powers of dose.

Experiments with human peripheral lymphocytes irradiated with neutrons of fission spectrum and somewhat higher energies in vitro have generally confirmed this expectation for mammalian cells (Gooch et al., 1964; Bender and Gooch, 1966; Scott et al., 1967). One would also expect that neutrons would be more efficient on an absorbed energy basis than X or γ rays; that is, the R.B.E. for neutrons should be greater than one. This expectation was also confirmed. For human lymphocytes the R.B.E. for deletions appears to be about 5; no simple value can be stated for exchange aberrations, because of the change in kinetics.

With dose protraction or fractionation the curves for multiple-break aberrations are non-linear. The breaks induced by radiation have short lifetimes during which they remain able to interact with other breaks, so that some time after their induction (usually a matter of a few hours) they cease to be available for recombination. Thus, if two doses are separated by an interval of many hours, those breaks induced by the first dose have no opportunity to interact with those induced by the second dose, and the yields are accordingly much lower (to be precise, they would be the sum of the dose-square function of each of the two half-doses, instead of a function of the square of the whole dose). To carry this to its extreme, one would expect an exposure at a sufficiently low dose rate to yield virtually no multiple-break aberrations.

There are only a few pertinent observations on mammalian cells. These confirm the expectations regarding multiple-break aberrations and also provide some new insight into the nature of single-break aberrations. Nowell and Cole (1963) demonstrated a dose rate effect for multiple-break aberrations induced in mice; though they apparently did not expect this effect, it is of course exactly what prior experience predicts. Scott et al. (1967) looked for but, as expected, did not find a dose rate effect in neutron-irradiated human lymphocytes.

Brewen (1963) looked for and successfully demonstrated a small dose rate effect on chromatid deletions in the corneal epithelium of the Chinese hamster. This, of course, was not to be expected on the basis of strictly linear (i.e. strictly "one-hit") dose effect kinetics. On the basis of experiments with an inhibitor of protein synthesis, Brewen concluded that this effect was the result of an influence of dose rate on the chromosomal rejoining system, rather than on primary breakage.

As already mentioned, Brewen and Brock (1968) found a very large dose-square component in the dose-effect curve for terminal deletions induced by γ rays in wallaby lymphocytes. In fractionation experiments they demonstrated a dose fractionation effect on the yields of these aberrations and, not surprisingly, on ring and dicentric yields. They postulate that a large fraction of what are scored as terminal deletions in the wallaby are actually the result of incomplete asymmetrical exchanges. Some degree of incompleteness in the formation of exchange aberrations probably accounts for the observed non-linearity of chromosome deletion dose-effect curves in human lymphocytes. One might anticipate a dose rate effect there, too, but this has not yet been demonstrated.

Summary

I have tried to point out how classical radiation cytogenetics actually predicts most of the phenomena observed in the study of chromosomal aberrations induced in mammalian cells. Most of the observations that have been made in mammalian radiation cytogenetics have simply confirmed these expectations. There are a few areas, however, in which unexpected results have been reported. The virtually linear dose-effect curves reported by Evans for two-break aberrations induced by X-irradiation of human lymphocytes are a particularly important case. Although other workers have not been able to demonstrate such kinetics, Evans' result would have important consequences for our thinking about human radiation hazards, especially with regard to chronic exposures, should they be confirmed. Similarly, the demonstrations of Brewen and of Brewen and Brock of dose-rate effects for deletions force us to revise our predictions regarding the importance of chronic exposures. Another important result is Brooks and Lengemann's demonstration of the significantly greater radiosensitivity of Chinese hamster spermatogonia than of somatic cells in the same species. If this turns out to be a general phenomenon, it will certainly have an extremely great influence on our thinking about radiation hazards. It thus strikes me as the most urgent single area for future work in mammalian radiation cytogenetics.

References

Bell, A.G., and Baker, D.G. Irradiation-induced chromosome aberrations in normal human leukocytes in culture. Can. J. Genet. Cytol., 4, 340-351, 1962.

Bender, M.A. X-ray-induced chromosome aberrations in normal diploid human tissue cultures. Science, N.Y., 126, 974-975, 1957.

Bender, M.A. X-ray-induced chromosome aberrations in mammalian cells in vivo and in vitro. In Immediate and Low Level Effects of Ionizing Radiations, edited by A.A. Buzzati-Traverso, Taylor and Francis, London, pp. 103-118, 1960.

Bender, M.A. Human radiation cytogenetics. In Advances in Radiation Biology, Vol. III, edited by L. Augenstein, R. Mason and M. Zelle, Academic Press, New York, pp. 215-275, 1969.

Bender, M.A., and Barcinski, M.A. Kinetics of two-break aberration produced by X rays in human leukocytes. Cytogenetics 8, 241-246, 1969.

Bender, M.A., and Brewen, J.G. Factors influencing chromosome aberration yields in the human peripheral leukocyte system. Mutation Res. 8, 383-399, 1969.

Bender, M.A., and Gooch, P.C. Spontaneous and X-ray-induced somatic-chromosome aberrations in the Chinese hamster. Int. J. Radiat. Biol., 4, 175-184, 1961.

Bender, M.A., and Gooch, P.C. Types and rates of X-ray-induced chromosome aberrations in human blood irradiated in vitro. Proc. Natn. Acad. Sci., U.S.A., 48, 522-532, 1962.

Bender, M.A., and Gooch, P.C. Somatic chromosome aberrations induced by human whole-body irradiation: The "Recuplex" criticality accident. Radiat. Res., 29, 568-582, 1966.

Bloom, A.D., Neriishi, S., Kamada, N., Iseki, T., and R.J. Keehn. Cytogenetic investigation of survivors of the atomic bombings of Hiroshima and Nagasaki. Lancet, ii, 672-674, 1966.

Bloom, A.D., Neriishi, S., Awa, A.A., Honda, T., and Archer, P.G. Chromosome aberrations in leukocytes of older survivors of the atomic bombings of Hiroshima and Nagasaki. Lancet, ii, 802-805, 1967.

Brewen, J.G. X-ray-induced chromosome aberrations in the corneal epithelium of the Chinese hamster. Science, N.Y., 138, 820-822, 1962.

Brewen, J.G. Dependence of frequency of X-ray-induced chromosome aberrations on dose rate in the Chinese hamster. Proc. Natn. Acad. Sci., U.S.A., 50, 322-329, 1963.

Brewen, J.G., and Brock, R.D. The exchange hypothesis and chromosome-type aberrations. Mutation Res., 6, 245-255, 1968.

Brooks, A.L., and Lengemann, F.W. Comparison of radiation-induced aberrations in the testes and bone marrow of Chinese hamsters. Radiat. Res., 32, 587-595, 1967.

Brooks, A.L., and Lengemann, F.W. Determining the repair rate for radiation-induced chromatid deletions during the first 24 hours after irradiation. Radiat. Res., 36, 181-192, 1968.

Buckton, K.E., Jacobs, P.A., Court Brown, W.M., and Doll, R. A study of the chromosome damage persisting after X-ray therapy for ankylosing spondylitis. Lancet, ii, 676-682, 1962.

Buckton, K.E., Court Brown, W.M., and Smith, P.G. Lymphocyte survival in men treated with X rays for ankylosing spondylitis. Nature, Lond., 214, 470–473, 1967.

Buckton, K.E., Langlands, A.O., and Smith, P.G. Chromosome aberrations following partial- and whole-body X irradiation in man. Dose response relationships. In Human Radiation Cytogenetics, edited by H.J. Evans, W.M. Court Brown and A.S. McLean, North-Holland Publishing Company, Amsterdam, pp. 122-135, 1967.

Chu, E.H.Y., Giles, N.H., and Passano, K. Types and frequencies of human chromosome aberrations induced by X rays. Proc. Natn. Acad. Sci., U.S.A., 47, 830-839, 1961.

Court Brown, W.M., Buckton, K.E., and McLean, A.S. Quantitative studies of chromosome aberrations in man following acute and chronic exposure to X rays and gamma rays. Lancet, i, 1239-1241, 1965.

Court Brown, W.M., Buckton, K.E., and Langlands, A.O. The identification of lymphocyte clones, with chromosome structural aberrations, in irradiated men and women. Int. J. Radiat. Biol., 13, 155-168, 1967.

Curtis, H.J. Biological mechanisms underlying the aging process. Science, N.Y., 141, 686-694, 1963.

Evans, H.J. Repair and recovery from chromosome damage after fractionated X-ray dosage. In Genetical Aspects of Radiosensitivity: Mechanism of Repair, International Atomic Energy Agency, Vienna, pp. 31-48, 1966.

Evans, H.J. Repair and recovery from chromosome damage induced by fractionated X-ray exposures. Radiation Research, 1966, North-Holland Publishing Co., Amsterdam, pp. 482-501, 1967a.

Evans, H.J. Dose-response relations from in vitro studies. In Human Radiation Cytogenetics, edited by H.J. Evans, W.M. Court Brown and A.S. McLean, North-Holland Publishing Co., Amsterdam, pp. 20-36, 1967b.

Evans, H.J. Actions of radiations on chromosomes. The Scientific Bases of Medicine Annual Reviews, Athlone Press, London, pp. 321-339, 1967c.

Evans, H.J. The response of human chromosomes to ionizing radiations: in vitro. Proc. R. Soc. Edinb., B, 70, 132-151, 1968.

Ford, C.E., Ilbery, P.L.T., and Loutit, J.F. Further cytological observations on radiation chimeras. J. cell. comp. Physiol., (Suppl. 1) 50, 109-121, 1957.

Goh, K.-O. Total-body irradiation in human chromosomes. Cytogenetic studies of the peripheral blood and bone marrow leukocytes seven years after total-body irradiation. Radiat. Res., 35, 155-170, 1968.

Gooch, P.C., Bender, M.A., and Randolph, M.L. Chromosome aberrations induced in human somatic cells by neutrons. Biological Effects of Neutron and Proton Irradiation, Vol. I, International Atomic Energy Agency, Vienna, pp. 325-342, 1964.

Grouchy, J. de, Vallee, G., and Lamy, M. Analyse chromosomique de cellules humaines sanguines et médullaires après irradiation in vitro. C. r. Seanc. Soc. Biol., 257, 278-281, 1963.

Grouchy, J. de, Vallee, G., Nava, C., and Lamy, M. Analyse chromosomique de cellules cancereuses et de cellules médullaires et sanguines iradiées in vitro. Ann. Genet., 6, 9-20, 1963.

Heddle, J.A., Evans, H.J., and Scott, D. Sampling time and the complexity of the human leukocyte culture system. In Human Radiation Cytogenetics, edited by H.J. Evans, W.M. Court Brown and A.S. McLean, North-Holland Publishing Co., Amsterdam, pp. 6-19, 1967.

Kelly, S., and Brown, C.D. Chromosome aberrations as a biological dosimeter. Am. J. Publ. Hlth, 55, 1419-1429, 1965.

Langlands, A.O., Smith, P.G., Buckton, K.E., Woodcock, G.E., and McLelland, J. Chromosome damage induced by radiation. Nature, Lond., 218, 1133-1135, 1968.

Norman, A., and Sasaki, M.S. Chromosome-exchange aberrations in human lymphocytes. Int. J. Radiat. Biol., 11, 321-328, 1966.

Norman, A., Sasaki, M.S., Ottoman, R.E., and Fingerhut, A. Lymphocyte lifetime in women. Science, Lond., 147, 745, 1965.

Norman, A., Sasaki, M.S., Ottoman, R.E., and Fingerhut, A. Elimination of chromosome aberrations from human lymphocytes. Blood, 27, 706-714, 1966.

Nowell, P.C. Unstable chromosome changes in tuberculin-stimulated leukocyte cultures from irradiated patients. Blood, 26, 798-804, 1965.

Nowell, P.C. Chromosome aberrations and immunological memory. In Human Radiation Cytogenetics, edited by H.J. Evans, W.M. Court Brown and A.S. McLean, North-Holland Publishing Co., Amsterdam, pp. 99-105, 1967.

Nowell, P.C., and Cole, L.J. Reduced incidence of persistent chromosome aberrations in mice irradiated at low dose rates. Science, N.Y., 141, 524-526, 1963.

Puck, T.T. Action of radiation on mammalian cells. III. Relationship between reproductive death and induction of chromosome anomalies by X-irradiation of euploid human cells in vitro. Proc. Natn. Acad. Sci., U.S.A., 44, 772-780, 1958.

Revell, S.H. The accurate estimation of chromatid aberrations induced by ionizing radiation. Proc. R. Soc., B, 150, 562-589, 1959.

Sasaki, M.S., and Norman, Amos. Selection against chromosome aberrations in human lymphocytes. Nature, Lond., 214, 502-503, 1967.

Sasaki, M., Ottoman, R.E., and Norman, A. Radiation-induced chromosome aberrations in man. Radiology, 81, 652-656, 1963.

Sax, K. Chromosome aberrations induced by X rays. Genetics, 23, 494-516, 1938.

Schmickel, R. Chromosome aberrations in leukocytes exposed in vitro to diagnostic levels of X rays. Am. J. human Genet., 19, 1-11, 1967.

Scott, D., Sharpe, H.B.A., Batchelor, A.L., and Evans, H.J. RBE for fast neutrons and dose rate studies using fast neutron irradiation. In Human Radiation Cytogenetics, edited by H.J. Evans, W.M. Court Brown and A.S. McLean, North-Holland Publishing Co., Amsterdam, pp. 37-53, 1967.

Sharpe, H.B.A., Dolphin, G.W., Dawson, K.B., and Field, E.O. Chromosomal aberration in lymphocytes from an extracorporeally irradiated patient. Lancet, ii, 1338-1339, 1967.

Sharpe, H.B.A., Dolphin, G.W., Dawson, K.B., and Field, E.O. Methods of computing lymphocyte kinetics in man by analysis of chromosomal aberrations sustained during extracorporeal irradiation of the blood. Cell Tissue Kinetics, 1, 263-271, 1968

Stadler, L.J. The experimental modification of heredity in crop plants, I. Induced chromosomal irregularities. Sci. Agr., 11, 557-572, 1931.

Weber, W.T., and Nowell, P.C. Studies on long-lived small lymphocytes in the Rhesus monkey and some other mammals. J. Reticuloendothelial Soc., 2, 326-342, 1965.

CHAPTER VII

POPULATION GENETICS AFTER RADIATION EXPOSURE IN MAN

William J. Schull

Mutations induced as a consequence of exposure to ionizing radiation are linearly related to dose and dependent upon the intensity of the irradiation. These two assertions are the cornerstones of the current dogma which describes the effects on mammals of exposure to irradiation. To them may be added, somewhat tentatively, a third, namely, that the yield in mutations is inversely related to ionizing density. The latter is known to be true for *Drosophila melanogaster*, but has not been adequately documented in vertebrates. Mutations, induced or spontaneous, are deleterious in the main; this belief rests partially upon experimental evidence and partially upon the supposition that in an already highly adapted organism, a product of prolonged evolution, random changes will rarely improve adaptation. The evidence which supports the dogma is so extensive and involves such disparate levels of cellular and organismal complexity (viruses, bacteria, flies, and the mouse) that it has been generally accepted that human beings, more properly human genes will behave in a qualitatively similar, albeit possibly quantitatively different manner. I should like to emphasize at this point that as yet the applicability of the dogma to man is, *in sensu stricto*, a conjecture, though a sound one; otherwise stated, on the evidence from man alone, it would be foolhardy scientifically to maintain that ionizing radiation is mutagenic. But, as previously stated, the evidence on infra-human forms is so voluminous that the burden of proof rests on him who would believe otherwise with respect to man.

If the applicability of the dogma to man is accepted, as I believe it should be, two problems confront radiation geneticists, namely, (1) to produce the best possible estimate (or estimates) of the increased probability of a mutation per locus per generation per roentgen or some other suitable physical constant, and (2) to measure the fate of induced mutations in natural populations, that is, to assay the impact upon a human population of the burden of disease and disability accruing from increasing exposure to ionizing radiation. Let us consider the first of these two problems and the one to which I will address most of my time.

Efforts to estimate the radiation sensitivity of human genes can, in theory, proceed in either of two ways. One can undertake to estimate the mutability resident in specific, previously designated, and presumably representative genetic loci. This has been termed the specific locus approach, and it has been widely used in *Drosophila* and the house mouse. Alternatively, one might attempt to determine the increase in frequency per unit dose of certain common attributes which, though possibly not wholly genetic in origin, have a substantial genetic component. Though the former alternative is genetically more appealing, the latter, the so-called "population characteristics" approach, has been the more common in man. This reflects the general belief that successful implementation of the specific locus approach involves children in numbers that are unobtainable; somewhat later we shall examine whether this belief is justified in view of recent, technological innovations.

The possible observable genetic effects of irradiation upon the first generation born after exposure to ionizing radiation or, if you will, the choices of "population characteristics" to be measured, are many and varied. These include changes in the sex ratio, an increase in the frequency of stillbirths, an increase in the frequency of congenital malformations, an increase in infant mortality, and in growth and development, mental as well as physical. Each of these possible indicators of genetic damage is also influenced by a number of other factors, generally environmental; there are no known unique yardsticks of genetic damage. Clearly, under these circumstances, selection of the control, or better the comparison material is especially critical. Unfortunately, selection of this latter material seems often to have been perfunctory, or at least poorly thought out.

All of the studies to date on man's genetic radiosensitivity incorporate an element of opportunism in the choice of the irradiated as well as the comparison group, and as a consequence vary greatly from one to another in a variety of respects. The samples range from several individuals to tens of thousands, and doses have varied from one or two to over a thousand roentgens above background. Data have been collected on chronic low levels as well as acute episodes of exposure. Observations have been obtained by skilled observers, on the one hand, and, on the other, through questionnaires completed by the recipients. Few of the populations which have been studied can be viewed as "normal". Most groups were irradiated for some underlying disease, the effects of which may have been confounded with the radiation damage. Furthermore, since, as previously stated, no single genetic metric of radiation damage is known, the contribution that a study makes to the ultimate resolution of the problem under discussion is directly proportional to the success with which that study has been able to control the effects of concomitant variation on the "experimental" variables, either through the choice of the comparison population or through appropriate statistical techniques. Few, if any, studies can claim to have removed all extraneous variation.

Of the dozen or so investigative efforts which have been published, that of the Atomic Bomb Casualty Commission (ABCC) remains unique in the number and scope of its observations (Neel and Schull, 1956). Since this study embraces the bulk of the observations presently available on man, and since it continues, incidentally, now in its twenty-first year, a brief look at the genetics programme of the ABCC seems warranted. It consists of three distinct phases or types of activities. The first of these, a clinical phase, concerns some 75,000 children who were born and examined, on more than one occasion in many instances, in Hiroshima or Nagasaki in the years 1948-1953. This aspect of the programme terminated in March 1954; with its termination emphasis shifted to an increased use of routine vital observations and the collating and colligating of these observations with ABCC's exposure records. Two somewhat different studies were begun during this second, vital statistical phase. One of these is directed toward the continuing collection of information on the sex ratio, and utilizes the records of births in Hiroshima and Nagasaki to those individuals who comprise ABCC's Master Sample of irradiated persons. The second one consists of a cohort of 54,000 children born in one or the other of these cities in the years 1946-1958 whose mortality experiences are under scrutiny. Here, the koseki, the household censuses required by law since 1871, are the crucial governmental records. All vital events which affect the composition of a family must be duly recorded in the koseki of which that family is a part. It is thus possible through periodic examination of the 54,000 koseki in which these children are recorded to determine their life status at any particular time. The third and most recent phase, one on which Dr. Arthur Bloom will enlarge, involves cytogenetic studies of a subset of children, the so-called F_1.

The findings of the clinical phase have been summarized elsewhere as follows (Nee and Schull, 1956):

1. "No significant effect of either mother's or father's exposure on the

frequency of congenital malformations." In this context, the word "malformation" is used to describe those individuals with conspicuous departures from normality which are either incompatible with life, life threatening, or seriously impinge upon one's ability to perform effectively in the society of which he or she is a member. It is further assumed that these departures are readily recognized in a new-born infant without special diagnostic procedures. As so defined, one would expect, as a rule of thumb, that approximately one pregnancy in every 100 persisting for at least seven months of gestation would terminate in a child that was malformed.

2. "No consistent effect of either maternal or paternal exposure on the frequency of stillbirths."

3. "Both with and without allowance for differences in parity among the mothers falling into the various radiation categories, there is no significant effect of mother's exposure or father's exposure on the frequency of neonatal deaths."

4. "When allowances are made for differences between exposure cells in maternal age and parity, there exists no significant difference between classes of father's exposure or classes of mother's exposure in mean birth weight. Furthermore, it was not possible to demonstrate a consistent effect of parental exposure on (a) the relationship between birth weight and concomitant variables, notably maternal age or parity, and finally, (b) the residual birth weight variances following removal of maternal age and parity effects are not significantly different one from another."

5. "Neither the generalized means nor the generalized variances of a series of four anthropometric yardsticks of physical growth and development can be shown to differ among classes of paternal or maternal exposure."

Insofar as the effect of radiation upon quantitative characteristics of man is concerned, two observations from other animals seem pertinent. First, the large study of the effect of radiation upon swine at Iowa State University has failed to disclose a significant effect of paternal exposure upon birth weight (Cox, 1968). Second, there are the results of a rather ingenious experiment performed at the Institute of Animal Genetics in Edinburgh (Clayton and Robertson, 1964). The latter experiment concerns the continuing exposure of two populations of Drosophila melanogaster, and the effect of this continuing exposure upon two quantitative characteristics, namely, the sternital and the sternal pleural bristles, both yardsticks commonly used by the quantitative geneticist who works with Drosophila. Two different populations, as I have stated, were used. In one, the flies had been inbred until all members of the population were homozygous or nearly so. The second consisted of a population which had plateaued following selection, that is to say, a population in which further selection failed to diminish variability. Two questions were asked, namely, how much irradiation would be necessary to restore to the plateaued population the same variability that it had initially, i.e. before selection, or to the inbred population the same amount of variability that one would anticipate in a normal, outbred population? The rate of change in the variance was found to be about 10^{-5} variance units per roentgen. Alternatively stated, it took a half million roentgens to restore to these populations their original, known variability. This may very well account for why we find no effect at the quantitative level in man; inordinately large amounts of radiation are required to produce a detectable effect.

The observations on man enumerated above admit of certain dose-effect conjectures. Before I go into these, however, several reservations should be noted. First, the exposures of most of the parents whom we have just cited were not precisely known at the time of the clinical study, nor for that matter, are most of them precisely known now. The estimates which we have are fairly gross, and may differ from the true exposures by as much as a factor of two. Second, to ease the arithmetic, a number of assumptions are made such as linearity of effect, additivity of paternal and maternal exposure, equal attenuation factors in the sexes, etc. which are known not to apply in some instances and may not be satisfied in others as well.

Against this background, it may be observed that malformations could have been increased by as much as 1% (absolute) per 100 reps and pass undetected under the conditions of the study. Stillbirths could be increased by about 1.3% absolute per 100 reps, and neonatal deaths by a similar value. Thus, 100 reps would closely approximate the "doubling dose" of all three of these metrics of genetic damage. I hasten to add that no one of these events is solely genetic, but if we presume that all of the increase really is resident in that component which is genetic, then the amount of radiation necessary to double the genetic component would clearly be less.

These estimates, it must be emphasized, are based upon the maximum differences which might pass undetected under the circumstances of the study that ABCC conducted in a comparison of two groups of parents, i.e. one where both were exposed, and the other where neither was exposed. Alternatively put, these estimates stem from considerations of the confidence limits to be placed upon the studies in Hiroshima and Nagasaki and are not regression coefficients obtained directly from the data. The latter are somewhat smaller than the values I have just cited.

Let us return now to the ABCC studies enumerated earlier, and more specifically to mortality in the F_1 cohort. Mortality experiences in this group have thus far been assayed only once. At that time, all deaths of members of the cohorts prior to 1 January 1961, were recorded. The average number of years of risk of death was nine, but varied from 3 to 15 years.

The cohort itself can be divided into three subgroups on the basis of parental exposure (a high exposure dose group, a low exposure dose group, and an unexposed group). Comparison of these groups failed to disclose significant differences either in age specific death rates (based upon all causes of death) or in cause specific death rates including leukaemia (Kato et al., 1966).

Again, an estimate of the dose-effect relationship along lines previously described is possible. Since the cohort is adequate to detect a 10% deviation from the standard, i.e. the death rate in the comparison cohort, and since the mean total parental dose in the "heavily exposed" group is less than 200 rads, one is led to an upper estimate of a 5% increase in mortality per 100 rads, and by some further calculation to a doubling dose of the order of 100 roentgens.

Finally, the sex ratio studies. As most of you are aware, much of the data on the effect of ionizing radiation on the sex ratio was collected prior to the recognition that chromosomal abnormalities exist which give rise to individuals whose sex can be misclassified, an error which presumably would lead to an erroneous sex ratio.

These karyotypic abnormalities themselves are, moreover, probably dose dependent. At least, we have known for more than 40 years that nondisjunction increases in frequency in Drosophila as a function of the irradiation of the parent.

The earlier data, that is those collected before the present explosion in human cytogenetic information, were interpreted in a more simplistic frame of reference than would now be acceptable, one which held that the sex ratio should diminish with increasing maternal exposure, and increase with increasing paternal exposure.

If both parents were exposed, it was presumed that the sex ratio would reflect additively the conjoint parental exposures.

It was further believed that one might estimate the probability of inducing a sex-linked lethal mutant per unit exposure more or less directly from the observed changes in the sex ratio with changing dose. We have estimated, for example, the yield in sex-linked lethal mutations to be approximately 1% per 100 rads (Schull and Neel, 1958). The latter value, although it is an order of magnitude greater than the comparable figures for Drosophila, seemed reasonable at the time, for it was consonant with the then new evidence that specific locus mutation rates in the mouse were an order of magnitude greater than those in Drosophila.

While arguments can be adduced which lead to the conclusion that the loss or gain of sex chromosomes which one associates with Turner's and Klinefelter's syndromes should not alter the direction of the deviations stated above, the very existence of these chromosomal abnormalities does compromose the interpretation of a given set of data.

This state of affairs will undoubtedly persist until such time as either the genic or the chromosomal contribution to sex ratio changes can be separately estimated. The only substantial effort of which I am aware to relate abnormalities of the sex chromosomes to ionizing radiation faltered on technical and statistical difficulties. This was a study of buccal smears of Hiroshima school-children undertaken some years ago.

Time has created another difficulty in the interpretation of sex ratio changes in the Japanese data which arises as follows: Data on the sex ratio in Hiroshima and Nagasaki collected in the years 1948 through 1953, i.e. through the clinical phase, were generally consistent in suggesting small, but seemingly "reasonable" changes in the sex ratio of the nature previously indicated. Unfortunately, few of the some twelve estimates of the dose-effect response possible were significantly different from zero. Since the sex ratio is an unsatisfactory variable from a number of points of view, the temptation to collect further data was irresistible, but in retrospect, regrettable.

Observations collected in the years 1956 through 1962 were analysed and described in 1966 (Schull et al., 1966). These latter data did not bear out in any of the particulars the earlier findings. Two interpretations are obviously possible. One is, of course, that the earlier findings were fortuitous and had no biological meaning. The other is that the small earlier effects were real but have disappeared, or somewhat differently stated, the later observations are not in pari materia with those from 1948 to 1955.

Some experimental support exists for this notion. Russell, in 1965, for example, has presented fairly extensive evidence on the house mouse which suggests that the yield in mutations, following an exposure experience, may diminish with time either as a consequence of the repair of certain mutations, of cell selection, or both . It is conceivable, therefore, that the number of potentially recoverable sex-linked mutations in Hiroshima and Nagasaki has actually diminished with time, whether this is or is not so is admittedly moot; however, the ambiguity in the present status of the sex ratio should be apparent to every one.

To some my disregard of other studies in the literature of the genetic effects of ionizing radiations will appear cavalier, to say the least. There are, however, numerous reviews of these studies, and little is served by still another review. Of greater importance, it seemed, was an attempt to come to grips with the issue of "where do we go from here?" The Japanese study is, in this context, an illustration, and I believe a particularly good one of past efforts. But at this juncture we should ask ourselves, "What is to be learned from the studies in Japan and elsewhere which is relevant to future investigations?" The lessons are numerous.

Firstly, we should clearly look askance at those small studies involving at most a few hundred children which report significant differences, and particularly those where parental exposures are 5 to 10 roentgens, as appears so frequently the case. Dose-effect extrapolations from these studies are incompatible with most other radio-genetic information. To put it another way, these findings usually cannot pass a test of "reasonableness" when the observed effect is placed upon a unit dose basis.

Secondly, it should be recognized that we should not dissipate our funds and energies on studies so small that on prior grounds alone it is apparent that they will add little to our accumulated fund of information. Ludicrous as it may seem, there are reports in the literature where the number of authors exceeds the number of children or pregnancies studied. The numbers required to detect effects of the order of magnitude which are reasonable are large. For example, the number of observations required to compare two proportions, a "standard" and an "experimental", if it is assumed that Type I errors will occur five times in 100 judgments and Type II errors one in ten, is about 20,000 (equally divided between "standard" and "experimental" populations) if one expects to demonstrate a doubling in an event with a frequency of approximately 1%.

Thirdly, there is patently merit to studies on as broad a scope as possible; i.e. which embrace as many "population characteristics", as one can conveniently measure.

Finally, greater attention should obviously be paid to the use of cohorts than has been in the past, where these cohorts are examined repeatedly in time. Only in this manner is it likely that the accumulated impact of induced mutations upon a population will be adequately assayed.

The remarks which I have just made assume tacitly that studies of "population characteristics" will continue. Clearly, however, we should ask ourselves whether there are other alternatives, and it is to some of these that we now turn.

In the long haul, all of us presumably hope that at least as much information on the mutability of human genes will exist as now exists for *Drosophila* and the mouse. At the moment, one can hardly hazard a guess as to when this might possibly be true, but in the meantime, decisions which profoundly affect man's corporate genetic structure must and will be made. The more immediate task, therefore, is to enhance the value of the experimental evidence in its applicability to man through the establishment of "benchmarks" which will permit more meaningful extrapolations. The easiest possible means whereby these benchmarks may be achieved is through greater efforts to delineate the kinds and frequencies of chromosomal abnormalities which are to be seen in the first generation offspring of individuals exposed to ionizing radiation.

Again two sorts of studies suggest themselves. The most appealing one involves careful cytogenetic examinations of the tissues of such offspring; in most instances, this will undoubtedly involve short-term culture of peripheral leukocytes, but may on occasion involve other tissues, skin, for example. As stated earlier, the ABCC is already engaged in studies of this kind, and Dr. Bloom will, I am sure, describe their present status. Undertakings of this variety are costly and time-consuming, and this seems likely to continue to be so until some degree of automation of the techniques necessary is feasible. This may be near at hand, fortunately.

The second study that one might anticipate utilizes phenotypes known to be the result of chromosomal abnormalities, and relates the frequencies of these phenotypes to ionizing radiation. Such phenotypes would, of course, include Down's, Klinefelter's, and Turner's syndromes and possibly even Trisomy-D.

Cytogenetic observations need not necessarily be part of such a study, and it might be argued that an investment of an equivalent time in dose estimates would ultimately be more rewarding. Again, emphasis should be upon the best unbiased estimate of dose-effect rather than upon a test of significance. A number of studies of this latter variety do, of course, exist. The results are, however, inconsistent and often frankly contradictory. But let us turn to another kind of study which may now be feasible.

As previously stated, there has been as yet no large-scale effort to relate ionizing radiation to mutation at specific genetic loci in man despite the success of this approach in other animals. Objections to this tack have rested largely on estimates of its feasibility. The time may now be ripe, however, for such studies; an argument in support of this position might proceed somewhat as follows: we begin with the premise that the study under discussion will be, in essence, an attempt to measure inherited biochemical variants recognizable either in blood, urine, or saliva; there will be no major round of clinical examinations involved, and that, in fact, clinical examinations would be contemplated only in those instances where they contributed to the proper biochemical characterization of a given specimen of blood, urine, or saliva. Attention is to be focused specifically on those genetic loci at which measurable gene-controlled changes in the quality or quantity of proteins are known to occur.

Illustrative of the types of loci are those associated with the blood groups (more than fourteen); serum proteins such as the haptoglobins, transferrins, Gm, Gc, or rare ones such as the immunoglobins, albumins, ceruloplasmin, C_1 esterase inhibitor, alpha anti-trypsin, beta lipoprotein, alpha lipoprotein, coagulation components (possibly a dozen), cholinesterases; intraerythrocytic proteins such as hemoglobin (some six loci), G-6-PD, 6-PGD, catalase, carbonic anhydrase, proteins associated with congenital non-spherocytic hemolytic anaemia (pyruvate kinase, etc.), methemoglobin reductase, ATP; white cell variants; and platelet types. This list, of course, is not intended to be exhaustive, but as stated, merely illustrative. A generous estimate of the number of loci known to be involved in the control of the type of genetic variability under discussion would be 50. Ideally, one would be interested in loci where all genes were co-dominant so that each and every genotype would correspond to a unique phenotype. Under these circumstances the maximum number of mutational events would be detectable. An important consideration is the number of such loci where the change in the protein is recognizable by techniques which lend themselves to automation, for the examination of tens of thousands of specimens is envisaged, a task possible only if the requisite biochemical procedures can be automated and delegated to an automatic analyser of some type.

Among the 50 loci previously estimated, the biochemical procedures have actually already been automated in a number of instances, and in the remainder could be readily automated by present means provided that the demonstration of a particular protein variant does not necessarily involve electrophoresis.

While it may be possible in the not too distant future to automate even tests of the latter type, this is not now feasible.

Possibly 25 to 30 of the aforementioned loci give rise to changes which could be measured in a fully automated system.

Technological advances could be incorporated as they arise, needless to say, and since storage of specimens in liquid nitrogen is anticipated, the study would not necessari be restricted to the state of the art at its initiation.

It is pertinent to observe at this point, perhaps, that Herbert Scheinberg at Albert Einstein College of Medicine is already engaged in a very similar programme of study, called Genetic Alert, whose purpose is the early recognition of certain inherited diseases with manifest biochemical changes.

The requirements of such a study do not appear prohibitive. A 10 cm^3 specimen of blood plus saliva and urine on all children in the base population and on their fathers and mothers would be more than adequate for the tests conjectured. If the F_1 mortality study were to constitute the base, for example, this would imply specimens from approximately 162,000 individuals. Ten persons with transportation could fairly readily obtain 20,000 sets of blood, saliva, and urine per annum. Six autoanalysers could perform all presently automated tests on the 20,000 specimens per year and the hardware necessary to permit the passage from autoanalyser to stored digitized information already exists.

Viewed solely in these lights, an undertaking of this kind is feasible, and it is not financially prohibitive. But it should be contemplated presumably only if it stands a reasonably large prior probability of materially enhancing our knowledge of the mutability of human genes.

Let us examine this latter, critical issue.

The purpose is, it will be recalled, to identify individual events which may be interpreted as mutations. In its simplest form this implies that one is looking for children whose genotypes are conspicuously at variance with their parents.

Obviously, this could occur for a number of other reasons of which the most conspicuous is nonpaternity or nonmaternity. Presumably, however, the bulk of such cases, i.e. actual nonpaternity or nonmaternity, would give rise to parental exclusion at more than one lo an unlikely mutational event. There is also the tacit assumption that one's genotype (or phenotype) can be measured without error, and this is patently not so. Misclassification in the bloo group systems may be as frequent as 1% for a system such as the ABO or over 40% in the case of the P system. These figures, mind you, are based upon the comparison of results of testin the same persons at two different but highly professional laboratories. Much of this error apparently reflects variability in antisera rather than in the technicians themselves, and thus even automated systems would be sensitive to the error.

It must also be borne in mind that not all mutations would give rise to genotypes or phenotypes recognizably different from those of the parents, and hence would not be detectable.

Thus, for example, if at a particular locus two alternative states, say M and N, exist and mutations were interpreted as a change of M to N, or N to M, mutations arising in either parent in a mating of MN by MN would be undetectable, since the only genetic constitutions which could arise would be those which arise normally from segregation.

Intuitively it seems clear that the proportion of mutations which would be undetectable would vary with the frequencies of the various alleles at the locus in question. At worst, 50% of the mutations at one particular locus would be undetectable; i.e. would not give rise to discordant or discrepant children. There are other difficulties such as death of parents, etc. which would diminish the information in a given case, but let us assume that these difficulties are surmountable, or nearly so, and consider the size of the needle for which we would be searching.

Suppose this study was to be undertaken in Japan and suppose further that the population of inquiry was the cohort of F_1 children previously referred to. This cohort, it will be recalled, is subdivisible into three groups of children, each of approximately 20,000 in number. One group is the offspring of unexposed parents, one of parents neither of whom was closer than 2,500 metres to ground zero, and the last of parents one or both of whom were within 2,000 metres of the hypocentre at the time of the bombing. The estimated average parental exposures associated with these three groups are 0, 5, and 100 reps. To determine the number of mutant phenotypes in a given group, we need merely multiply the number of loci under scrutiny, say 30, by the number of children examined, 20,000, by the average exposure by the probability of a mutation per locus per roentgen, say 2×10^{-7} (the value appropriate to the mouse). We expect one mutant phenotype among the 20,000 in the 2,500 metre group and beyond, and 20 mutant phenotypes among the 20,000 in the 2,000 metre and closer group. Possibly half of these would occur in circumstances such that they would be recognizable. The needle, then consists of 0.5 and 10 children, respectively. Variations on the approach outline are possible, of course, which may increase the sensitivity of the study somewhat, but not by as much as an order of magnitude. I leave to each of you the task of making a value judgment as to whether a search for numbers this small merits the cost. In this appraisal it should be borne in mind that the rate of increase in information about inherited biochemical variants in man has been logarithmic since World War II; each decade has seen the number of variants double.

In the very few moments which remain, let us examine briefly the second of the two tasks cited at the outset of this presentation. What is the fate of these mutations in a human population? Clearly without such information one cannot interpret the impact of increased exposure. I presume we all accept that benefits can accrue to mankind from the use of ionizing radiation, but there are risks as well. The issue which thus confronts us is the price which society is prepared to pay in disease and disability to achieve the benefits. Of immediate concern is the estimation of the disease and disability which will accrue. We have unfortunately little solid information from which to generate the estimate required, but several observations are relevant here.

One of these concerns the probability of the survival of a mutant gene in a population. Given a population of stable size, we can determine the probability that a mutation induced at a particular instant in time will persist indefinitely, i.e. will contribute descendants to all succeeding generations. If the trait bearer, the individual who is heterozygous for the mutant gene, is at the reproductive norm, or will produce fewer children on the average than an individual without the gene, the probability of the indefinite survival of the mutation is zero. It will not perpetuate itself in a stable population. We do not really know, however, what will happen in an expanding population. It is quite conceivable that numerous disadvantageous genes could be carried along in the latter situation. Now, since we can calculate the probability of survival, we can obviously also calculate the half-life of a mutant. Under the conditions of human reproduction, i.e. where family sizes are distributed in the negative binomial fashion, the half-life of a neutral mutation is about 1.3 generations; the half-life is, of course, even shorter for disadvantageous genes. It is worth noting also that even favourable mutations have generally small probabilities of indefinite persistence. To a close approximation, the probability of their indefinite survival is only twice their selective advantage. That is to say, if a mutation increases reproduction on the part of the mutant-bearer by 1% as contrasted with the norm, the likelihood of indefinite persistence of the mutant is about one chance in fifty.

While some insight exists into the survival of mutant genes, we cannot as yet estimate their impact, for this ultimately depends upon the way in which genetic variability is maintained in population. There are at least half a dozen different models of the way in which genetic variability may be maintained, and for each of these at least one good illustration exists. But their relative contributions to the maintenance of the totality of genetic variability is still unknown despite the great deal of effort which has been expended in this direction. Intuitively one presumes we are closer to an appraisal than we were two decades ago, but not yet at the point where meaningful calculations can be made.

References

Clayton, G.A., and Robertson, A. The effect of X rays on quantitative characters. Genetical Res., 5, 410-422, 1964.

Cox, D.F. The effect of paternal irradiation on body weight and depth of fat. Genetics, 58, 271-274, 1968.

Kato, H., Schull, W.J., and Neel, J.V. A cohort-type study of survival in children of parents exposed to atomic bombings. Am. J. hum. Genet, 18, 339-374, 1966.

Neel, J.V., and Schull, W.J. The effect of exposure to the atomic bombings on pregnancy terminations in Hiroshima and Nagasaki. Washington, D.C., National Academy of Sciences-National Research Council Publication No. 461, 241 pp, 1956.

Russell, W.L. Effect of the interval between irradiation and conception on mutation frequency in female mice. Proc. natn. Acad. Sci. U.S.A., 54, 1552-1557, 196

Schull, W.J., and Neel, J.V. Radiation and the sex ratio in man. Science, N.Y., 128, 343-348, 1958.

Schull, W.J., Neel, J.V., and Hashizume, A. Some further observations on the sex ratio among infants born to survivors of the atomic bombings of Hiroshima and Nagasaki. Am. J. hum. Genet., 18, 328-338, 1966.

DISCUSSION OF CHAPTERS VI AND VII

Dr. Bloom: The papers of Drs. Bender and Schull deal with different aspects of the same problem, namely, the effect of radiation on the genetic material of the cells.

Dr. Bender's emphasis has been on somatic cells and alterations of groups of genes therein, while Dr. Schull's focus has been to a considerable extent on point mutations and the problem of their detection. The issues raised in these papers are exemplified by the exposed Japanese populations at Hiroshima and Nagasaki, for there both somatic cell aberrations and the implications of these aberrations, and germ cell effects are clearly of major concern.

I should, therefore, like to discuss the two papers in the framework of the Hiroshima and Nagasaki studies, feeling that our scientific experience there may serve both as a model and as a guide to the kinds of problems we will have in man in attempting to assess the mutagenic effects of drugs and chemicals, viruses and radiations.

Before beginning, I should like to acknowledge the indebtedness which all of us feel to the late Dr. Court Brown for his leadership in the field of human radiation cytogenetics.

Let us briefly consider, then, three groups of A-bomb involved persons. The F_1 generation; those exposed *in utero*; and the heavily exposed survivors themselves.

Dr. Schull has indicated that the initial attempts to study the population characteristics of this group were essentially negative with regard to radiation effects. One has to agree with his statement that ionizing radiation must be mutagenic in man. But the problem of how one detects mutations in man is still with us. The specific locus approach holds promise in that qualitative variations in proteins as well as quantitative variations may now be detected. However, the technology is perhaps not quite ready for the mass screening of 50 or more loci.

Our cytogenetic approach to the F_1 generation in Hiroshima and Nagasaki lies somewhere between the population characteristics and the specific locus approaches which Dr. Schull has outlined. That is, we have embarked on a programme to look for either a structural re-arrangement which has been induced in a parental germ cell and which has subsequently been transmitted, or for an increase in the frequency of abnormalities of chromosome number (losses or additions) which may result from primary non-disjunction.

Now, the limitations of such an approach are readily apparent. First of all, affected germ cells may well have been killed at the time of the bombings; and if they survived, they may have been selected against. Further, the zygote which was formed may have been non-viable and have passed, unknown to the mother, very soon after fertilization. Thus, we have three limitations to the present approach to the F_1 generation. In any event, we have begun this work and have selected F_1's from the mortality sample which Dr. Schull described.

We have been concerned particularly with parents whose exposure dose was well over 100 rads. Special interest in those born soon after maternal exposure is mandatory because of Russell's suggestion that in mammals, mutations resulting from maternal irradiation diminish with time after exposure. To date some 100 F_1's of heavily exposed parents have been studied and two abnormalities have been found in this group. The first was a short arm deletion of one of the small acrocentric chromosomes, which, on examination of the family, turned out to be transmitted from the mother and grandmother. This was clearly, then, not the result of any structural abnormality induced by the gamma and neutron radiations of the A-bombs.

The second abnormality which has been thus far detected in this small sample was an XO/XX mosaic. This kind of error probably results from a non-disjunctional error in mitosis, and, therefore, is likely to be a postzygotic error.

We anticipate studying some 1,000 to 2,000 F_1 persons. The precise number is open-ended at the present time. Our chances of detecting, in this relatively small number of individuals, any radiation effect on the meiotic chromosomes are obviously slim. But, it does seem eminently worth the effort. We are also saving sera so that should the day arise when we can study the F_1 generation using a specific locus approach, by doing biochemical studies, we will have this material on hand.

The in utero exposed has been another group with which we have been concerned. As indicated by previous speakers, there has been no increased incidence of leukaemia in this group. On the other hand, the group is very small. While we are following clinically a total in utero group of some 1,600 individuals, a fraction of those had estimated maternal dose exposures of 100 rads, or more.

Among 39% of the in utero exposed studied cytogenetically, we did find small numbers of cells with rings, dicentrics, acentric fragments and translocations. We studied 38 heavily exposed individuals, that is, individuals whose maternal dose was in excess of 100 rads, and compared them with a group of 48 controls who were in utero, but whose mothers were not exposed.

These findings suggest either that the lymphocytes we examined had survived and essentially not divided since exposure; or that, in fact, the lymphocytes which we examined were the progeny of affected precursor cells. In any event, the clinical significance of these residual chromosome aberrations is unclear.

Among the survivors themselves, we have a group of carefully selected individuals, in whom residual chromosome aberrations are frequently present, perhaps in 10% or more of cells in any given subject. There are differences by age which I will not discuss, but it is now clear that we have a sizable increase in the proportion of residual aberrations in the heavily irradiated survivors. This is no surprise. On the other hand, up to 61% of heavily exposed individuals have these aberrations, and it is this high proportion of individuals with whom we are particularly concerned. The sample size, I should mention, in the exposed individual study is just under 200 patients at the present time.

Dr. Bender has specified that, "We have no reason to believe that radiation does not produce chromosome aberrations of all the expected types of cells of all tissues of all mammals including man". I have shown you that the in utero exposed and the exposed survivors have lymphocyte aberrations. We are currently looking at other tissues from autopsy specimens; but, indirectly, Dr. Bender's statement is supported by recent clinical and pathological findings at ABCC*. For, not only leukaemia but now also carcinoma of the thyroid (and possibly also of lung and breast) has been shown to be significantly increased in proximally exposed survivors.

---

* Atomic Bomb Casualty Commission.

I have made an assumption here which I hope will evoke some discussion; namely, that where one has chromosome aberrations, one may also find malignant disease. Dr. Fialkow has summarized some of these relationships in a scheme which suggests that not only do viruses, radiations, and drugs produce neoplasia, but that their effects may be mediated by chromosomal aberrations. We used to believe that, in fact, individuals who had neoplastic diseases developed the chromosomal aberrations in the neoplastic tissues as a result of whatever the neoplastic process was. On the other hand, there is increasing evidence of late that there are individuals with chromosomal abnormalities, persons with Fanconi's anaemia, Bloom's syndrome and other clinical entities in which we have a high frequency of chromosomal aberrations, who are at high risk in terms of the development of solid neoplasms or leukaemia.

The cell death-proliferation cycle of Fialkow illustrates one possible mechanism by which chromosomal aberrations may give rise to neoplasia. That is, if sufficient chromosome damage is produced in a cell population, with a high proportion of the cells dying, then on proliferation and regeneration of this damaged population, one may have an increased risk of spontaneous mutation in the direction of neoplastic disease.

There is clearly a need for more cytogenetic data on normal human populations in order for us to be able to draw reasonable conclusions as to the possible effects of chromosome damage. An opportunity to obtain some of this information arose fairly recently when Drs. Neel and Chagnon from Ann Arbor went to South America to study some primitive Indians with whom they have been working for several years now. I thought that this would represent a group of cytogenetically normal individuals, essentially non-exposed to the insults of civilization, such as diagnostic radiation. I anticipated that we might be able, by studying them, to get some very baseline cytogenetic data with which to compare, for example, the irradiated populations of Hiroshima and Nagasaki.

Instead, we have found a whole host of cells with bizarre chromosomal aberrations. Cells with multiple dicentric chromosomes, tricentric chromosomes, and many fragments have been found. Here we have the beginning, I think, of what is probably a new chapter in human population cytogenetics, and the same question of biological and clinical significance came up. Why do these individuals have these chromosomal abnormalities? What effects will these chromosomal abnormalities have on the soma, and can this damage be transmitted?

I think that Drs. Bender and Schull have shown multiple ways in which we can approach some of these questions. I will stop here and open up the discussion period to get your reactions to some of the things which you have seen in our Hiroshima and Nagasaki work and in the previous two papers.

Dr. Brent: Are there no individuals in whom you studied chromosomes where you do not see breaks in the controls?

Dr. Bloom: In general, most controls studied have some degree of chromosome damage, though usually in 1% or less of cells.

Dr. Brent: What is the range of aberrations in the controls, and what is the range of aberrations in the exposed?

Dr. Bloom: The frequency of aberrations of the chromosome type, as Dr. Bender has defined them, is extremely low, particularly in younger individuals. That is, one rarely sees things like ring chromosomes and dicentrics in individuals at a relatively young age, and by that I mean individuals under the age of about 50. This assumes that the control population has been screened to eliminate recent diagnostic X-ray and recent viral infection. The frequency of aberrations in the exposed is, overall, from 0.6 to 1.5% of all cells examined, again the frequency being both dose and age dependent.

Dr. Grahn: I would like to discuss the genetic analysis of sex ratio changes, as this was the first positive measure of a genetic effect in the Japanese study.

The best way to study this experimentally and in human populations is to use the three-generation procedure. It was first tried by Cavalli-Sforza with an Italian populatior You identify a population of grand-sires, their daughters, and then the grandchildren. Now if there is an increasing probability of a lethal occurring spontaneously in the grand-sire with increasing age, one should expect to find, with increasing grand-sire age, a decrease in sex ratio among the grandchildren. More and more of the expected grandsons die as a result of the lethal gene transmitted by the mother from grandfather to grandson. Initial studies gave a positive result.

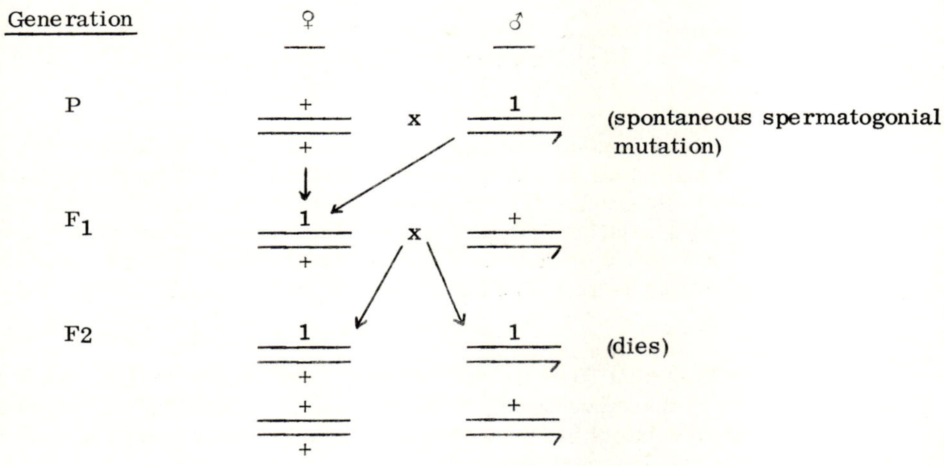

Another study, from Minnesota, on foetal death used the same procedure, only now looking at the sex ratio of the foetal deaths where one would expect more and more males to die with increasing grand-sire age. This was observed in terms of foetal sex ratio.

On the other hand, Cavalli-Sforza's follow-up efforts have been negative along with the follow-up efforts in Japan by Neel and Schull. This should not be too discouraging because, one, the mammalian sex chromosome is not fully understood in terms of its genetic behaviour; and two, in the mouse we do have some evidence that would suggest that mutation is predominantly to detrimental or sublethal gene changes that can only be measured as lethal equivalents; substantially what was estimated in the Japanese data.

I have done this in the mouse with the use of a marker gene to eliminate the problem of F_1 XO females. On the basis of about 600 chromosomes tested, I obtain a difference that would lead to an estimated mutation rate for lethal equivalents in the X-chromosome of the mouse of approximately 6.7×10^{-5}/X/R.

The difficulty in all this is in the generations after you ascertain that you do have a significant sex ratio deviation in the F_2. When you attempt to follow this to the F_3 and subsequent generations, the presumed lethals tend to just disappear, as if they were really only transiently detrimental to begin with. They are certainly not categorical lethals as we learned to understand lethal mutations in Drosophila, but they may only be acting as lethals in a temporarily imbalanced genetic system. Since we do not know exactly the genetic behaviour of these lethals in our mouse populations under controlled conditions, the observation that they seem to come and go in human populations should not really discourage us.

Dr. Lamerton: Dr. Bender said, I think, that there was no possibility of chromosomal repair except immediately following radiation.

Dr. Bender: That is an oversimplification. The point I was trying to make is that once you have a chromosome that is broken and committed, it does not rejoin. In the first few hours perhaps, it is a question of what really came apart; but once it is broken, the break is fixed.

Dr. Lamerton: This general concept has worried me, because otherwise one could expect continued irradiation to be much more effective than it is on the tissues of the body, and one does not find this. Either there has been repair of damage without cell turnover, or those cells for some reason are much more resistant to the effects of radiation.

Dr. Bender: I am not sure I know why you say that. Curtis' data, for example, on the regenerating liver seems consistent to me in terms of the effects of chronic, radiation on chromosome aberration frequencies. His data was very largely on bridge formation and anaphases.

Dr. Lindop: Coggle (1968) has done experiments assaying anaphase bridges and fragments in mouse liver cells using single and fractionated doses of X-rays given at various times before and after surgical partial hepatectomy. The liver cells before the surgical stimulus are in G_0, resting phase; the cells after the surgery are actively in cell cycle G_1, S and so on. The dose-response curve for cells irradiated in G_0 (24 hours before partial hepatectomy) is given in fig. 1, curve A. A series of fractionated doses given in G_0 liver cells reveals that they are unable to repair chromosomal damage between the fractions (see fig. 2, curve A).

The dose-response curve for liver cells given a series of X-ray doses 24 hours after partial hepatectomy (cells in late G_1) is given in fig. 1, curve B. Fractionated X-ray doses given to cells between 24 and 48 hours after partial hepatectomy (cells in late

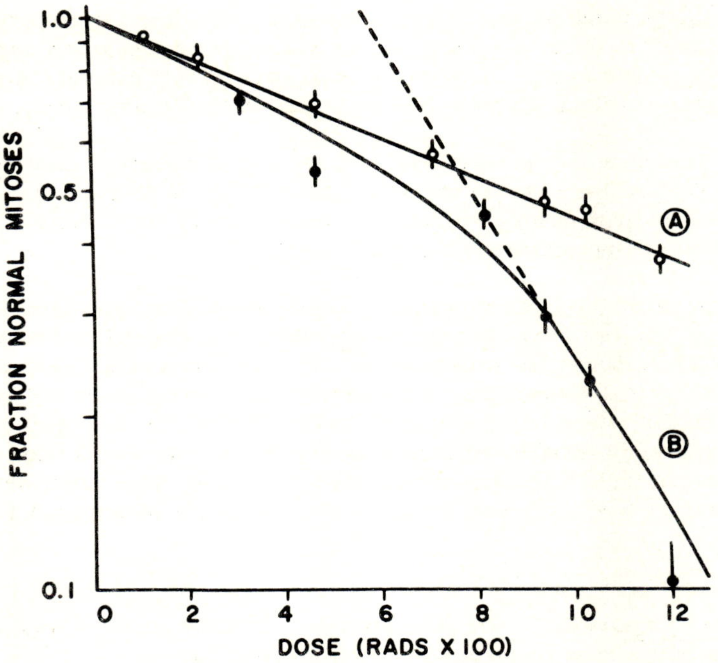

Fig. 1. A plot of the logarithm of fraction normal mitotic figures against doses of X rays. O (A), Doses given 24 hours before partial hepatectomy; ● (B), Doses given 24 hours after partial hepatectomy. More points would be desirable for the latter fitted line; this is, however, technically very difficult. (with permission from Nature, Lond., 217, 180-182, 1968.)

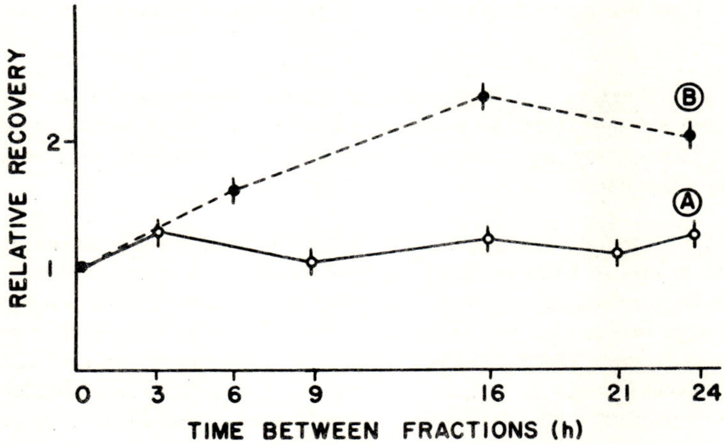

Fig. 2. Relative recovery factor for chromosomal damage induced by radiation against time between two fractions of 475 rads each. ● (B), Doses given after partial hepatectomy; O (A), doses given before partial hepatectomy. (with permission from Nature, Lond., 217, 180-182, 1968.)

G_1, S and G_2) reveals an increased proportion of normal mitoses, interpreted as "recovery", relative to a single large X-ray dose (see fig. 2, curve B). The use of Actinomycin D to depress DNA directed RNA synthesis has no inhibiting effect on the chromosomal repair processes. It may be suggested that the mechanisms that keep cells in G_0 also inhibit the metabolic pathways required for the repair of radiation damage. Such pathways appear operative in cells actively in cell cycle.

Reference

Coggle, J.E. Effect of cell cycle on recovery from radiation damage in the mouse liver. Nature (Lond.) 217, 180-182, 1968.

CHAPTER VIII

LATE EFFECTS OF RADIUM DEPOSITION IN MAN

R.J. Hasterlik*, A.J. Finkel‡ and
C.E. Miller‡

The proper subject for the study of the late and subtle effects of ionizing radiation on man is man himself. Although several large-scale studies on animals have yielded confirmatory evidence concerning the mechanism involved in the induction of certain types of tumour seen in radium-bearing man, in the last analysis extrapolations from the experimental animal to man concerning "dose-effect" relationships may not be reasonable or tenable. Instead, therefore, of discussing the late and subtle effects of all of the alpha-particle emitters in man, we shall confine ourselves to a discussion of the effects of one alpha emitter, ^{226}Ra, in the series of patients we have been fortunate enough to have been able to observe for a very long period of time, and attempt to derive certain dose-effect relationships for the effects we have observed.

For the past 20 years investigators at Argonne National Laboratory and Argonne Cancer Research Hospital have studied the long-term effects of radium deposited in the skeletal tissues of man and experimental animals. The consequences of radium deposition in man were reported by Martland in a series of papers (1931) and later by other investigators (Aub et al., 1952; Evans, 1966) for a group of dial painters in eastern United States and by Looney et al. (1955) for a series of patients in the Chicago area, and most recently at the Symposium on Radiation-induced Cancer in Athens (Finkel et al., 1969 a, b).

In 1957 the Argonne studies were intensified after the discovery of a photograph of 98 dial painters taken in October 1924, in front of the factory where they worked. These women were identified and most of those living were located. Other photographs were discovered and a successful field investigation yielded a list of approximately 400 names. Many of these individuals have been persuaded to participate in our studies during the past 12 years and the data derived from these investigations form a substantial basis of this report.

Meanwhile, we have also studied a number of persons who received radium orally or intravenously from their physicians. One group of 41 patients were given a variable number of weekly intravenous radium injections during 1931-33 at a state mental hospital in Illinois, not far from Chicago, and we have studied most of the living patients (Schlundt et al., 1933; Miller and Finkel, 1968). Another group of patients who received radium orally or intravenously from their personal physicians from 1920 to 1933 has also come to our attention, largely as a result of the symptoms of serious disease that eventually ensued.

---

* From the Department of Medicine and the Argonne Cancer Research Hospital, University of Chicago, Chicago, Ill. 60637.

‡ From the Health Division, Argonne National Laboratory, Argonne, Ill. 60349.

The radium patients that we have studied, then, comprise the following population:

Occupational exposure	
Dial painting industry	208
Radium chemists	4
Iatrogenic cases	
State mental hospital	41
Private patients	40

These numbers represent those cases that we have either studied in some detail or about whose radium body burden and medical fate we have some knowledge. Many of the 400 persons whose names we have acquired have worked in recent years under conditions of reasonably good industrial hygiene and have consequently acquired negligible burdens of radium. We have deliberately refrained from extensive studies of these persons and we have concentrated instead largely on the older populations of persons who worked in the early 1920's.

The basic data relating to the occupational exposure, medical history, radium burden measurements, skeletal radiography, and other pertinent items for these patients recently have been published in a joint report from Argonne National Laboratory and Argonne Cancer Research Hospital (Miller et al., 1969).

Malignant Tumours in Radium Dial Painters

The malignant tumour experience of our radium patients was discussed in some detail at the University of Utah Symposium on "Delayed Effects of Bone-seeking Radionuclides" in September, 1967 (Finkel, Miller and Hasterlik, 1969a). The data in the present report are somewhat different, having been modified by the addition of a newly developed case of osteogenic sarcoma (Case 03-429) and the deletion of a much debated case of questionable carcinoma of the maxilla (Case 03-685). The tissues of the latter patient have been examined widely and the opinion of competent oral pathologists is that the lesion most probably is not a malignant tumour but instead may be a benign tumour of the odontogenic epithelium or may represent a stage in the healing of a tooth socket affected by periodontal disease. For this reason we have removed it from our list of established malignancies attributable to radium deposition in bone.

The malignant tumours of skeletal tissues in radium dial painters who have had radium body burden determinations are given in table 1. Similarly, table 2 lists carcinomas, principally of the mastoids and the jaw and a case of "splenic leukaemia" (chronic myelogenous leukaemia), that have developed in dial painters. The cases of malignant tumours, without body burden measurements have been omitted since they cannot contribute to an analysis of the radiation dose and radiobiological parameters that may be involved in radiation carcinogenesis. In our experience, the development of carcinomas of the mastoids, paranasal sinuses, and other locations close to the bones of the skull is largely a phenomenon of the 1960's and has generally occurred much later than most of the osteosarcomas and the aplastic anaemias and leukaemias.

For the present purposes, the presence or absence of radium-induced malignancies will be discussed in terms of these radiobiological indices: (1) current or preterminal radium body burden, (2) retrospectively estimated maximum body burden (i.e. peak initial burden), (3) estimated amounts of radium absorbed daily into the blood stream from

Table 1

Malignant tumours of skeletal tissues attributable to radium in dial painters

Case No.	Yr of birth	Work period		Diagnosis and year of diagnosis	Mean current or preterminal radium burden	Date of measurement
		Dates	Days[a]		μCi	
03-455	1906	7/22-8/23	395	Fibrosarcoma, left radius, 1935	0.81	1958
03-402[b]	1905	7/23-7/26	914	Fibrosarcoma, left femur, 1954	1.06	1962
03-649[c]	1906	10/24-10/50	455	Fibrosarcoma, right ischium, 1954	1.30	1951
03-619	1903	8/22-4/23	242	Fibrosarcoma, left femur, 1962	1.50	1962
03-429	1908	8/23-8/27	883	Osteosarcoma, right 3rd metacarpal, 1967	1.70	1966
03-401	1900	6/23-4/25	669	Fibrosarcoma, left leg, 1963	2.29	1960
03-671	1906	7/22-9/22	61	Fibrosarcoma, left femur, 1953	3.82	1952
03-648[d]	1903	9/21-9/22	1090	Fibrosarcomas, left femur and right humerus, 1956	7.61	1955

[a]Work period F computed to 1 January, 1926.
[b]Each of these two cases also had malignant tumour of mastoid; see table 2.
[c]Case 03-649 also listed as 01-023 (M.I.T. series).
[d]Case 03-648 also listed as 01-013 (M.I.T. series).

Table 2

Other malignant tumours attributable to radium in dial painters

Case No.	Yr of birth	Work period		Diagnosis and year of diagnosis	Mean current or preterminal radium burden	Date of measurement
		Dates	Days[a]			
					μCi	
03-417	1909	7/24-9/25	426	Carcinoma, right gingiva, 1962	0.62	1964
03-402[b]	1905	7/23-7/26	914	Carcinoma, right mastoid, 1964	1.06	1965
03-407	1905	6/23-6/46	944	Carcinoma, right mastoid, 1959	1.40	1957
03-648[c]	1903	1/22-12/24	1090	Mixed carcinosarcoma, right mastoid, 1955	7.61	1955
03-657	1906	7/22-7/36	1279	Splenic leukaemia, 1934	18.00[d]	1936

[a]Work period F computed to 1 January 1926.

[b]Also had a malignant tumour of bone, see table 1.

[c]Also had a malignant tumour of bone, see table 1. Listed as 01-013 (M.I.T. series).

[d]Measurement by R.D. Evans; also listed as 01-002 (M.I.T. series).

the gastro-intestinal tract, and (4) estimated total amount of radium absorbed into the blood stream during the critical work period.

Patterns of Radium Retention

The computation of the values for three of the four radiobiological indices proposed above depends on our notions of the patterns of radium retention in the skeleton during the years after various routes of administration. Two principal mathematical models have been proposed to describe the course of retention of radium and other bone-seeking radionuclides. These are the power function and the sum of a series of exponentials. In a recent paper we have evaluated both approaches in an analysis of the existing data for the state mental hospital patients who were given intravenous injections of radium in 1931-33 (Schlundt et al., 1933).

The power function, as proposed by Norris et al. (1955, 1958), gives the value of retained radium at time t after a single intravenous injection by

$$R = a\,t^{-b} \tag{1}$$

where a is the vertical intercept or amount of retained radium at unit time, and b is the slope of the straight line that this function produces on a log-log grid.

Where radium is acquired orally and where it can be assumed that the same amount was absorbed each day, the amount of radium retained at t days after cessation of unit daily absorption during F days is given by

$$R_{oral}\,(F,\ t) = \frac{a}{b+1}\quad (t+F)^{b+1} - t^{b+1} \tag{2}$$

The family of curves generated by equation (2) for selected ingestion periods is given in fig.1, where the power function parameters used are: $a = 0.30$, and $b = 0.44$. The latter values have been used instead of those proposed by Norris et al. (1955, 1958) on the basis of restudy of the same patients that Norris used and a re-computation based on additional data (Miller and Finkel, 1968). It can be seen in fig. 1 that the curve for one day's ingestion is very close to that expected for a single intravenous injection. As the ingestion period becomes longer, the earlier portion of the retention curve becomes flatter, but eventually the slopes of the curves bend down and approach that for a single injection.

Maximum retention, which occurs at the end of the feeding period, F, is given by

$$R_{oral}\ (F,\ 0) = \frac{a}{b+1}\ F^{b+1} \tag{3}$$

since this is at the end of the ingestion period when $t = 0$. Again, this computation is based on the assumption of absorption into the blood stream of a unit amount of radium during the ingestion period. For each case where radium was acquired orally, as in the case of the radium dial painters, we computed a ratio, Q, in which the estimated radium burden at the end of the ingestion period was divided by the radium calculated to be present at time, t, after cessation of ingestion:

$$Q = \frac{R_{oral}(F,\ 0)}{R_{oral}(F,\ t)} \tag{4}$$

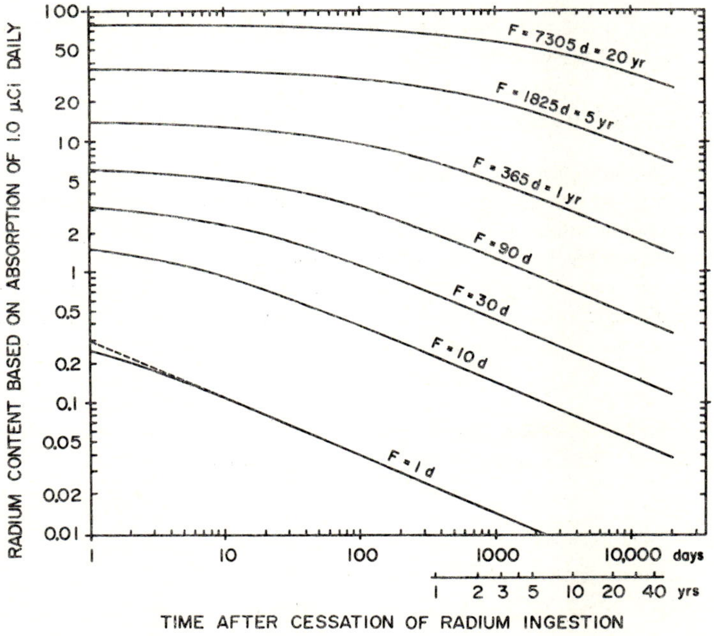

Fig. 1. Log-log plot of radium retention after cessation of oral ingestion for ingestion periods (F) of selected lengths of time. Daily incorporation of 1.0 μCi is arbitrarily assumed. Power function parameters: a = 0.30, b = 0.44.

This quotient represents the ratio of the maximum radium burden to any measured burden at time t thereafter, and in this way provides a factor by which the maximum burden estimated for each patient is greater than the subsequently measured amount. Values of Q are shown in fig. 2 for selected F periods and t days after cessation of ingestion. Sample retention values of retained radium and the accompanying Q ratios computed for t days after cessation of periods of ingestion F days in duration were given in a previous paper (Finkel et al., 1969 a, b).

For specific cases, then, the maximum radium burden at t = 0 can be estimated from the magnitude of Q (which depends upon F, t, a, and b) and the whole-body radium measurement at time t:

Estimated maximum burden = Q x (measured radium burden at t) (5)

This estimated maximum burden represents a value for peak initial burden computed separatel for each whole-body radium measurement for each patient.

For the radium dial painters whose work-history was known, the length of the ingestion period, F, was computed in days on the assumption that ingestion occurred throughout the period at the same rate because of consistency in personal work habits. This computation does not correct for absence from work on weekends, holidays and vacations, but is nevertheless a reasonable approximation. In the cases of those dail painters whose work-history straddled 1 January 1926, we have ignored any work-period subsequent to that data on the assumption that the bulk of the ingestion occurred before the practice of pointing the brushes between the lips was discontinued.

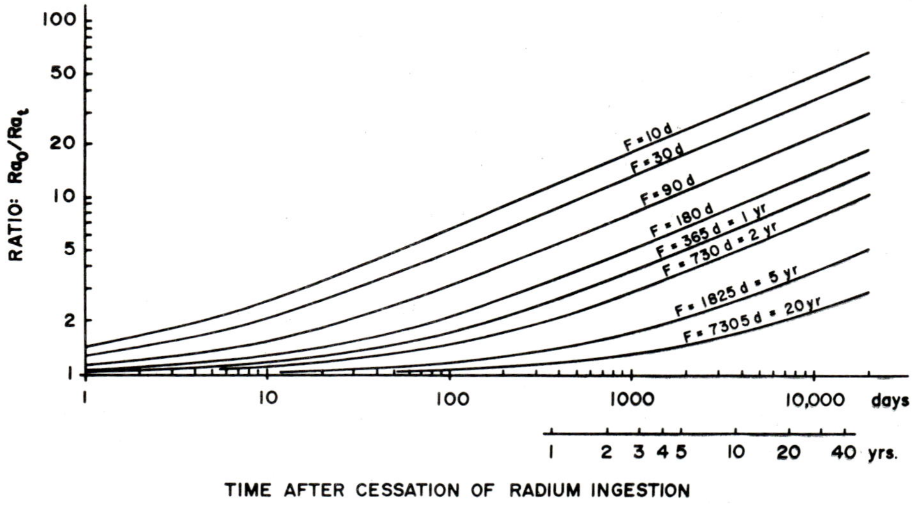

Fig. 2. Ratio of estimated maximum radium burden to calculated measured radium burden at time t, both computed on the assumption of unit daily absorption of radium from gut. Power function parameters: a = 0.30, b = 0.44.

Another index that can be computed is the amount of radium absorbed daily from the gut. This value is the ratio of the measured body radium at time t to the radium computed to be retained in accordance with equation (2). We have termed this the <u>Ingestion Q</u>:

$$\text{Ingestion Q} = \frac{\text{Measured radium at t}}{\text{Computed retained radium at t}} \qquad (6)$$

Since the computed retained radium is estimated on the assumption of <u>unit</u> absorption of radium daily from the gastrointestinal tract, the <u>Ingestion Q</u> value is a measure of the amount actually <u>absorbed</u> daily (rather than ingested in the sense of swallowed). The <u>Ingestion Q</u> value presumably varied from person to person depending on work-practices (tipping the brushes between the lips and general personal hygiene) as well as individual physiological factors. Again, on the assumption that these physiological factors remained reasonably constant during the period of employment, with the major exception of the January 1926 change in work-procedures mentioned above, the total amount of radium absorbed into the blood stream from the gut is given by the product of F and Q:

$$\text{Total absorbed radium} = F \times Q \qquad (7)$$

The computed values of FQ constitute the fourth of the measures used in this paper for evaluating the long-term effects of radium deposition.

Similar computations can be made on the basis of radium retention described by a sum of a number of exponential terms. Analysis of long-term retention data of the State mental hospital patients already alluded to (Miller and Finkel, 1968) has established that average radium retention during the period beginning with the first year after administration can be described by a single exponential term. This exponential equation has the form $R = 0.0246\ Ae^{-0.693t/5472}$, where t is given in days and A is the total amount administered.

This expression implies that 2.46% of the injected radium (and hence also of radium absorbed into the blood from the gut) is retained with a 14.98 year half-time. The early portions of the retention curve cannot be reconstructed from this single exponential term but can perhaps be approximated in the following way. Maletskos et al. (1968) reported some experimental work with ^{224}Ra that indicated a 2.4 day half-time for 85% of injected radium. We have assumed a 30-day half-time for the remaining 12.5% of administered radium since there is no indication of more than one remaining exponential term after one year.

Maximum radium retention, then, can be computed by the sum of three exponentials given by

$$R = 0.85\ Ae^{-0.693t/2.4} + 0.125\ Ae^{-0.693t/30} + 0.025\ Ae^{-0.693t/5472}$$

Here again a Q ratio can be computed and a peak initial burden can be estimated for each whole-body measurement made years later. Similarly, values can be computed for <u>Ingestion Q</u> and for total radium absorbed from the gut during the critical work-period.

These several measures of radium retention and radium metabolism have been computed for all our patients for whom suitable data are available. These indices have then been examined for their pertinence in characterizing the conditions in which radium-induced malignant change has occurred and may be expected to occur in the future.

Radiobiological Indices for Malignant Tumours in Dial Painters

Table 3 presents the estimates of maximum body burden, the amount of radium absorbed daily, and the total amount of radium absorbed during the critical work-period for those cases of malignant tumours of skeletal tissue that are listed in table 1. Where more than one whole-body measurement was made, the value listed is in each case the mean of the computed index. Estimates have been made by both the power function, $R = 0.30\ t^{-0.44}$ and the sum of the three exponentials given above. Table 4 presents similar data for the carcinomas and for the case of leukaemia presented in table 2. From these tables it can be seen that the lowest <u>mean</u> values for any malignancy attributable to radium are:

Current or preterminal radium burden	0.62 μCi
Estimated maximum radium burden	5.72 μCi
Estimated daily absorbed radium	0.29 μCi
Estimated total absorbed radium	153.33 μCi

These minimum values are based on a specific power function and are very close to those independently estimated from the sum of three exponentials.

Radiobiological Indices and Degrees of Radiographic Change

Most of the dial painters whom we have discussed have had skeletal radiography along with whole-body measurements of radium by gamma-ray spectrometry. The radiographic changes typical of radium deposition were found to be, in increasing order of severity: coarsening of traveculation, localized areas of bone resorption in the cortices of long bones and skull, spotty areas of sclerosis, aseptic necrosis, pathological fracture, and development of malignant tumours of bone and adjacent tissues. A quantitative scoring system was utilized to grade the severity of the radiographic changes. An overall impression, that characterized the general degree of skeletal damage attributable to radium, was recorded

Table 3

Estimates of radiobiological indices for cases of malignant tumour of skeletal tissue attributable to radium in dial painters

Case No.	Power function $0.30\ t^{-0.44}$			Sum of three exponentials		
	Estimated mean maximum radium burden	Estimated mean daily absorption	Estimated mean total absorption during critical work period	Estimated mean maximum radium burden	Estimated mean daily absorption	Estimated mean total absorption during critical work period
	μCi	μCi	μCi	μCi	μCi	μCi
03-455	6.72	0.441	174.16	7.96	0.461	181.93
03-402	6.99	0.287	262.09	8.87	0.314	287.14
03-649	8.89	0.539	245.31	7.83	0.421	191.55
03-619	16.14	1.393	337.17	23.02	1.658	401.12
03-429	11.21	0.469	413.83	15.10	0.547	483.05
03-401	15.38	0.751	502.65	17.62	0.761	509.02
03-671	66.49	12.418	757.49	90.56	10.674	651.14
03-648	38.63[a]	1.435	1564.62	42.54	1.338	1458.09

[a]Recomputed since previous publication (Finkel et al., 1969b).

Table 4

Estimates of radiobiological indices for cases of carcinoma and leukaemia attributable to radium in dial painters

Case No.	Power function $0.30\ t^{-0.44}$			Sums of three exponentials		
	Estimated mean maximum radium burden	Estimated mean daily absorption	Estimated mean total absorption during critical work period	Estimated mean maximum radium burden	Estimated mean daily absorption	Estimated mean total absorption during critical work period
	μCi	μCi	μCi	μCi	μCi	μCi
03-417	5.72	0.360	153.33	7.16	0.399	169.77
03-402	6.99	0.287	262.09	8.87	0.314	287.14
03-407	7.67	0.309	291.49	8.56	0.297	280.06
03-648	38.63[a]	1.435	1564.62	42.54	1.338	1458.09
03-657	55.64	1.891	2418.43	38.25	1.077	1377.92

[a]Recomputed since previous publication (Finkel et al., 1969b).

for each set of roentgenograms. These impressions were recorded in the following categories: negative, minimal, mild, moderate, advanced, and malignant changes due to radium deposition. These broad categories were closely related to the quantitative score for the entire skeleton and in general they expressed not only the extent of radiographically detectable damage but also the degree of orthopaedic disability.

In a number of cases, periodic radiography at intervals of 3 or 4 years demonstrated a progression of changes in the direction of increasing severity. For the purpose of the present analysis, all the cases were reclassified, where necessary, so as to reflect the most severe category of change that had developed by January 1969. By this procedure the various parameters or radiobiological indices were applied to the most severe degree of pathological change that had manifested itself at that time.

For 207 dial painters there were 313 independent determinations of radium body burden. When these measurements are sorted in terms of the most recent diagnosis, the magnitude of the body burden increases with increasing severity of radiographic change (table 5).

Table 5

Measured radium body burden in dial painters
sorted by latest diagnosis

Latest X ray or clinical diagnosis	No. of Patients	No. of measurements	Measured body radium μCi	
			Range	Median
Negative	146	168	0.001- 0.500	0.018
Minimal	21	33	0.001- 0.761	0.150
Mild	10	29	0.041- 1.743	0.523
Moderate	9	29	0.115- 1.622	0.900
Advanced	10	29	0.574- 2.200	1.170
Malignant	11	25	0.597-18.000	1.420

In many ways the measured radium burden is among the least satisfactory of the indices for characterizing radium damage because its magnitude depends largely upon whether it is determined soon after the burden is acquired or at long time intervals thereafter. Furthermore, the rate of change of this value also depends on the route and time-scale of administration, i.e. whether the radium was received as a single intravenous injection or over a protracted period of time by ingestion of repeated injections.

It would seem then that the radium burden measurements made 35 to 50 years after exposure or administration have only a limited applicability to the delineation of conditions of radium-induced carcinogenesis. Yet, despite these considerations, there is a persistent association between the level of current or preterminal body burdens of radium and the severity of skeletal damage set forth in table 5, principally because most of the measurements were made in a relatively narrow time-band many years after exposure. Nevertheless, such values as are presented in table 5 cannot be used for evaluating the hazard of a freshly acquire radium burden. For such purposes the estimated peak initial burden, or maximum burden, may be much more valuable. This view is fortified by the finding of Finkel et al. (1961) that the dose rate during the first days after injection of ^{90}Sr into mice provided the amount of radiation necessary to induce malignant bone tumours.

Table 6 presents values estimated retrospectively for the maximum radium burdens in dial painters. These values have been computed for each whole-body measurement, and have been calculated by various methods, as indicated, and have been sorted by latest diagnosis. Three sets of computations, each by a different power function, are listed. In addition to the power function $R = 0.30\ t^{-0.44}$ we have also used $R = 0.20\ t^{-0.35}$ which may also be a valid average function as shown by recent studies (Miller and Finkel, 1968). For purposes of comparison, we have also included values computed by the power function proposed by Norris et al. (1955, 1958), $R = 0.54\ t^{-0.52}$. Calculations were also made with a sum three exponentials whose values have already been presented.

The significant point of table 6 is the indication that malignancies have not developed in those cases where the computed maximum radium burden was less than 5.0 μCi when $R = 0.30\ t^{-0.44}$ was used for the calculations. Use of the function $R = 0.54\ t^{-0.52}$ would place this lower limit at about 7.7μCi, while the other computations vary with the parameters and mathematical functions used. The former power function leads to an estimate of 3.0 μCi for peak initial burden as the level below which serious orthopaedic difficulties are not likely to ensue, even after 40 years. These values should be evaluated against the maximum permissible level of 0.1 μCi for radium body burden that has been the standard for many years (ICRP, 1960).

Table 7 similarly presents computations of the estimated daily amount absorbed into the blood stream from the gut by the dial painters, again computed for each body burden measurement for each patient by several methods and sorted by latest diagnosis. Here, although there is an increase in the amounts absorbed as one proceeds from the negative radiography group to those with advanced changes and with malignancy, the progression is not smooth and the separation of the groups is not as clear as it was with estimated values for maximum burden. The principal reason for this finding is the variation in the length of the work-period, which is not taken into direct consideration in this computation. Despite the unevenness of the data, the development of a malignancy seems to have required a minimum absorption of 0.26 μCi daily (calculated either by the power function with $a = 0.30$ and $b = 0.44$ or by three exponentials).

When Ingestion Q is multiplied by F, the total radium absorbed during the critical work period is computed. Here there appear to be three clusters of values: (a) cases with minimal or no changes, (b) those with mild or moderate changes, and (c) those with advanced orthopaedic difficulties and/or malignant neoplasms. The latter appear to develop only in those cases in which the total amount of absorbed radium is computed to have exceeded 130 μCi either by the standard power function that we have been using or the sum of three exponentials. These values generally agree with the data for the four State mental hospital patients who developed malignant tumours attributable to radium. These four patients had received from 11 to 41 weekly intravenous injections of radium in amounts of 10 μCi each, so that the total amount introduced into the blood ranged from 110 to

Table 6

Estimated maximum radium burden in dial painters, computed by various methods and sorted by latest diagnosis

Latest X ray or clinical diagnosis	Power function $0.30\ t^{-0.44}$		Three exponentials		Power function $0.20\ t^{-0.35}$		Power function $0.54\ t^{-0.52}$	
	Range	Median	Range	Median	Range	Median	Range	Median
	μCi	μCi	μCi	μCi	μCi	μCi	μCi	μCi
Negative	0.00- 4.51	0.20	0.002- 5.69	0.18	0.00- 2.66	0.11	0.00- 7.37	0.35
Minimal	0.00- 6.20	1.23	0.006- 7.25	1.91	0.00- 3.91	0.83	0.00- 9.53	1.81
Mild	0.35- 9.47	3.48	0.448-13.61	4.65	0.22- 6.49	2.29	0.55- 13.52	5.20
Moderate	1.83-12.12	7.08	2.40 -17.66	9.35	1.00- 7.62	4.58	2.77- 18.73	10.64
Advanced	3.09-15.29	7.18	5.31 -21.93	9.91	2.12- 9.78	4.90	4.41- 23.24	10.34
Malignant	4.99-66.49	8.89	6.64 -90.56	10.77	3.13-42.85	5.82	7.71-117.36	13.24

Table 7

Estimated daily amount absorbed by dial painters, computed by various methods, and sorted by latest diagnosis

Latest X ray or clinical diagnosis	Power function $0.30\ t^{-0.44}$		Three exponentials		Power function $0.20\ t^{-0.35}$		Power function $0.54\ t^{-0.52}$	
	Range	Median	Range	Median	Range	Median	Range	Median
	μCi	μCi	μCi	μCi	μCi	μCi	μCi	μCi
Negative	0.000- 0.849	0.018	0.000- 0.858	0.019	0.000-0.544	0.011	0.000- 1.004	0.021
Minimal	0.000- 0.407	0.064	0.000- 0.420	0.073	0.000-0.261	0.040	0.000- 0.481	0.077
Mild	0.024- 0.599	0.174	0.027- 0.596	0.206	0.016-0.387	0.112	0.029- 0.704	0.219
Moderate	0.044- 0.803	0.343	0.062- 0.949	0.418	0.028-0.516	0.224	0.054- 0.948	0.412
Advanced	0.104- 1.388	0.279	0.147- 1.754	0.294	0.065-0.876	0.177	0.125- 1.664	0.330
Malignant	0.265-12.418	0.441	0.261-10.674	0.461	0.167-8.076	0.281	0.318-14.502	0.523

410 μCi (Finkel et al., Hasterlik, 1969a). On the other hand, the computed maximum radium body burdens at the end of the injection period for these same four patients ranged from 16.9 to 26.5 μCi (Finkel et al., 1969a), amounts that are generally higher than those given in table 6 for the dial painters who developed radium-induced malignant disease.

The radiobiological indices evaluated here for 207 radium dial painters, to date, set lower limits on the observed radium-induced malignancies in respect to the various "dose" parameters discussed. Such lower limits, based on individual measurements rather than on the mean values for the affected patients noted earlier, would have these values:

Measured radium burden after at least 35 years	0.6 μCi
Estimated maximum (i.e. peak initial)burden	5.0 μCi
Total amount of radium absorbed from the gut	130.0 μCi

These levels can roughly be used to establish the probability of developing a radium-induced malignancy in the population already studied. It would appear that none of those now negative radiographically will develop a malignancy attributable to radium, while one of the 21 persons now classified as having minimal changes may be so affected eventually. For the mild group, 40% of the patients now have indices that fall within the range of the malignant group, while for the moderate group this proportion ranges from 44 to 78%, depending upon the index used. The group with advanced changes practically overlaps with the malignant group and might be expected to have a high likelihood of developing radium-induced neoplasm.

These admittedly crude probability estimates reinforce our conviction that the patients in the high risk groups should be maintained under reasonably close medical surveillance as long as they are alive and as long as it is feasible to do so. For these reasons, the present study cannot be considered closed, and the data and conclusions presented here are still somewhat tentative.

The sarcomas in radium-bearing patients, arising in connective tissue in or adjacent to bone and the carcinomas arising in epithelial tissue lying in close opposition to bone, especially in such sites as the mastoids, paranasal sinuses, and gingival tissues, have been described. Their pathogenesis is not difficult to envisage, although "dose" calculations at the site of neoplastic change are at present imprecise and may not be meaningful. A recent analysis of death certificate data and of hospital records of former radium dial painters summarized in our recent study (Miller et al., 1969), and who may or may not have been studied by us according to our methods, disclosed that the incidence of central nervous system tumours was significantly higher than could be expected in this small population group. The specific tumour types and body burdens, where known, are listed in table 8. Of the four patients dying of central nervous system tumours, only two had been seen by us and the total body burden of ^{226}Ra determined, and in one the terminal body burden was 0.16 μ g ^{226}Ra and in the other 0.012 μ g.

Central nervous system tumours in the past have not been considered to be sequelae of radium deposition in man. Not, until recently, was attention focused on the mastoid, paranasal sinus, and gingival tumours. A rough estimate of the incidence of the central nervous system tumours in our group of dial painters in the 43-year period since the cessation of significant exposure to radium would indicate that it approaches between 25 and 50 times the expected incidence. Intracranial neoplasms following roentgen ray therapy of acromegaly have been described by Goldberg et al. (1963).

Table 8

Central nervous system tumours

Patient No.	Diagnosis and date of death	Terminal body burden of ^{226}Ra and date of measurement	Period from last significant radium exposure to date of tumour diagnosis
03-408	Glioblastoma multiforme frontal lobe Died 8.7.1959	0.16 μg ^{226}Ra 9.25.1957	33 years
03-507	Malignant acoustic neurinoma Died 11.14.1962	0.012 μg ^{226}Ra 2.26.1959	36 years
03-654	Glioma Died 2.1.1954	Not studied	Probably 26 years
03-768	Malignant astrocytoma Died 3.23.1964	Not studied	40 years

The body burdens observed for two of the patients with intracranial neoplasms in our series are well below that for other hithertofore described radium-related malignant tumours; in fact, one is a factor of 8 below the present permissible level. One can postulate that the present method of determining "body burden" which essentially measures radium deposited in the skeleton does not give an estimate of the quantity of radon and its daughter deposited in the lipid-rich cells of the central nervous system and in which, we propose, radon may be soluble by a factor considerably higher than in non-lipid-rich tissues. The "skeletal" body burden may not, therefore, reflect a comparable "dose" to the cells of the central nervous system.

All groups of radium-bearing patients in this country and abroad must be observed to confirm or refute whether the incidence of nervous system tumours in radium-bearing patients is in fact higher than expected in a comparable control population and whether these tumours are appearing at body burdens below the present permissible levels for ^{226}Ra.

Finally, it should be pointed out that the radiobiological indices discussed here are only one set of the many that can be used. Evans (1966) has proposed measures such as residual average skeletal rad/day, cumulative rads, cumulative μCi-years, cumulative rad-years, and others. Evaluations in terms of delivered dose to the entire skeleton have special problems, principally those concerned with the lack of knowledge of the precise duration of the induction and latent periods as well as of the precise volume of sensitive tissue and requires irradiation for malignant transformation. Furthermore, there is considerable evidence that radium deposition in the skeleton is highly non-uniform in its distribution so that the concentration of radium in bone varies widely even in persons who had acquired their burdens over a substantial ingestion period. This non-uniformity exists between major areas of the skeleton as well as on a microscopic level within each bone (Goldbert et al., 1963).

Despite these difficulties, we are currently evaluating our data for each patient in terms of daily dose rates and cumulative doses to the skeleton at selected times during and after exposure in an effort to illumine the problem. We hope that when these dose calculations are considered together with the indices presented here, some contribution will have been made in understanding the conditions of radium-induced carcinogenesis in man.

Conclusions

A mixed population of about 300 persons that acquired appreciable body burdens of radium 35 to 50 years ago has been followed by our group for the past 20 years. Radium was acquired by these patients by occupational exposure and from administration orally and intravenously by their physicians. To date, a number of these patients have developed fibrosarcomas and osteogenic sarcomas of skeletal tissues, carcinomas and sarcomas of the mastoids and paranasal sinuses, and serious blood dyscrasias. In many cases, analysis of the exposure history and of contemporary body burdens has enabled us to reconstruct the patterns of radium retention. From these computations, we have been able to analyse the appearance of neoplasms in terms of: (1) contemporary or terminal radium burdens, (2) estimated maximum (i.e. peak initial) radium burdens, and (3) estimated daily and total amounts of radium entering the blood stream during exposure. The ranges of values of these various indices that characterize the groups of patients with and without malignant disease and other disabling conditions can be used roughly to predict the likelihood of radiation carcinogenesis in these and similar patients.

The incidence of central nervous system tumours appears to be markedly higher than expected in our radium-bearing population. Another late and subtle effect of the deposition of ^{226}Ra in man may be at hand and points up the importance of careful clinical observation and epidemiological studies of all patients and groups bearing a body burden of ^{226}Ra significantly above background levels.

Acknowledgments

This work was supported by the United States Atomic Energy Commission. We wish to thank Mrs. Irene Sweet for her contributions to this investigation by her assistance in the tracing of patients, and the collection and organization of the data.

References

Aub, J.C., Evans, R.D., Hempelmann, L.H., and Martland, H.S. The late effects of internally-deposited radioactive materials in man. Medicine, 31, (3), 221, 1952.

Evans, R.D. The effect of skeletally deposited alpha-ray emitters in man. Br. J. Radiol., 39, 881, 1966.

Finkel, M.P., Bergstrand, P.J., and Biskis, B.O. The latent period, incidence, and growth of Sr^{90}-induced osteosarcomas in CF_1 and CBA mice. Radiology, 77, 269, 1961

Finkel, A.J., Miller, C.E., and Hasterlik, R.J. "Radium-induced malignant tumours in man", In: Delayed Effects of Bone-seeking Radionuclides, edited by C.W. Mays et al., University of Utah Press, Salt Lake City, p. 195, 1969a.

Finkel, A.J., Miller, C.E., and Hasterlik, R.J. "Radiobiological parameter in human cancers attributable to long-term radium deposition", In: Radiation-Induced Can International Atomic Energy Agency, Vienna, p. 183, 1969b.

Goldberg, M.B., Sheline, G.E., and Malamud, N. Malignant intracranial neoplasms following radiation therapy for acromegaly. Radiology, 80, 465-470, 1963.

International Commission on Radiological Protection. Report of Committee II on permissible dose for internal radiation (1959). Hlth Phys., 3, 1, 1960.

Looney, W.B., Hasterlik, R.J., Brues, A.M., and Skirmont, E. A clinical investigation of the chronic effects of radium salts administered therapeutically. Am. J. Roentgen., Radium Therapy and Nucl. Med., 73, 1006, 1955.

Maletskos, C.J., Keane, A.T., Telles, N.C., and Evans, R.D. "Retention and absorption of ^{224}Ra and ^{234}Th and some dosimetric considerations of ^{224}Ra in human beings", In: Delayed Effects of Bone-seeking Radionuclides, edited by C.W. Mays et al., University of Utah Press, Salt Lake City, p. 29, 1968.

Martland, H.S. The occurrence of malignancy in radioactive persons. Am. J. Cancer, 15, 2433, 1931.

Miller, C.E. "An experimental evaluation of multiple-crystal arrays and single-crystal techniques", In: Whole Body Counting, International Atomic Energy Authority, Vienna, p. 81, 1962.

Miller, C.E., and Finkel, A.J. Radium retention in man after multiple injections; the power function re-evaluated. Am. J. Roentgen. Radium Therapy and Nucl. Med. 103, 871, 1968.

Miller, C.E., Hasterlik, R.J., and Finkel, A.J. The Argonne Radium Studies; Summary of Fundamental Data. ANL-7531 and ACRH-106, 1969.

Norris, W.P., Speckman, T.W., and Gustafson, P.F. Studies of the metabolism of radium in man. Am. J. Roentgen., Radium Therapy and Nucl. Med., 73, 785, 1955.

Norris, W.P., Tyler, S.A., and Brues, A.M. Retention of radio-active bone seekers. Science, N.Y., 128, 456, 1958.

Schlundt, R., Nerancy, J.T., and Morris, J.P. Detection and estimation of radium in living persons. IV. Retention of soluble radium salts administered intravenously Am. J. Roentgen., Radium Therapy and Nucl. Med., 30, 515, 1933.

CHAPTER IX

LATE EFFECTS OF RADIATION FROM INTERNAL GAMMA AND BETA RAY EMITTERS

Arne Nelson

Introduction

The increasing amount of radioactive wastes from the peaceful use of atomic energy and the possibility of resumption of nuclear weapons tests make it necessary to prepare and discuss a current review of the late and subtle effects of exposure to ionizing radiation. The recommended MPD and MPC values* for radionuclides have often been calculated under simplified presumptions which only partially take into account all the complicated conditions of the uptake of the radionuclides. Repeated reconsiderations of the MPD and MPC values based on further radiobiological investigations of the late effects of internal contamination are, therefore, of the greatest importance. A survey of the literature provides us with a large amount of data on radioactivity in the air, in the water and in food, as well as in plants, animals, and man. This gives us good information on the presence, behaviour, and quantitative distribution of various radionuclides in the human sphere. The number of investigations on the late and gross effects of internal contamination with radionuclides is also great; the number of studies on such low concentrations that give no or only subtle effects is, however, limited. It is necessary to review the obvious late effects as a basis for a discussion of the most subtle effects observable.

In a review of this kind, the main emphasis must be laid on ^{90}Sr, ^{137}Cs and ^{131}I, which are the three most important fission products with regard to their appearance in the environment and their potential effect on the health of man, complemented with some other radionuclides of significance in fall-out and in research.

The Effect of the Radionuclides

Radiostrontium

Due to its relatively long physical half-life, its high and rapid uptake into the skeleton, and, its long retention time, ^{90}Sr is considered to be especially dangerous to man and his biosphere.

The critical organs are the skeleton, the bone marrow, and some tissues in close contact with the bone tissue. The circulation of ^{90}Sr in the body before fixation into the skeleton, while of short duration, is sufficient, however, to cause lesions to certain radiosensitive organs. The most obvious consequence, however, of internal contamination

---

* MPD = maximum permissible dose; MPC = maximum permissible concentration.

with ^{90}Sr is the development of malignant tumours in the bone tissue, i.e. osteosarcomas.

Mice

The induction of the osteosarcomas has especially been studied in mice (Cosgrove and Upton, 1962; Finkel et al., 1958, 1959, 1961; Finkel and Biskis, 1968; Nilsson, 1962). The development of the tumour starts, in the majority of cases, from endosteal cells or, in some cases, as islets from the reticular cells in the bone marrow; the former usually giving rise to osteoblastic, the latter to fibroblastic osteosarcomas (Nilsson, 1962). It is unanimously agreed that the tumours never originate from periosteal cells. The tumour buds, which often start simultaneously in several places, grow and fill up the bone-marrow cavity before they break through the bone.

The optimum dose for tumour induction varies with animal species. For mice 0.7 - 0.9 μCi/g body weight results in an incidence of 90 to 95% in both male and female mice (Finkel et al., 1958; Nilsson, 1962). No osteogenic sarcomas have been seen with 4.5 μCi/g or more and on the other end of the scale the tumour incidence after injections of 0.001 to 0.009 μCi/g was within the range found in the controls.

The latent time between the administration of ^{90}Sr and the appearance of a tumour in mice is variable. The induction time after an optimal tumour dose is on the average 240 to 270 days, the shortest time being 150 (Nilsson, 1962) to 168 days (Finkel et al., 1958) in CBA mice and 98 days in CF_1 mice (Finkel et al., 1958). Microscopically intra-medullary tumours, however, have been seen after 90 days (Nilsson, 1962). The most common localization of the tumours is the lower part of the femur and the upper part of the tibia, followed by the lumbar spine, the pelvis and the skull. The tumours induced by ^{90}Sr and other radionuclides are, with very few exceptions, osteosarcomas. The majority, about 80%, are osteoblastic and about 20% are fibroblastic. In single cases, angiosarcomas develop in the bone marrow cavity. In very rare cases, chondroblastic osteosarcomas are seen. The mucous membranes of the skull are subject to continuous irradiation from the underlying bone which may result in squamous cell carcinomas. The most common site seems to be the mucous membrane covering the palatine bone (Nilsson, 1968).

There is an obvious dose dependence. The tumour incidence decreases with decreasing dose. At 1.6 μCi/g, 33% of the animals developed carcinomas, at 0.3 μCi/g, 14% and at 0.4 μCi/g only 2.5%. The latency period was shorter in the highest dose group, 235 days, than in the other groups, 340 and 465 days respectively (Nilsson, 1968).

Leukaemia of the lymphatic type is also a long-term effect of ^{90}Sr. The optimal dose, which causes leukaemia in 10 to 12% of the exposed mice, seems to be only about half of the optimum osteosarcoma producing dose (Nilsson, to be published). A case of leukaemia after ^{85}Sr injections of 0.1 μCi/g twice a week, 7 to 8 times, has been reported (Watanabe, 1957, 1958). A dose of 0.2 μCi ^{90}Sr/g increased the incidence of thymic lymphosarcomas but did not increase the incidence of myeloid leukaemia. Other leukaemias also increased in numbers and occurred earlier (Cosgrove and Upton, 1962).

Apparent effects of ^{90}Sr on testes in mice have been seen after 0.1 - 0.7 μCi/g body weight. The testes weight decreases and there is a temporary inhibition of the spermat genesis (Henricson et al., 1962). The effects of 0.7 μCi ^{90}Sr/g correspond to about 12 R (Henricson and Nilsson, 1964, 1967). The weight of the testes was still significantly decreas after 60 days. After 0.7 μCi/g body weight, an increased rate of development of oocytes intc follicles and of those into later follicular stages has been observed (Henricson and Nilsson,

1965). The possibility of a certain lethal effect on young oocytes cannot be excluded. The oocytes of mouse embryos are extremely sensitive to ^{90}Sr (Rönnbäck, personal communication).

The question of a possible genetic effect of ^{90}Sr is of great importance. In some investigations (Lüning et al., 1963, 1965) the intra-uterine mortality was increased in progeny of ^{90}Sr-treated fathers when compared to saline-treated controls. This was considered to be due to disturbances in the pre and peri-meiotic phases of spermatogenesis.

Rats

The carcinogenic effect of ^{89}Sr and ^{90}Sr in rats has been demonstrated by several investigators (Baxter and Tuttle, 1962; Boegler and Kriegel, 1968 a, b; Budkov and Strel'tsova, 1959; Cassarett et al., 1961; Kuzma and Zander, 1957; Thomas and Scott, 1968). A total of 1.0 and 0.5 μCi $^{89}Sr/g$ in ten daily doses induced malignant tumours in 60% of the animals, mainly bone tumours, but also squamous cell carcinomas of the snout. After total doses of 330 μCi to 790 μCi of ^{90}Sr per rat, a high incidence of osteosarcomas, an increased incidence of certain soft tissue malignant tumours including leukaemia, and facial skin carcinomas were observed within about 5 months (Cassarett et al., 1961).

At a dose of 0.15 μCi of $^{90}Sr/g$, which is regarded to be the lower limit for induction of bone tumours, seven leukaemias (five lymphocytic, two myelogenous) among 160 rats were observed (Boegler and Kriegel, 1968a, b). With a body burden of 0.2 μCi/g through inhalation no life-span shortening was observed but several cases of leukaemia were noted. With a body burden of 0.75 μCi/g, 50% of the animals developed osteosarcomas (Thomas and Scott, 1968).

After single and chronic administration by way of the gastrointestinal tract, with doses not greater than 100 to 1,000 MPC, haematopoiesis was inhibited with marked pathological regeneration and leukosis (Strel'tsova and Moskalev, 1957). After doses as low as 1.5 pCi/g of ^{90}Sr, which is calculated to give an accumulated dose of 10 to 20 mrads, a reduced cellularity in the bone marrow has been reported (Stokke et al., 1968).

A dose of 0.4 μCi/g induced morphological changes in the ovaries which was expressed as cell destruction, increased follicular dimensions, reduced corpora luteae and increased connective tissue to to 8 months after injection. Functional changes appeared before the morphological ones (Vorozheikina, 1961).

Microscopic and functional changes have been observed in the pancreatic islets after exposure to ^{89}Sr and ^{90}Sr (Khomutovskii, 1966).

Rabbits

Radiation-induced osteosarcomas develop in rabbits (Downie et al., 1959) and are localized in the growing ends of their long bones and in the bone surrounding the maxillary and mandibular teeth. Several cases of squamous cell carcinomas of the external auditory meatus have been observed after single ^{90}Sr doses of 0.2 to 0.6 μCi/g given at the age of 5 to 8 weeks (Sissons and Vaughan, 1960). In no instance was a true leukaemia blood picture seen though a white cell count of 27,000 per mm^3, without an increase of abnormal white cells, was found in a rabbit (Downie et al., 1959).

The data reported so far from studies performed on mice, rats and rabbits indicate that there is a potential hazard of ^{90}Sr to man, but the obvious differences between man and small laboratory animals with respect to body size, life-span, size of bone and other physiological features preclude a direct extrapolation. Several extensive large animal studies using dogs or miniature swine have, therefore, been carried out at the University of Utah, the Argonne National Laboratory, the University of California at Davis, and the Battelle Northwest Laboratories at Hanford, Washington.

Swine

An extensive series of investigations in swine carried out at Hanford has been reported (Clarke and colleagues, 1959, 1960a, b, c, 1967; McClellan and colleagues, 1961, 1964, 1965, 1966). The study was initiated in 1958 in order to ascertain the biological effect of daily ingestion of ^{90}Sr in miniature swine. During the course of this continuing experiment, a total of 718 animals representing three generations have been exposed to ^{90}Sr in their food at levels ranging from 1 to 3,100 μCi/day of ^{90}Sr. At ingestion levels of 25 μCi or less per day for 7 to 10 years, except for those swine developing leukaemia, no definite changes were observed in the formed elements of the blood. The cumulative skeletal radiation dose received by these animals ranged from 300 to 14,000 rads. At levels greater than 25 μCi/day, there was a progressive decline in the number of leukocytes and platelets and a terminal precipitous drop in red blood cells which was associated with a platelet loss.

Radiographic surveys of the skeletons of the swine fed 1 to 25 μCi/day have failed to reveal definite osseous changes.

By 1967, i.e. after 9 years, 53 (7%) of the ^{90}Sr fed swine had developed haemic or lymphatic disorders, of which 35 (67%) have been myeloproliferative and 18 (33%) lymphoproliferative. The lowest dose level in the parent generation in which a case of lymphoproliferation was observed was at the 5 μCi/day level. In the offspring of ^{90}Sr fed swine, three cases of lymphoproliferation, however, have appeared at the low level of 1 μCi/day. The leukaemogenic process observed in the swine of this experiment in certain respects mimics the spontaneous leukaemias occurring in man and animals, especially the myelosclerosmyeloid metaplasia-granulocytic leukaemia syndrome.

Bone tumours have developed thus far in five of the swine fed 125 μCi ^{90}Sr/day since conception. Four of the five also exhibited granulocytic leukaemia.

Dogs

The long-term ^{90}Sr feeding programme in dogs at Davis has been extensively reported (Andersen and colleagues, 1963, 1964 a, b, 1965 a, b). The feeding levels were between 0.007 and 3.33 μCi ^{90}Sr/g Ca.

One case of soft tissue neoplasm (lymphosarcoma) at the highest ingestion level caused death at 827 days of age. At the two highest dose levels, the animals continued to show depressed leukocyte values for some $1\frac{1}{2}$ years after ^{90}Sr feeding stopped. No decrease in erythrocytic elements or thrombocytes has been observed.

In contrast to the results reported from the Davis programme, a great number of osteosarcomas was observed in the Argonne National project (Biskis et al., 1964) when 0.05 μCi ^{90}Sr/g was given to dogs in one injection or in daily injections throughout one year. Leukaemia, however, was not observed among the 45 dogs so treated. On the other hand, no osteosarcomas had appeared among 39 dogs that had received 0.015 μCi/g in 278 divided injections, but one had died from chronic myeloid leukaemia and another had died with acute reticulosis. These cases are particularly interesting because myeloid leukaemia is very rare in dogs.

The Argonne results were confirmed particularly by similar investigations at the University of Utah (Dougherty and colleagues, 1962, 1964). After a single injection of 0.1 μCi/g in 14 dogs, six developed osteosarcomas, two haemangiosarcomas in the skeleton, and one squamous cell carcinoma in the gingiva.

At the Lovelace Foundation beagle dogs have been exposed by inhalation to aerosols of $^{90}SrCl_2$ resulting in initial body burdens ranging from 0.0028 to 0.28 μCi/g. One dog, with an initial body burden of 0.082 μCi/g, died 585 days after exposure with leukaemia of the acute type (McClellan and Rupprecht, 1967). Dogs which have received acute exposure to ^{90}Sr have shown a large number of neoplasms but no haematopoietic tissue neoplasms in contrast to miniature swine. On the other hand, some animals with chronic exposure to moderate radiation dose rates from ^{90}Sr starting early in life, have developed haematopoietic tissue neoplasms (McClellan, 1966).

Several investigators in the U.S.S.R. have reported effects of ^{90}Sr on the functional activity of the central nervous system in dogs (Klimova and Alekseeva, 1960; Nazarov, 1962). They found in the early stages a disturbance of higher nervous activity which was partially restored when the administration of ^{90}Sr was stopped. In one investigation, female dogs received a total amount of 0.140 μCi/g of ^{90}Sr prior to parturition. This dose does not cause signs of radiation sickness in the irradiated dogs but produces the development of functional disturbances in the cerebral cortex of the offspring of these animals both in the first and second generation. Disturbances of the conditioned reflex activity, reactivity of the organism, and external behaviour were qualitatively of the same type in the first and second generation.

Disturbances in the spermatogenesis have also been reported (Burykina and Trusova, 1963; Trusova, 1956). After administration of ^{90}Sr with food in amounts of 0.02 or 0.2 μCi/kg/day during 24 to 40 months, the first changes in the spermatogenesis were found after 5 to 12 months and consisted of an instability in the functional activity of the glands and an increase in the number of atypical forms of spermatozoa. A consistent inhibition of spermatogenesis was observed after 14 months. No recovery could be observed 2 years after the interruption of the administration of ^{90}Sr.

Sheep

In contrast to the results reported in dogs, there seems to be a remarkable ability of recovery of spermatogenesis in sheep. When 31.5 mCi of ^{90}Sr was intravenously administered to a ram, the sperm cells were dead between the forty-fifth and the fifty-second day. Eight weeks after administration, the sperm cell picture was normal (Åberg and Gillner, 1966).

Monkeys

After the imbibition of 500 or 1,000 μCi of ^{90}Sr, only one of seven rhesus monkeys survived 80 months. One died of osteosarcoma, one of chondrosarcoma, one of monocytic leukaemia, and the others of haematopoietic tissue damage (Cassarett et al., 1961). In another investigation, monkeys (Macaca mulatta) of varying age and sex were exposed to irradiation by ^{90}Sr deposited skeletally for time periods ranging from $3\frac{1}{2}$ to $6\frac{1}{2}$ years

(Tuttle, 1967). The animals are currently receiving radiation doses at a calculated dose rate ranging from 80 to 1,200 rads per year. Minimal changes have been noted at the extremities of the long bones in some animals. The minimal changes did not correlate with dose rate or cumulative dose and indicate a high degree of variability in radiosensitivity of individual animals.

No chromosome aberrations in cultured peripheral lymphocytes that could be definitely attributed to radiation injury were found in preparations from ^{90}Sr treated animals, which had received doses from 100 to 4,000 rads over time periods of 2 to 6 years (Tuttle, 1967).

Man

The human data for ^{90}Sr are limited to investigations on luminous-dial painters. One complicating factor in these studies is that the paints used contain not only ^{90}Sr but also ^{226}Ra, which, of course, makes it impossible to separate the effects of the two radionuclides.

In a Czech investigation (Müller and colleagues, 1961, 1966), a follow-up was made of 103 workers, in a luminizing industry, who had used a paint containing up to 1.2 mCi ^{90}Sr/g of paint as well as a small amount of ^{226}Ra. The highest body burden of ^{90}Sr was estimated to be on the order of tens of microcuries.

Haematological studies revealed signs of alteration or stimulation of erythropoiesis, such as reticulocytosis and hyperplasia of the erythroblast series in bone marrow. A comparison of the exposed group with a control group of 100 healthy prospective blood donors showed significantly higher haematocrit, haemoglobin, and erythrocyte values in the exposed group.

There was a significant increase in the occurrence of aneuploid cells in the exposed group. A significant number of chromosomal aberrations could be detected in patient carrying body burdens higher than 10% of the maximum permissible level. According to the investigator, however, no conclusions could be drawn at present as to the validity of present-day, internationally agreed upon maximum permissible body burden.

Yttrium

Yttrium-90, as well as yttrium-91, induces osteogenic tumours in mice (Finkel et al., 1964) and rats (Litvinov, 1958). Quite unlike the usually rapid growth of ^{90}Sr-induced osteogenic sarcomas, there is a slow growth and a semblance of healing during the early stages of tumour evolution when injected ^{90}Y is the carcinogen. These differences might be associated with the presence and then the absence of continuing irradiation, since ^{90}Y has a half-life of only 64 hours.

Mice

In mice, different kinds of malignant tumours have been observed after intramuscular and subcutaneous administration of 1.5 to 10 μCi of ^{91}Y (Finkel et al., 1956; Lisco et al., 1956).

Rats

Osteogenic sarcomas developed in more than 50% of the rats after intraperitonea injection of 0.6 μCi ^{91}Y/kg (Litvinov, 1958).

After chronic irradiation of rats by the addition of ^{90}Y (91 to 410 μCi/day) to their drinking water, there was a remarkable paucity of tumours of the gastrointestinal tract. Only one adenocarcinoma of the colon was observed. Several tumours of the uterus and the oral region were observed (Sullivan et al., 1963).

Calcium

Investigations in rats have demonstrated that ^{45}Ca is able to produce osteogenic sarcomas. It is, however, not so effective as ^{89}Sr (Kuzma and Zander, 1957). It appears that the ^{45}Ca osteogenic sarcoma has a "benign" phase for some significant period of time. In the ^{89}Sr-induced tumours, it is not quite the same, and it appears that the borderline between repair and neoplasia is much sharper and narrower. Squamous cell carcinomas have not been seen after ^{45}Ca, which is apparently not of sufficient energy to cause radiation-induced carcinomas in mucosa closely aligned to bone tissue.

Caesium

The effect of radiocaesium could be expected to be similar to that of external irradiation.

Mice

A relatively consistent concentration of ^{137}Cs in testes (Nelson et al., 1961) seems to cause some injury. In mice, the sexual activity of the male decreased after 4 μCi ^{137}Cs/g with a diminished number of spermatogonia, a decreased pregnancy (insemination) rate and smaller litter sizes. The testes gradually recovered to about 90% of their normal state by the seventieth day of observation (Tamura, 1965a, b). Disturbances in the development of germ cells occurred in mice slightly, but obviously, even at doses of 0.05 μCi/g.

Histopathological changes such as atrophy and pyknosis of cells in the liver, but not in the spleen or kidney, were noticed after a dose of 1 μCi/g (Kameta et al., 1962).

There was a significant increase of post-natal deaths among the offspring of mice which had been given a dose of 2 μCi/g of ^{137}Cs on the fourth day of pregnancy (Tabuchi et al., 1962).

Rats

After a dose of 0.05 μCi/g body weight in rats giving a calculated dose of less than 10 rads to the animal, the "Germ Cell Tubulus Ratio of the Testis" was calculated. A diminution of this ratio of each type of germ cells was slight but statistically significant with the exception of sperm cells. The exception was the sperm cells which kept a stationary level of 90 to 100% throughout the observation period (Kitabatake, 1961).

The activity of serum GPT*, but not of GOT*, was increased after 0.16 μCi/g in rats (Stojadinovic and Jovanovic, 1966).

---

* GPT = glutamic pyruvic transaminase; GOT = glutamic oxaloacetic transaminase.

Man

A man ingested, by accident, a solution containing about 4 mCi of ^{137}Cs. The changes in the human organs and system seemed to develop slowly. No acute or subacute effects were observed, this apparently being due to the low dose of the ingested element. After about 6 months, the man developed symptoms of the vegetative nervous system. The blood values changed. The leucocyte count decreased, due to a fall in the granulocyte values, as well as in the lymphocyte values. Eosinopaenia was also observed. The thrombocyte values remained normal. The man was working one year later, but his working capacity was decreased (Fateeva et al., 1960).

Iodine

Radioisotopes of iodine, especially ^{131}I, are the dominating risks in the first few weeks after a nuclear detonation within an area affected by radioactive fall-out. It might possibly be of concern in accidents associated with a nuclear reactor.

Iodine compounds of various kinds, which reach the gastrointestinal tract or the lungs, are to a great extent taken up by the blood and accumulated in the thyroid glands. A high concentration of ^{131}I in the gland could be expected to cause permanent damage or even malignant transformation of the thyroid tissue. The epithelial cells of the thyroid seem to be extremely radioresistant so long as they do not divide. Doses near the level that will cause necrosis are required to affect the function of the thyroid. The reproductive integrity of the thyroid epithelium is much more sensitive. The high proliferation rate of the thyroid epithelium of young animals makes it more sensitive to radioiodine than that of adult animals.

Mice

A dose of about 3,000 rads to adult CBA mice causes a significant decrease of the volume of the thyroid epithelium within one year after the exposure. Doses of about 10,000 rads practically stop the epithelial regeneration of the gland whereas much higher doses are required to give corresponding effects in growing animals and fetuses (Walinder, 1969).

Rats

Investigations in rats have shown that there is no gross difference in response to goitrogens after administration of ^{131}I in weanling and adult animals (Doniach, 1957). The post-natal metabolism of radioiodine administered pre-natally has also been studied. Alterations in the thyroid physiology, notably a low thyroid reserve, has been induced in animals after administration of iodine at dose levels which produce little or no other changes (Sikov, 1965).

Thyroid adenomas have been observed in several rat experiments with Wistar rats, but only in Long Evans rats have malignant tumours been observed after single ^{131}I injections. After three monthly doses of 10 μCi of ^{131}I, benign thyroid nodules or adenomas were observed in 39% of the rats and papillary carcinomas of low-grade malignancy were observed in 3 of 49 female rats. The incidence of thyroid neoplasms was lower in the females than in males (Lindsay et al., 1963).

Sheep

An extensive investigation was carried out at Hanford in order to find out the biological effects of chronically administered ^{131}I in sheep. The feeding levels ranged from 0.005 to 1,800 μCi/day (Bustad and colleagues, 1955, 1957, 1958, 1962, 1963; Hackett et al., 1960; Horstman and colleagues, 1959, 1961; Marks and Bustad, 1963). Observations made over a period of 10 years have been reported.

No damage was observed in adult ewes fed 0.15 μCi/day for 4 years or in their offspring fed 0.15 μCi/day for 5 years. This feeding level resulted in a thyroid dose of about 3 rads/week. After 10 years, however, a thyroid adenoma appeared in one ewe fed on this level. This finding was regarded as a reflection of the naturally occurring incidence in these sheep since thyroid adenomas had been observed in aged control ewes previously. A thyroid carcinoma was observed in an animal fed 1.5 μCi ^{131}I/day for 7 years. A depression of thyroid ^{131}I uptake occurred in all sheep fed 5.0 μCi/day or more, and in some sheep fed 0.5 to 5.0 μCi/day. Two ewes fed 1.5 μCi/day for $4\frac{1}{2}$ years manifested thyroid tumours at autopsy. The accumulated thyroid dose was estimated to be between 5,000 and 10,000 rads.

Six of seven sheep fed 5 μCi/day throughout their lifetime developed thyroid tumours. A decrease in PBI* values was the first change in a blood constituent that could be attributed to ^{131}I feeding at all levels above 5 μCi/day. This effect was then followed by an increase in creatinine values in all sheep receiving above the 15 μCi level. A depression in leukocyte count was observed at all high levels. No thyroidal, histological, or functional changes occurred in sheep at less than a calculated 600 rads of exposure to ^{131}I.

Swine

Swine fed 5 μCi ^{131}I/day for 3 years, including ^{131}I exposure in utero and in milk during the suckling period, showed no evidence of thyroid damage; but after 5 years feeding, the mean thyroid weights were less than one-half that of the controls (Bustad et al., 1963; Horstman et al., 1961).

Man

The thyroid gland in adult man does not appear to be an especially radiosensitive organ. Among the great number of patients who have been treated with ^{131}I since the end of the 1940's, no case of cancer of the thyroid has been reported, except for a single invasive adenoma in a 9 year old girl (Sheline et al., 1962). In order to disturb significantly the function of a healthy thyroid gland in an adult man, a dose of more than 5,000 rads is required. The developing thyroid gland is, however, much more radiosensitive and more extensive damage can be observed than in the adult thyroid with the same dose.

The report from the medical survey of the people of Rongelap and Utirik Islands 11 and 12 years after exposure to fall-out radiation attracted great attention (Conard et al., 1967). Thyroid abnormalities were not observed until 1963, when an exposed girl, who had reached the age of 10 years, was found to have a nodule in her thyroid. In 1964, two further nodules were observed in two other 10 year old girls. These two cases were diagnosed as benign adenomatoid goitres. The abnormalities were considered to be caused by the exposure of the thyroid to radioiodine from the fall-out and from the external total-body gamma radiation. The doses to the thyroid glands of the children were calculated to be between 700 and 1,400 rads from radioiodine, and, in addition, there was 175 rads total-body exposure from gamma radiation. No nodules were found in unexposed children.

---

* PBI = protein-bound iodine.

By 1966, the number of thyroid abnormalities had increased to eighteen; 16 cases with nodules and two with hypothyroidism. It is noteworthy that in the higher exposure group thyroid abnormalities occurred in 79% of the children exposed at less than 10 years of age, as compared with no cases in the children of the lower exposure or unexposed group. Only one adult in the lower exposure group developed a thyroid nodule. Several nodules were noted in the thyroid glands of older Utirik inhabitants and unexposed adults of Rongelap. Surgery was performed in 11 cases. Nine children and one adult were found to have adenomatous goitres, and one adult a mixed papillary and follicular carcinoma of the thyroid gland with localized metastasis. Correlation of growth retardation in exposed children with thyroid pathology was indicated by recent findings of definite hypothyroidism in two boys with most retardation of growth. There was subsequent resumption of growth with thyroid hormone treatment.

Man, like most mammals, appears to react similarly to the mice with regard to the radiation inhibited regeneration of the thyroid epithelia. Patients who have been treated with various ^{131}I doses and who, during the period immediately after the treatment, have been euthyroid, develop after a period of time a hypothyroidism which increases in frequency with the time after treatment. One significant exception to this rule appears to be the Long Evans rat. In these animals, even after rather high doses, the weight of the thyroid is only slightly altered by the irradiation exposure. The Long Evans rat appears, however, to be the only mammalian species in which a single dose of ^{131}I to the adult can induce thyroid cancer. The reason for the induction of thyroid cancer after a single dose of ^{131}I in Long Evans rats may only depend on the fact that thyroid growth is inhibited substantially in all other species.

It is obvious, however, that induction of tumours is not the only problem in this connection. The experience gained at Rongelap also indicates that relatively small doses of radioiodine in combination with external total-body irradiation can damage the thyroid tissue in children to such a great extent that the production of hormone will be insufficient to give a normal body growth.

Cerium

Mice

Cerium (^{144}Ce), like yttrium (^{90}Y and ^{91}Y), produces sarcoma of the skeletal system in mice, primarily in the long bones. Leukaemia has also been observed in one study in a group of mice which had received 0.3 μCi of ^{144}Ce/g body weight twice a week intratracheally (Watanabe, 1957, 1958). The fertility of mice, but not of their offspring, was affected by 0.5 μCi/g (Lisco et al., 1961).

Rats

In rats, after intratracheal insufflation of $^{144}CeF_3$, bronchogenic carcinomas have been observed (Cember et al., 1959; Cember, 1963; Cember and Stemmer, 1964). At the lowest dose level, 0.5 μCi, the first death due to a lung tumour, a lymphosarcoma, occurred 528 days after exposure. The radiation dose to the lungs was calculated to be 600 rads.

Liver tumours have also been reported after parenteral administration of various doses of ^{144}Ce. The incidence of neoplasms was proportional to the quantity of ^{144}Ce and the time of their occurrence was inversely proportional to the dose. The lowest dose used was

0.005 μCi/g (Strel'tsova, 1961). Neoplasms were also induced in the gastrointestinal tract after doses of 9 to 18 μCi/g of ^{144}Ce. Adenomas, papillomas, leiomyomas, sarcomas, and carcinomas were also seen. The most frequent site of tumours was the large intestine (Lebedeva, 1963).

Rabbits

After intra-tracheal administration of a dose of 25 μCi $^{144}CeF_3$ to rabbits, lung tumours were found in 30%of the animals (Krushakova and Ivanov, 1963).

Dogs

After inhalation of ^{144}Ce-^{144}Pr particles by dogs with initial depositions of 0.05 to 2.2 mCi, only a decreased lymphocyte count and a slight neutrophil depression were observed. No clinical or biochemical changes were observed 21 months after a deposition of up to 0.9 mCi (Stuart, 1964; Stuart et al., 1964).

Doses of ^{144}Ce as low as 25 μCi/kg body weight given intravenously can induce bone tumours in dogs. The time of appearance seems to be related to the dose (Fritz et al., 1967).

Ruthenium

Six months after an injection of 1.4 μCi ^{106}Ru/g of body weight in mice, an increased density of the long bones has been observed on radiographs which resembles the changes characteristically seen in mice treated with carcinogenic doses of bone-seeking radioelements (Walton and Brues, 1954).

After peroral administration to rats of ^{106}Ru for 100 days with daily doses of 1.6 μCi to 800 μCi, i.e. 10 to 5,000 times the MPC, a chronic lesion, which was observed, was characterized by colonic ulcers and bleedings in other organs such as kidneys, uterus, mammae and lungs (Strel'tsova and Moskalev, 1957).

Rabbits, which had received daily doses of 3.9 μCi ^{106}Ru/kg, were observed for 22 months. No outward signs of disease appeared. Disorders of the erythropoiesis, myelopoiesis and changes in the lymphoid system were, however, found (Beloborodova and Baranova, 1959).

Zirconium

In mice, apparent histological changes were recognized in the spleen and lymph nodes after 1 μCi or 3 μCi of ^{95}Zr. Some changes remain after 2 months only in the liver (Fukunda, 1961).

The late effects in dogs of small quantities of ^{95}Zr (0.2 μCi/kg daily) administered with food for 17 months have also been reported. Disturbances of the haematopoietic system were noted. The impaired functions of the leuko and myelopoiesis were not restored even 16 months following the cessation of ^{95}Zr administration (Tikhaya, 1959).

Sulphur

After weekly intra-tracheal insufflations of 375 μCi of ^{35}S in the form of

$BaSO_4$ particles, rats developed severe squamous metaplasia and bronchogenic squamous cell carcinomas. Since the insufflated dose corresponded to an atmospheric concentration which was only 900 times the recommended MPC, it has been suggested that a more conservative value should be considered for exposure to ^{35}S (Cember and Watson, 1958).

Phosphorus

Mice

In mice given ^{32}P twice weekly, 7 to 16 times as many cases of leukaemia developed as in controls at an average rate of 17.4%. In such cases, the total dose of ^{32}P was from 14.1 to 98 μCi. The survival time was between 175 and 602 days after the start of administration. The incidence of leukaemia was nearly parallel to the dose delivered. However, no leukaemia was seen in animals given less than 1.0 μCi/g (Hirose, 1959; Watanabe, 1957). A leukaemogenic effect of ^{32}P has also been seen in adult females and foetally exposed male and female mice (Holmberg et al., 1964).

The administration of ^{32}P to mice on the eighth day of pregnancy in doses of 2 to 20 μCi/g of maternal body weight exerts selective and permanent disturbances to the highly sensitive central nervous system of the foetuses. It was found that with doses of more than 15 μCi/g foetal death occurred in all cases. From 24% to 66% of all embryos with doses ranging from 2 to 15 μCi/g died and morphologic anomalies occurred in 25% to 47% (Kameyama, 1961).

Rats

A very high incidence of tumours, about 40%, was observed in rats after a single dose of 4.5 μCi of ^{32}P/g, with an average latent period of 290 days, and after repeated doses of 1.5 μCi/g, an average latent period of 165 days. The majority of the tumours were osteogenic sarcomas but squamous cell carcinomas were also observed (Koletsky, 1950). After such a small dose as 0.031 μCi/g body weight in rats, the dynamics of changes of white blood cells resembled those after external radiation with a progressive fall of leukocyte and especially lymphocyte counts in the third and fourth week (Dienstbier and Vitek, 1960). Morphological changes in rats have been reported (Reiher and Lang, 1955) after 1.2 μCi ^{32}P/g but not after 0.3 and 0.6 μCi/g. A daily dose of 2 μCi of ^{32}P for a year changed the estrous cycle; the number of maturing follicles decreased, and in many the ova perished at various stages of development (Dobrovolskii, 1964).

Tritium

Thymidine labelled with tritium, or with ^{14}C, when incorporated into DNA of proliferating cells produces a selective mode of irradiation of cells and cell nuclei. Single and multiple injections of radioactive thymidine have been found to shorten life-span and to produce an increased incidence of tumours in mice. The incidence of rare tumours was particularly increased while tumours that are relatively frequent in the breed of mice used, such as lung tumours and lymphomas, showed a shorter induction time (Baserga et al., 1962, 1966; Lisco et al., 1961). After administration of 1 μCi of ^3H/g of body weight into newborn, 2 months old, 6 to 7 months old, and 12 to 14 months old mice, a significant increase in the tumour rate was observed among the exposed animals in comparison with the controls. In the 12 to 14 months group, 43 of 84 dead animals had tumours of different kinds, thymic lymphoma, non-thymic disseminated lymphoma, salivary gland tumours, carcinomas of the skin, lungs and liver. Labelling of embryos in utero with tritiated thymidine likewise increased the incidence of malignant tumours. Dose levels of 0.1 μCi of ^{3}H-thymidine or of 0.02 μCi of ^{14}C-thymidine/g body weight have so far failed to show an increased incidence of tumours but the death rate was noticeably higher in the latter group.

In one investigation, lymphoid leukaemia but no other leukaemias or malignant tumours appeared after administration of 0.3 μCi of ^{3}H-thymidine/g body weight (Méwissen, 1965).

All the results of investigations on the effects of ^{3}H-thymidine are, however, not in accord. In one investigation at Brookhaven National Laboratory, no significant increase either in tumour incidence or in mortality rate has been observed at levels of 1 μCi or 5 μCi/g of ^{3}H (Johnson and Cronkite, 1966, 1967).

Carbon-14

Besides the above-mentioned investigation (Baserga et al., 1962), a study of the effects of the incorporation by the mouse embryo of high levels of ^{14}C (100 or 175 μCi/g) using sodium formate-^{14}C has been carried out. The litters produced were normal in all respects when compared with litters from non-radioactive controls. When mice that had received ^{14}C during their embryonic development were mated, no evidence was obtained of a lowered fertility.

Cobalt

Cobalt is a part of the organic complex of vitamin B_{12} and is a microelement which participates in haemopoiesis by assisting in erythropoiesis. This property of stable cobalt makes the study of its radioisotope particularly interesting when considering the effect of ionizing radiation on the haematopoietic processes.

After daily administration of 150 μCi of ^{60}Co/kg body weight to rates before, during, and after pregnancy, the level of radioactivity in the new-born rats was 0.03 to 0.07 μCi/kg. The number of young rats in the litter, duration of pregnancy, weight, and their general condition and development were normal (Beloborodova et al., 1963).

In rabbits which had received 1.25 μCi of ^{60}Co/kg of body weight, an impairment of lymphopoiesis was expressed as a retardation of lymphocyte maturation. Under ordinary experimental conditions that treatment does not produce an absolute decline of lymphocyte numbers in the peripheral blood. Lymphopenia was detected by functional stress which also revealed impairment of erythropoiesis (Beloborodova, 1963).

Summary of the late effects

It is obvious from a review of the research reported, that the late effects of internal contamination with radionuclides in general are dose-dependent not only with regard to the magnitude of effects but also as to the variety of effects.

Carcinogenic effects

Considering the carcinogenic effects, there seems, however, to be an optimum dose. When the dose is too high, the life-span will be too short to allow for development of malignant tumours. After too low a dose, no tumours will be observed due to the very low incidence or possibly a threshold value.

The most effective carcinogenic dose varies with animal species. With ^{90}Sr the optimum dose for osteosarcomas in mice is ~ 0.8 μCi/g of body weight which produces a tumour incidence of 90 to 95%. The comparable dose in rats is 0.4 μCi/g, and in the dog 0.15 μCi/g (Finkel and colleagues, 1959, 1961, 1968; Nilsson, 1968). One reason for the decrease in the optimum carcinogenic dose with size of the animal is the relatively long range of the β radiation from ^{90}Sr-^{90}Y. A greater part of the radiant energy is absorbed within the bone tissue in the animals with a large skeleton. It has been calculated that 32% of the radiation is absorbed by bone tissue in mice, 54% in rats, 79% in dogs, and 88% in man (Parmley et al., 1962).

Doses higher than the optimum carcinogenic dose seem to produce epithelial cell carcinomas in the mucous membranes of the head due to the close contact between bone tissue and the mucous membranes. Doses lower than for the optimum carcinogenic effect induce higher incidences of leukaemias. No osteogenic sarcoma has been seen in mice at 4.5 μCi ^{90}Sr/g of body weight or more, and on the other end of the scale the tumour incidence after injection of 0.001 to 0.009 μCi/g was within the range of the controls (Finkel et al., 1958).

Carcinomas

Squamous cell carcinomas in the soft tissues of the head have been observed in mice, rats, and rabbits after high doses of ^{90}Sr but not after ^{45}Ca, apparently due to the lower energy of the radiation from the latter (Cassarett et al., 1961; Kuzma and Zander, 1957; Nilsson, 1968; Sissons and Vaughan, 1960).

After chronic irradiation of rats by addition of ^{90}Y (91 to 410 μCi/day) to their drinking-water, a remarkable paucity of tumours, originating from the gastrointestinal tract, has been noted. Only one adenocarcinoma of the colon after ^{90}Y in drinking-water to rats has been noted (Sullivan et al., 1963).

A number of thyroid abnormalities have been observed after internal contamination with ^{131}I. But very few of them have been malignant (vide supra). In mice, no malignant thyroid tumour has been observed and in rats only the Long Evans strain develop thyroid carcinomas (Doniach, 1957; Lindsay et al., 1963; Walinder, 1969). In sheep, one single case of thyroid carcinoma has appeared. And in man only two cases have been reported; one adult from the Marshall Islands in a group with an estimated dose of only 69 rads, had a mixed papillary and follicular carcinoma, and a 9 year old girl had what has been called an invasive adenoma (Conard, 1967; Sheline et al., 1962).

Insufflation of ^{144}Ce and ^{35}S in rats has caused bronchiogenic carcinomas (Cember and colleagues, 1958, 1959, 1963, 1964). Different kinds of malignant tumours have, however, been seen in the gastrointestinal tract after 9 to 18 μCi/g of Ce (Lebedeva, 1963). A squamous cell carcinoma in rats after treatment with ^{32}P has been noted (Koletsky et al., 1950). Different kinds of malignant tumours, among other carcinomas of the skin, lungs, and liver, have been observed in mice after ^{3}H-labelled thymidine (1 μCi ^{3}H/g body weight) (Baserga et al., 1962, 1966; Lisco et al., 1947; Méwissen, 1965).

Osteosarcomas

The optimum dose for osteosarcoma production in mice is ~ 0.8 μCi/g of ^{90}Sr (Finkel and colleagues, 1961, 1964, 1968; Nilsson, 1962). In higher dose groups, the osteoblastic osteosarcomas predominate, and in the lower dose groups the fibroblastic osteosarcomas (Nilsson, 1962). In rats, osteosarcomas are observed in 50 to 60% of the animals at dose levels of 0.5 to 1.0 μCi/g of ^{90}Sr (Kuzma and Zander, 1957). In rabbits, multiple osteosarcomas are noticed after 8 to 11.8 μCi of ^{90}Sr daily (Downie et al., 1959).

In the larger animals, osteosarcomas are rarer. Thus, in swine only a few osteosarcomas developed in a group fed 125 μCi $^{90}Sr/g$ daily since conception (Clarke and colleagues, 1959, 1960a, b, c, 1967; McClellan and colleagues, 1961, 1962, 1963, 1964, 1965, 1966, 1967). In dogs, osteosarcomas have been observed when 0.05 μCi/g in a single injection (Biskis et al., 1964).

After imbibition of 500 or 1,000 μCi of ^{90}Sr, single cases of osteosarcoma and chondrosarcoma have been observed in monkeys (Cassarett et al., 1961). In mice, osteosarcomas have appeared after administration of 1.5 μCi ^{90}Y and in rats after 0.6 μCi/g (Finkel et al., 1956; Lisco et al., 1956; Litvinov, 1958). There seems, however, to be a slower growth rate of osteosarcomas induced by radioyttrium. Similarly, it appears that ^{45}Ca induced osteogenic sarcomas in rats have a "benign" phase for some significant period of time (Kuzma and Zander, 1957). After ^{144}Ce osteosarcomas have been seen in mice and after doses of 25 μCi/kg body weight in dogs (Lisco et al., 1947). A high incidence of osteogenic sarcomas was observed in rats after a single dose of 4.5 μCi/g of ^{32}P (Koletsky et al., 1950).

Leukaemia

Due to the apparent relation between radiation and leukaemia in man, the leukaemogenic effects of internal contamination of radionuclides are of special importance and interest. In mice, the rate of leukaemia of the lymphatic type increased after doses of ^{90}Sr above about 0.1 μCi/g (Nilsson, unpublished; Watanabe, 1958). Also, in rats at doses above 0.15 μCi/g an increased rate of leukaemia, lymphatic as well as myelogenous, has been observed (Boegler and Kriegel, 1968 a, b). In rabbits, no true case of leukaemia has been reported (Downie et al., 1959).

In swine, leukaemogenesis after ^{90}Sr feeding mimics in certain respects the spontaneous leukaemias in man. Granulocytic leukaemias have been observed after feeding levels of 125 μCi ^{90}Sr/day. But lympho-proliferation appeared at as low levels as 1 μCi/day (Clarke and colleagues, 1959, 1960a, b, c, 1967; McClellan and colleagues, 1961, 1962, 1964, 1965, 1966, 1967). In dogs, a few cases of haematopoietic tissue neoplasms have been observed after chronic exposure to ^{90}Sr, for example, one case of chronic myeloid leukaemia, one of lymphosarcoma, and one of acute leukaemia (Anderson et al., 1965a; Dougherty, 1962, 1964). The acute leukaemia developed after a low initial body burden of 0.082 μCi/g (McClellan, 1967). Monocytic leukaemia and haematopoietic tissue damage have been noticed in monkeys after imbibition of 500 to 1,000 μCi ^{90}Sr (Cassarett et al., 1961). Caesium-144 has induced leukaemia in one case in a group of mice after repeated intra-tracheal administration of 0.3 μCi/g (Watanabe, 1957, 1958). The incidence of leukaemia has also increased in mice after administration of 1.0 μCi/g of ^{32}P (Hirose, 1959; Holmberg et al., 1964; Watanabe, 1957).

Dose levels of 0.1 μCi of ^{3}H-thymidine or of 0.02 μCi of ^{14}C-thymidine/g have failed to increase the tumour incidence in mice, but after 1 μCi/g of ^{3}H at least 50% of the animals died from various kinds of tumours (Baserga et al., 1962, 1966; Lisco et al., 1961). After 0.3 μCi/g of ^{3}H-thymidine, only the incidence of lymphoid leukaemia appeared to be increased (Méwissen, 1965).

Other haematopoietic disorders

Haematopoiesis in the bone marrow was inhibited in rats after doses not greater than 100 to 1,000 MPC of ^{144}Ce, ^{106}Ru, and ^{89}Sr and ^{90}Sr (Strel'tsova and Moskalev, 1957). Also, the cellularity in the bone marrow after such low doses as 1.5 pCi ^{90}Sr/g was stated to be reduced (Stokke et al., 1968). In man, luminous-dial painters who had used a paint containing ^{90}Sr, as well as ^{226}Ra, showed higher haematocrit, haemoglobin, and erythrocyte values. There was a significant increase in the occurrence of aneuploid cells in the exposed group, and in those of them carrying body burdens higher than 10% of the maximum permissible level an increase in the occurrence of chromosomal aberrations was observed (Müller and colleagues, 1961, 1966). A technician in the U.S.S.R. who ingested 4 mCi of ^{137}Cs developed a leukopaenia after 6 months (Fateeva et al., 1960).

After inhalation of 0.05 to 2.2 mCi of ^{144}Ce-^{144}Pr, only a depression in leukocyte values was observed in dogs (Stuart, 1964; Stuart et al., 1964). The haematopoiesis in rabbits was affected after 3.9 μCi ^{106}Ru/kg per-orally (Beloborodova and Baranova, 1959). Also, after ^{95}Zr, disturbances in the haematopoiesis were seen in mice after 1 to 3 μCi and in dogs after 0.2 μCi/kg daily (Fukunda, 1961; Tikhaya, 1959). A reduction in lymphopoiesis was observed at 1.25 μCi ^{60}Co/kg body weight in rabbits (Beloborodova, 1963).

Non-malignant changes in different organs

Gonads

Changes in the testes weight and spermatogenesis, as well as the development of oocytes into follicles and a certain lethal effect on young oocytes, have been observed in mice after 0.7 μCi ^{90}Sr/g (Henricson and Nilsson, 1962, 1965, 1966, 1967). Morphological changes in ovaries were observed in rats after 0.4 μCi ^{90}Sr/g (Vorozheikina, 1961). An inhibition of spermatogenesis was observed in dogs after daily administration of 0.02 or 0.2 μCi ^{90}Sr/kg/day for 14 months and no recovery was seen 2 years after the cessation of treatment (Burykina and Trusova, 1963; Trusova, 1956).

A diminution of germ cell ratio and injuries in development of germ cells have been observed in rats after such a low dose of 0.05 μCi/g (Kameta et al., 1962; Kitabatake, 1961). After 0.05 μCi/g of body weight of ^{137}Cs disturbances in the development of germ cells occurred (Kameta et al., 1962; Kitabatake, 1961).

The fertility of female mice was affected by 0.5 μCi of ^{144}Ce/g of body weight (Kulikova, 1960). Morphological changes in the ovaries of rats have been seen after 1.2 μCi ^{32}P/g but not after 0.3 μCi/g (Reiher and Lang, 1955).

Liver

The GPT activity in serum was increased in rats after 0.16 μCi ^{137}Cs/g (Stojadinovic and Jovanovic, 1966). Histopathological changes in the liver of mice after a dose of 1 μCi of ^{137}Cs/g (Kameta et al., 1962) and after a daily dose of 0.2 μCi ^{95}Zr/kg of body weight (Fukunda, 1961) in their food have been observed, and liver tumours occurred after parenteral administration of ^{144}Ce down to as little as 0.005 μCi/g of body weight in rats (Strel'tsova, 1961).

Pancreas

Changes in the pancreatic islets from radiostrontium have been reported in rats

(Khomutovskii, 1966).

Thyroid

Benign thyroid nodules or adenomas caused by radioiodine have been reported in different animal species and man (vide supra). In sheep no changes occurred at less than 600 rads of ^{131}I, and in man the thyroid abnormalities were caused by external irradiation and internal contamination with calculated doses of 700 to 1,400 rads from radioiodine and 175 rads from gamma radiation.

Skeleton

In monkeys which had received a radiation dose ranging from 80 to 1,200 rads/year from ^{90}Sr minimal changes were noted at the extremities of the long bones by radiography (Tuttle, 1967). An increased density of the long bones in mice was noted after 1.4 μCi ^{106}Ru/g of body weight (Walton and Brues, 1954).

Central nervous system

Disturbances of higher nervous activity of dogs have been observed after ^{90}Sr also in the offspring when the mother got a total amount of 0.14 $\mu Ci/g$ of ^{90}Sr (Nazarov, 1962). The Soviet technician, who by accident imbibed 4 mCi of ^{137}Cs, developed symptoms after 6 months from the vegetative nervous system. He was working one year after the accident but his working capacity was diminished (Fateeva et al., 1960).

Comments

Internal contamination with high doses of β- and γ-emitting radionuclides will, in man and other mammals, cause serious acute injuries ending in death. Lower doses, though not producing acute effects, will result in a shortening of life-span in relation to the dose. The life-span shortening is a complex picture of morphological and functional changes. Within the higher dose range, the carcinogenic effect is most apparent, especially after bone-seeking radionuclides.

The majority of the studies, however, have been carried out within the carcinogenic dose range. But at doses below 0.01 μCi ^{90}Sr/g of body weight, the tumour incidence is within the control range in mice. The testes weight is decreased after 0.1 μCi ^{90}Sr/g in mice but no lower dose has been used.

In the bone marrow, which is the most sensitive indicator, the cellularity is still decreased more than 1 year after the administration of 0.2 μCi ^{90}Sr/g in mice. In rats, a hyperplasia of the haematopoietic tissue of the bone marrow has been observed 13 to 23 months after 0.1 μCi ^{90}Sr/g but all the animals died within 2 years. In another investigation, reduced cellularity was said to be observed in rats 6 to 12 weeks after injection of as little as 1.5×10^{-3} μCi ^{90}Sr/kg (!) leading to accumulated doses of 10 to 20 mrads. It is, however, very likely that a mistake has been made in the reporting and in the calculations, since this dose is within the range of variation of the natural background radiation.

The lowest dose of ^{137}Cs reported to give an effect is 0.05 $\mu Ci/g$ in rats causing diminution of germ cell ratio and injuries in development of germ cells (Kameta et al., 1962; Kitabatake, 1961).

The thyroid is very radioresistant and to obtain functional disturbances such as hypothyroidism which may lead to retarded growth in the young, very high doses of radiation are required, i.e. approximately 500 rads X rays and on the order of 3,000 rads from ^{131}I in rodents. Human studies indicate that there is a similar effect in man.

The obvious effects of ^{90}Sr on the foetal gonads and the very strong indication that ^{90}Sr could cause genetic damage is a serious sign of warning and calls for an expansion of the research work on this topic.

Special attention must be directed towards the increasing use of ^{3}H and ^{14}C-labelled organic compounds in biomedical research. Dose levels of 0.1 μCi of ^{3}H-thymidine and of 0.07 μCi of ^{14}C-thymidine/g body weight have so far failed to show an increase in tumour rate, but great amounts of new, labelled organic compounds may in the future be used which through their localization in the DNA may cause great and unanticipated damage.

An enormous amount of work on the late effects of radionuclides in man and animals has been carried out as can be seen from the reference list. This does not pretend to be complete. All the cited reports, however, deal with the effects of single radionuclides. In the future, it will be necessary to carry out experiments with combinations of radionuclides since an amplified effect might well be expected as has happened with other combinations of injurious agents in man and animals.

References

Åberg, G., and Gillner, M. Radiostrontium, radiophosphorus, stable strontium, stable calcium, DNA and DNA-P in ram spermatozoa. Acta physiol. scand., 66, 106-114, 1966.

Anderson, A.C., and Gee, W. The effects of continued Sr^{90} ingestion during the growth period of the beagle and its relation to Ra^{226} toxicity. Blood values in Sr^{90} fed beagles at one year of age. Sixth Annual Progress Report, University of California, School of Veterinary Medicine, Davis, California, UCT-108, 1963.

Andersen, A.C., and Gee, W. The effects of continued Sr^{90} ingestion during the growth period of the beagle and its relation to Ra^{226} toxicity. Hematology report. Seventh Annual Progress Report, University of California, School of Veterinary Medicine, Davis, California, UCT-472-110, 1964a.

Andersen, A.C., and McKelvie, D.H. The effects of continued Sr^{90} ingestion during the growth period of the beagle and its relation to Ra^{226} toxicity. Pathology report. Seventh Annual Progress Report, University of California, School of Veterinary Medicine, Davis, California, UCT-472-110, 1964b.

Andersen, A.C., and Gee, W. The effects of continued Sr^{90} ingestion during the growth period of the beagle and its relation to Ra^{226} toxicity. Hematology report. Eighth Annual Progress Report, University of California, School of Veterinary Medicine, Davis, California, UCT-472-112, 1965a.

Andersen, A.C., and McKelvie, D.H. The effects of continued Sr^{90} ingestion during the growth period of the beagle and its relation to Ra^{226} toxicity. Pathology report. Eighth Annual Progress Report, University of California, School of Veterinary

Medicine, Davis, California, UCD-472-112, 1965b.

Baserga, R., Lisco, H., and Kisieleski, W. Further observations on induction of tumours in mice with radioactive thymidine. Proc. Soc. exp. Biol. Med., 110, 687-690, 1962.

Baserga, R., Lisco, H., and Kisieleski, W. Tumor induction in mice by radioactive thymidine. Radiat. Res., 29, 583-596, 1966.

Baxter, R.C., and Tuttle, L.W. The effect of x-irradiation and of morbidity on strontium-90 absorption and retention by rats. University of Rochester Report, UR-617, 1962.

Beloborodova, N.L., and Baranova, E.F. Effect of continuous peroral administration of radioactive ruthenium on the blood formation. U.S.A.E.C. Technical Information Service Report AEC-tr-3794, 1959.

Beloborodova, N.L. Changes in hemopoiesis during prolonged internal administration of ^{60}Co. The Toxicology of Radioactive Substances, 2, 44-60, 1963.

Beloborodova, N.L., Viktorova, V.L., and Red'kina, E.K. Hemopoiesis in the offspring of rats which have undergone prolonged ^{60}Co administration. The Toxicology of Radioactive Substances, 2, 61-73, 1963.

Biskis, B.O., Finkel, M.P., and Greco, I.L. Myelogenous leukemia and acute reticulosis in beagles after Sr^{90}. Radiat. Res., 22, 169, 1964.

Boegler, F., and Kriegel, H. Leukämoide Reaktion nach 90-Strontium-Inkorporation bei Ratten. Blut, Z. Schr. für die gesamte Blutforschung, 17, 345-350, 1968a.

Boegler, F., and Kriegel, H. Strahlenspätschaden nach 90-Strontium-Inkorporation bei Ratten. Deutsche Gesellschaft für Biophysik e.v. Österreich. Gesellschaft für reine und angewandt Biophysik. Gemeinsame Jahrestagung, Baden bei Wien, 1968b.

Budkov, L.N., and Strel'tsova, V.N. The influence of single and prolonged access to the rat organism of radioactive strontium through the gastrointestinal tract. Med. Radiol., 4, # 2, 20-29, 1959 (in Russian).

Burykina, L.N., and Trusova, N.E. Changes in spermatogenic function of dogs in chronic injury by strontium-90. Radiobiology, U.S.S.R., 3, # 3, 59-69, 1963 (English translation).

Bustad, L.K., George, L.A., Marks, S., Warner, D.E., Barnes, C.M., Herde, K.F., and Kornberg, H.A. Biological effects of I^{131} chronically administered to sheep. Hanford Atomic Products Operation, Richland, Report HW-38757, 1955.

Bustad, L.K., George, L.A., Warner, D.E., Barnes, C.M., Herde, K.F., and Kornberg, H.A. Biological effects of I^{131} continuously administered to sheep. Radiat. Res., 6, 380-413, 1957.

Bustad, L.K., George, L.A., Marks, S., Clarke, W.J., Seigneur, L.J., Horstman, V.G.,

Barnes, C.M., Hackett, P.L., and Kornberg, H.A. Biological effects of I^{131} in sheep and swine. Radiat. Res., 9, 97-98, 1958.

Bustad, L.K., Cable, J.W., Casey, H.W., Horstman, V.G., Kerr, M.E., and McKenney, J.R. Biological effects of I^{131} in sheep and swine. Hanford Atomic Products Operation, Richland, Report HW-72500, 1962.

Bustad, L.K., Horstman, V.G., Elefson, E.E., Wood, D.H., Ragan, H.A., Marks, S., and Clarke, W.J. Biological effects of radioiodine in sheep and swine. Hanford Atomic Products Operation, Richland, Report HW-76000, 1963.

Cassarett, G.W., Tuttle, L.W., and Baxter, R.C. Pathologic effects of ingested strontium-90 in rats and monkeys. University of Rochester, Report UR-597, 1961.

Cember, H., and Watson, J.A. Bronchogenic carcinoma from radioactive barium sulfate. A.M.A. Arch. Indust. Health, 17, 230-235, 1958.

Cember, H., and Watson, J.A., and Spritzer, A.A. Bronchogenic carcinoma from radioactive cerium fluoride. A.M.A. Arch. Indust. Health, 19, 14-23, 1959.

Cember, H. Further studies on lung cancer from $Ce^{144}F_3$. Hlth Phys., 9, 539-544, 1963.

Cember, H., and Stemmer, K. Lung cancer from radioactive cerium chloride. Hlth Phys., 10, 43-48, 1964.

Clarke, W.J., McKenney, J.R., Hackett, P.L., Horstman, V.G., and Bustad, L.K. Strontium metabolism and toxicity. Hanford Atomic Products Operation, Richland, Report HW-62638, 1959.

Clarke, W.J., and McKenney, J.R. Biological effects of Sr^{90} in miniature swine. I. Experimental designs and preliminary observations. Hanford Atomic Products Operation, Richland, Report HW-63499, 1960a.

Clarke, W.J., McKenney, J.R., Hackett, P.L., Horstman, V.G., and Bustad, L.K. Strontium metabolism and toxicity. Hanford Atomic Products Operation, Richland, Report HW-63643, 1960b.

Clarke, W.J., McKenney, J.R., McClellan, R.O., Hackett, P.L., Horstman, V.G., and Bustad, L.K. Strontium metabolism and toxicity. Hanford Atomic Products Operation, Richland, Report HW-66306, 1960c.

Clarke, W.J., Howard, E.B., and Hackett, P.L. Sr-90 induced neoplasia in swine (haematopoietic, lymphocytic, and bone tumors in Sr-90 swine). Report BNWL-SA-1418, 1967.

Conard, R.A., Meyer, L.M., Sutow, W.W., Robertson, J., Rall, J.E., Robbins, J., Jesseph, J.E., Deisher, J.B., Hicking, A., Lanwi, I., Gusmano, E.A., and Eicher, M. Medical survey of Rongelap and Utirik islands eleven and twelve years after exposure (March 1965 and March 1966). Brookhaven National Laboratory, Upton, Report BNL-50029 (T-446), 1967.

Cosgrove, G.E., and Upton, A.C. Some late effects of radiostrontium in RF male mice.

J. nucl. Med., 3, 293-299, 1962.

Dienstbier, Z., and Vitek, F. Peripheral blood changes after internal irradiation. I. The effect of the radiophosphorus P^{32}. Sb. lék., 62, 173-184, 1960 (in Czech).

Dobrovolskii, L.A. Change in the sexual cycle and the trend of ^{32}P concentration in the ovaries during repeated administration of small quantities of the isotope. Akush. Ginek., 5, 153-154, 1964 (in Russian).

Doniach, I. Sensitivity of the weanling rat thyroid to radiation. Br. J. Cancer, 11, 253, 1957.

Dougherty, T.F., Stover, B.J., Dougherty, J.H., Jee, W.S.S., Mays, C.W., Rehfeld, C.E., Christensen, W.R., and Goldthorpe, H.C. Studies of the biological effects of Ra^{226}, Pu^{239}, Ra^{228} ($MsTh_1$), Th^{228} (RdTh) and Sr^{90} in adult beagles. Radiat. Res., 17, 625-681, 1962.

Dougherty, T.F. (editor). Research in radiobiology. Annual report of work in progress on the chronic toxicity program. Injection tables. I. Toxicity animals. E. Strontium-90. University of Utah, College of Medicine, Radiobiological Division of the Department of Medicine, Report COO-119-229, 1964.

Downie, E.D., MacPherson, S., Ramsden, E.N., Sissons, H.A., and Vaughan, J. The effect of daily feeding of ^{90}Sr to rabbits. Br. J. Cancer, 13, 408-423, 1959.

Fateeva, M.N., Klimov, V.S., Ponizovskaya, A.I., Gorbaraenko, N.I., Sokolov, V.V., and Smirnova, M.I. The effect of radioactive cesium (Cs^{137}) on the human organism. Med. Radiol., 5, 14-19, 1960.

Finkel, M.P., Lisco, H., Lathrop, K.A., and Brues, A.M. Toxicity of locally deposited yttrium-91 in mice. I. Experimental design and gross pathology. Argonne National Laboratory Report ANL-5655, 1956.

Finkel, M.P., Bergstrand, P.J., and Biskis, B.O. Consequences of the continuous ingestion of Sr^{90} by mice. I. Experimental design and results up to 200 days. Argonne National Laboratory, Biol. and Med. Res. Div., Report ANL-6093, 1958.

Finkel, M.P., Bergstrand, P.J., and Biskis, B.O. Latency and growth of osteosarcomas induced by radiostrontium. Argonne National Laboratory, Biol. and Med. Res. Div., Report ANL-6264, 1959.

Finkel, M.P., Bergstrand, P.J., and Biskis, B.O. The latent period, incidence, and growth of ^{90}Sr-induced osteosarcomas in CF_1 and CBA mice. Radiology, 77, 269-281, 1961.

Finkel, M.P., Jinkins, P.B., and Biskis, B.O. The radiographic evolution of osteogenic sarcomas induced in mice by Y^{90}. Proc. Am. Ass. Cancer Res., 5, 18, 1964.

Finkel, M.P., and Biskis, B.O. Experimental induction of osteosarcomas. Prog. exp. Tumor Res., 10, 72-111, 1968.

Fritz, T.E., Norris, W.P., Rehfeld, C.E., and Poole, C.M. Cerium-144 toxic manifestations in beagle dogs. Argonne National Laboratory Report ANL-7409, 1967.

Fukunda, R.Z. Patho-histologic observations of various mouse organs internally radiated with minimum Zr^{95}. U.S.A.E.C. Technical Information Service Report AEC-tr-4482, 1961.

Hackett, P.L., Galgraith, T.A., Bennett, C.A., and Bustad, L.K. Changes in blood constituents in sheep following prolonged daily administration of iodine. Am. J. vet. Res., 21, 775-781, 1960.

Henricson, B., Knudsen, O., and Nilsson, A. The effect of radiostrontium on mouse testes. Acta radiol., 58, 52-64, 1962.

Henricson, B., and Nilsson, A. Chromosome investigations on the embryo progeny of male mice treated with ^{90}Sr. Acta Radiol. ther. Phys. Biol., 2, 315-320, 1964.

Henricson, B., and Nilsson, A. Effect of radiostrontium on oocytes and follicles of adult mice. Acta Radiol. ther. Phys. Biol., 3, 296-304, 1965.

Henricson, B., and Nilsson, A. Compared effects of radiostrontium and roentgen rays on germ cells of male mice. Acta Radiol. ther. Phys. Biol., 4, 26-32, 1966.

Henricson, B., and Nilsson, A. Effects of radiostrontium and roentgen rays on germ cells of male mice. Acta Radiol. ther. Phys. Biol., 6, 209-213, 1967.

Hirose, P. Pathological study on late effects of internal irradiation by P^{32} on the hematopoietic tissue of mice. J. Hiroshima Med. Ass., 7, 1941-2000, 1959.

Holmberg, E.A.D., Dosne de Pasqualini, C., Arini, E., Pavlovsky, A., and Rabasa, S.L. Leukemogenic effect of radioactive phosphorus in adult and fetally exposed BALB mice. Cancer Res., 24, 1745-1748, 1964.

Horstman, V.G., Persing, R.L., Hackett, P.L., Marks, S., McKenney, J.R., Clarke, W.J., and Bustad, L.K. Biological effects of I^{131} in sheep and swine. Hanford Atomic Products Operation, Richland, Report HW-69500, 1961.

Johnson, H.A., and Cronkite, E.P. Effect of tritiated thymidine on mortality and tumor incidence in mice. Radiat. Res., 27, 64, 1966.

Johnson, H.A., and Cronkite, E.P. The effect of tritiated thymidine on mortality and tumor incidence in mice. Radiat. Res., 30, 488-496, 1967.

Kameta, K., Katayama, K., and Kiyota, T. Studies on radioactive cesium. III. A histopathological study on injuries by Cs^{137} in organs of the mouse, particularly in testis. Kumamoto med. J., 15a, 90-91, 1962.

Kameyama, Y.O. Experimental anomaly of fetus produced by P^{32} internal radiation. U.S.A.E.C. Technical Information Service Report AEC-tr-4482, 1961.

Khomutovskii, O.A. Structural and functional disturbances of the pancreas islands of Langerhans in animals suffering from radiation sickness induced by radioactive strontium. Radiobiologiya, 6, 214-218, 1966.

Kitabatake, T. Spermatogenesis of rats injected with radioactive cesium-137. J. radiat. Res. (Japan), 2, 124-130, 1961.

Klimova, E.N., and Alekseeva, O.G. Certain features peculiar to the development of radiation affection in dogs in chronic action of Sr^{90}. Med. Radiol., 5, 3-7, 1960.

Koletsky, S., Bonte, F.J., and Friedell, H.L. Production of malignant tumors in rats with radioactive phosphorus. Cancer Res., 10, 129-138, 1950.

Kulikova, V.G. The effects of incorporated cerium-144 on the fertility of mice and the development of their offspring. Trudy Inst. biol.Sverdlovsk , 12, 34-45, 1960.

Kurshakova, N.N., and Ivanov, A.E. A model of experimental lung cancer caused by intra-tracheal introduction of radioactive cerium. Bull. exp. Biol. Med. U.S.S.R., 54, 787-793, 1963 (Eng. translation).

Kuzma, J.F., and Zander, G. Cancerogenic effects of Ca^{45} and Sr^{89} in Sprague-Dawley rats. Archs. Path., 63, 198-206, 1957.

Lebedeva, G.A. Data on the study of gastro-intestinal tumors induced by radioactive cerium (Ce^{144}). Arkh. Patol., 25, 40-44, 1963.

Lindsay, S., Potter, G.D., and Chaikoff, I.L. Radioiodine-induced thyroid carcinomas in female rats; induction by low doses of radioiodine. Archs. Path., 75, 8-12, 1963.

Lisco, H., Finkel, M.P., and Brues, A.M. Carcinogenic properties of radioactive fission products and of plutonium. Radiology, 49, 361-363, 1947.

Lisco, H., Finkel, M.P., and Brues, A.M. Local tumors following injection of $Y^{91}PO_4$. Argonne National Laboratory, Biol. and Med. Res. Div., Quarterly Report ANL-5518, 1956.

Lisco, H., Baserga, R., and Kisieleski, W.E. Induction of tumors in mice with tritiated thymidine. Nature, Lond., 192, 571-572, 1961.

Litvinov, N.N. Morphological changes in the bones of rats affected by radioactive yttrium-91. Med. Radiol., 3, 41-50, 1958.

Lüning, K.-G., Frölén, H., Nelson, A., and Rönnbäck, C. Genetic effects of strontium-90 injected into male mice. Nature, Lond., 197, 304, 1963.

Lüning, K.-G., Frölén, H., Rönnbäck, C., and Nelson, A. Further studies of the genetic effects of ^{90}Sr on various stages of the spermatogenesis in mice. A preliminary report. FOA 1 Internal Report C 1164-F17, 1965.

Marks, S., and Bustad, L.K. Thyroid neoplasms in sheep fed radioiodine. J. natn. Cancer Inst., 30, 661-674, 1963.

McClellan, R.O., Clarke, W.J., Hackett, P.L., Vogt, G.S., and Bustad, L.K. Biological effects of Sr^{90} in miniature swine. First progress report. II. Clinical observations. Hanford Atomic Products Operation,Richland, Report HW-69500, 1961.

McClellan, R.O., McKenney, J.R., Casey, H.W., Case, A.C., Dockrum, N.L., Vogt, G.S., and Bustad, L.K. Biological effects of Sr^{90} in miniature swine. Second progress report. Hanford Atomic Products Operation, Richland, Report HW-72500, 1962.

McClellan, R.O., Vogt, G.S., Clarke, W.J., McKenney, J.R., and Bustad, L.K. Biological effects of Sr^{90} in miniature swine. Third progress report. Hanford Atomic Products Operation, Richland, Report HW-76000, 1963.

McClellan, R.O., Clarke, W.J., Vogt, G.S., Ragan, H.A. Palotay, J.L., and Bustad, L.K Biological effects of Sr^{90} in miniature swine. Progress report. Hanford Atomic Products Operation, Richland, Report HW-80500, 1964.

MoClellan, R.O., Clarke, W.J., Palotay, J.L., Ragan, H.A., and Vogt, G.S. Biological effects of ^{90}Sr in miniature swine. Hanford Atomic Products Operation, Richland, Report BNWL-122, 1965.

McClellan, R.O. Hematopoietic tissue neoplasms in animals administered ^{90}Sr. Hlth Phys. 12, 1362-1365, 1966.

McClellan, R.O., and Rupprecht, F.C. (editors). Annual report of the fission product inhalation program 1966-1967. Section I: Dose-effect studies. Toxicity of inhaled $^{90}SrCl_2$ in beagle dogs. Lovelace Foundation, Albuquerque, Report LF-38, 1967.

Méwissen, D.J. Induction de leucémies chez la souris C57 BL au moyen de thymidine tritiée. Cot. r. Séanc. Soc. Biol., 159, 1005-1007, 1965.

Müller, J., David, A., Rejskova, M., and Brezikova, D. Chronic occupational exposure to strontium-90 and radium-226. Lancet, 2, 129-131, 1961.

Müller, J., Klener, V., Tuscany, R., Thomas, J., Brezikova, D., and Houskova, M. Study of internal contamination with strontium-90 and radium-226 in man in relation to clinical findings. Hlth Phys., 12, 993-1006, 1966.

Nazarov, V.A. Deviations of higher nervous activity in second generation of dogs subjected to chronic internal irradiation with Sr^{90} beta rays. U.S.A.E.C. Technical Information Service Report AEC-tr-5429, 1962.

Nelson, A., Ullberg, S., Kristoffersson, H., and Rönnbäck, C. Distribution of radiocesium in mice. An autoradiographic study. Acta radiol., 55, 374-384, 1961.

Nilsson, A. Strontium-90 induced bone and bone-marrow changes. An Experimental Study with Special Reference to the Histogenesis and Histopathology of Osteosarcomas. Almqvist and Wicksell, Uppsala, Sweden, 1962.

Nilsson, A. Pathologic effects of different doses of ^{90}Sr in mice. Development of carcinoma in the mucous membranes of the head. Acta Radiol. ther. Phys. Biol., 7, 27-41, 1968.

Nilsson, A., and Henricson, B. The effect of ^{90}Sr on the ovaries of the fetal mouse. Proc. of the symposium on Radiation Biology and Fetal and Juvenile Mammal, Richland, May 5-8, 1969.

Nilsson, A. Pathologic effects of different doses of ^{90}Sr. Dose effect relationship in ^{90}Sr-induced bone tumors. To be published.

Parmley, W.W., Jensen, J.B., and Mays, C.W. Skeletal self-absorption of beta-particle energy. Some Aspects of Internal Irradiation, Pergamon Press, New York, 1962.

Reiher, K.H., and Lang, G. Zur Frage der schädigenden Wirkung von P^{32} auf das Ovargewebe. Strahlentherapie, 98, 453-463, 1955 (in German).

Rönnbäck, C. Personal communication, 1969.

Sheline, G.E., Lindsay, S., McGormack, K.R., and Galante, K. Thyroid nodules occurring late after treatment of thyrotoxicosis with radioiodine. J. clin. Endocr. Metab., 22, 8, 1962.

Sikov, M.R. The pre-natal and post-natal sequellae of the intrauterine administration of ^{131}I in the rat. Final technical report June 1, 1963-February 28, 1965. AEC Report TID-22767, 1965.

Sissons, H.A., and Vaughan, J. Ear tumours in rabbits receiving strontium-90. Nature, Lond., 185, 399-401, 1960.

Stojadinovic, S., and Jovanovic, M. Activity of transaminases in the rat serum after internal contamination with ^{137}Cs and ^{90}Sr. Strahlentherapie, 131, 633-636, 1966, (in English).

Stokke, T., Oftedal, P., and Pappas, A. Effects of small doses of radioactive strontium on the rat bone. Acta Radiol. ther. Phys. Biol., 7, 321-329, 1968.

Strel'tsova, V.N., and Moskalev, Ju. I. Late effects of single and chronic gastro-intestinal administration of radioactive isotopes (^{144}Ce, ^{106}Ru, $^{89,90}Sr$). Med. Radiol., 2, 23-34, 1957 (in Russian).

Strel'tsova, V.N. Liver tumors developing under the influence of cerium-144. Report JPRS-9963, pp. 12-21. (Translation from Arkh. Patol., 23 (1961), pp. 9-16.)

Stuart, B.O. Whole-body retention and biological effects of inhaled ^{144}Ce-^{144}Pr and ^{106}Rh oxides in beagles. Hanford Biology Research Annual Report, BNWL-122, 1964.

Stuart, B.O., Casey, H.W., and Bair, W.J. Acute and chronic effects of inhaled $^{144}CeO_2$ in dogs. Hlth Phys., 10, 1203-1209, 1964.

Sullivan, M.F., Marks, S., and Thompson, R.C. β-irradiation of rat intestine. Long-term studies after daily yttrium-90 ingestion. Am. J. Path., 43, 527-537, 1963.

Tabuchi, A., Kinutani, K., Nkagawa, S., Hirata, M., Fujiwara, T., Yoshinaga, H., and Antoku, S. Fetal disturbances due to irradiation (neutron, X-ray, and Cs^{137}). Hiroshima J. med. Sci., 11, 101-115, 1962.

Takemoto, H. Long-term effects of internal irradiation by ^{131}I on the haematopoietic organs and hypophysis. Proc. Inst. nucl. Paediat. Res. Japan, 1, 71, 1960.

Tamura, T. Experimental studies on the effects of internal exposure of ^{137}Cs on the male reproductive organ. Report I. The effects of copulation, pregnancy, and litter size by mating male mice internally exposed to ^{137}Cs with normal females. Jap. J. Hyg., 20, 268-276, 1965a (in Japanese).

Tamura, T. Experimental studies on the effects of internal exposure of Cs^{137} on the male reproductive organ. Report II. The distribution of Cs^{137} in the body of mice and the histologic changes in the testis resulting from its exposure. Jap. J.Hyg. 20, 320-328, 1965b (in Japanese).

Thomas, R.L., and Scott, J.K. Toxicity of inhaled ^{90}Sr in rats. Hlth Phys., 15, 173,1968.

Tikhaya, M.G. The chronic action of small quantities of radioactive zirconium (Zr^{95}) on the organism of animals. Med. Radiol., 4, 62-67, 1959 (in Russian).

Trusova, N.E. Influence of ionizing radiation on the activity of dog spermatozoa. Summaries of papers presented at the Conference on the Remote Consequences of Injuries Caused by Action of Ionizing Radiation, State Medical Literature Press, Moscow, 1956. U.N. Doc. A/AC.82/G/R.49, Committee on Medical Radiology, Ministry of Health, U.S.S.R.

Tuttle, L.W. (editor). The late effects of Sr-90 in the monkey: Studies of carcinogenic, leukemogenic and cytogenic changes. Mechanisms of carcinogenesis and radiation injury. Report ORO-3297-3, 1967.

Vlasov, P.A. Reaction of the bone marrow to the influence of radioactive strontium. Radiobiologiya, 4, 163-166, 1964 (in Russian).

Vorozheikina, T.V. Sr^{90} induced morphologic changes in albino rat ovary and disturbances in fertility. Radiobiologiya, 2, 601-606, 1961 (in Russian).

Walinder, G. The effect of ^{131}I on thyroid growth in mouse fetuses. Proc. of the symposium on Radiation Biology and Fetal and Juvenile Mammal, Richland, 5-8 May, 1969.

Watanabe, S. Experimental studies on the development of leukemia in mice with frequent administrations of small doses of some radioactive isotopes (^{32}P, ^{89}Sr, ^{144}Ce). Gakujutsu Geppo, 10, 57-65, 1957.

Watanabe, S. Leucémies experimentales provoquées chez la souris par administration répété de petite doses de certains radioisotopes (^{32}P, ^{89}Sr et ^{144}Ce). Pathologie-Biologies (Extrait de la Sem. Hôp.) 34, 1833-1848, 1958.

DISCUSSION OF CHAPTERS VIII AND IX

Dr. Mays: Drs. Hasterlik and Nelson have introduced the topics of internally-deposited α and β-emitters, respectively. First, I will discuss the α-emitters, and then Dr. Goldman will discuss the β-emitters. My remarks on the α-emitters will be on two subjects: (1) Prediction of the toxic dose of ^{239}Pu in the skeleton of man, and (2) the toxicity of injected ^{224}Ra (Th X) in German patients. This last subject may be new to many of you because it is little known outside of Germany.

Studies of the American dial painters by Drs. Hasterlik, Finkel and Miller in Illinois, and by Dr. Robley Evans' group at M.I.T. have been of exceptional value. And so it is with great personal sadness that I have learned that Drs. Hasterlik and Miller have chosen to leave this field, and that Dr. Evans will soon be retiring. Thus, their efforts will have to be completed by other hands.

Although radium intake is no longer an industrial hazard, it is extremely important that the radium dial painters continue to be followed throughout their remaining life-spans. From the known toxicity of radium in the skeleton, the risk to bone can be predicted for present nuclear hazards, such as ^{239}Pu.

But the risk from ^{239}Pu is unequal to that from ^{226}Ra, because of their unequal deposition patterns. ^{239}Pu typically deposits on bone surfaces where half of its α-particles shoot out into soft tissues, whereas the ultimate deposition site of ^{226}Ra is throughout the volume of mineralized bone from which only a small fraction of the α-energy can escape. Thus, one would expect that in terms of the average dose in rads to the skeleton, ^{239}Pu would be much more toxic than ^{226}Ra, and indeed this has been found to be the case.

Our Radiobiology Laboratory at the University of Utah was established nearly 20 years ago to establish experimentally the relative biological effectiveness (RBE) of ^{239}Pu relative to ^{226}Ra. This study has recently been published in detail (Dougherty and Mays, 1969; Mays et al., 1969), and reprints are available from me, so I will only mention the RBE results which are shown in fig. 1.

For the radium dial painters, bone sarcomas have only been observed above about 1200 rads average skeletal dose at death, both in the M.I.T. series and also in the Illinois series. Thus, dividing by the RBE of 6 for ^{239}Pu relative to ^{226}Ra (experimentally determined in dogs) one would predict high incidences of bone cancer above 200 rads average skeletal dose from ^{239}Pu in humans. (A constant skeletal burden of 0.3 μCi ^{239}Pu gives an average dose of 200 rads to the 7-kg marrow-free wet skeleton of a 70-kg standard man during the typical occupational work period of 50 years.)

No bone cancers have yet occurred in dial painters whose average skeletal doses are below 1200 rads from ^{226}Ra or ^{228}Ra, but it is unknown whether or not a similar "practical threshold" relationship exists for ^{239}Pu.

Now I would like to tell you about the effect of short-lived 3.62-day ^{224}Ra injected into humans, and the remarkable man who pointed out its toxicity. The man is Heinz Spiess, a paediatrician. He is presently head of the Department of Paediatrics at the University of Munich, which is the largest University in Germany.

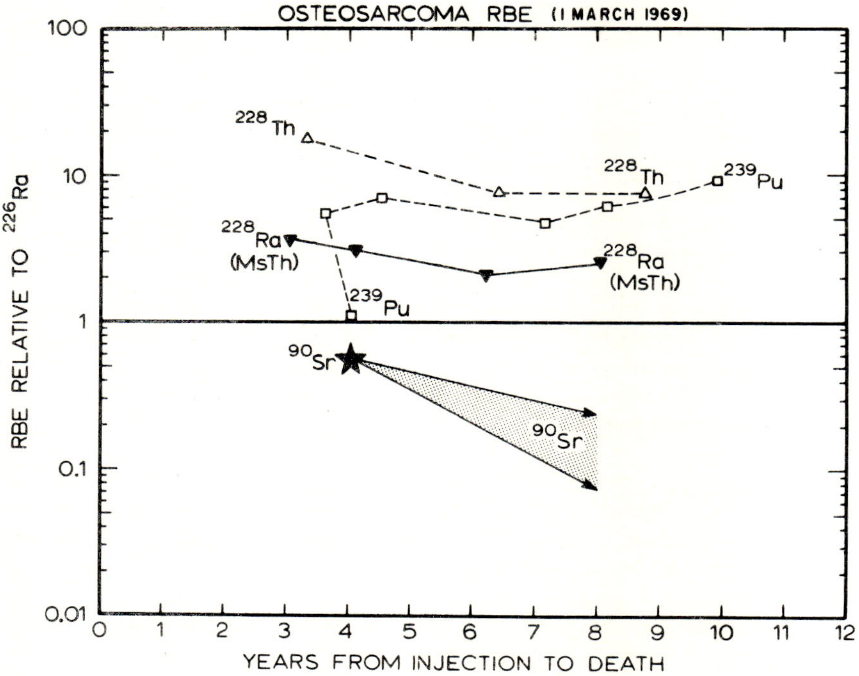

Fig. 1. RBE for death with osteosarcomas in beagles (March 1969) based on the cumulative average skeletal dose received up to 1 year preceding death. For death with osteosarcomas 8 years after injection, values for RBE relative to $^{226}Ra = 1$ are: $^{239}Pu = 6$; $^{228}Th = 8$; ^{228}Ra (MsTh) = 2.5; and $^{90}Sr = 0.07$ to 0.24. The bone-surface seekers ^{239}Pu and ^{228}Th are more effective than the bone-volume seekers ^{228}Ra and ^{226}Ra. The β-emitter ^{90}Sr is less effective than the emitters of α-radiation.

Shortly following World War II roughly 2000 patients were intravenously injected with ^{224}Ra in divided doses for the treatment of tuberculosis and ankylosing spondylitis. Spiess began following these patients over 20 years ago and now has in his series over 200 persons injected as juveniles plus over 700 injected as adults. Bone sarcomas have developed in 34 of the juveniles plus 15 of the adults, as of April 1969. To my knowledge, this study forms the only opportunity to compare the effects of a bone-seeking radionuclide in both children and adults. During April 1969 I worked with Spiess in Munich and computed the average skeletal doses to the patients in his series. The details are in a manuscript, preprints of which are available from me (Spiess and Mays, 1970). As shown in fig. 2 the total incidence of bone sarcomas increased with dose in approximately linear fashion at 1.4% per 100 rads average skeletal dose for the juveniles and 0.7% per 100 rads average skeletal dose for the adults. Among the 49 patients developing bone sarcomas, the lowest average skeletal dose was 90 rads and this patient was an adult. This is much less than the lowest average skeletal dose at death (1200 rads) among the American dial painters who developed bone sarcomas following ingestion of long-lived 1600-year ^{226}Ra. This difference seems mainly due to the short 3.62-day half-life of ^{224}Ra which causes a large fraction of the skeletal ^{224}Ra to decay while still on bone surfaces. In fact, the effectiveness of ^{224}Ra seems more similar to ^{239}Pu than it (^{224}Ra) does to ^{226}Ra.

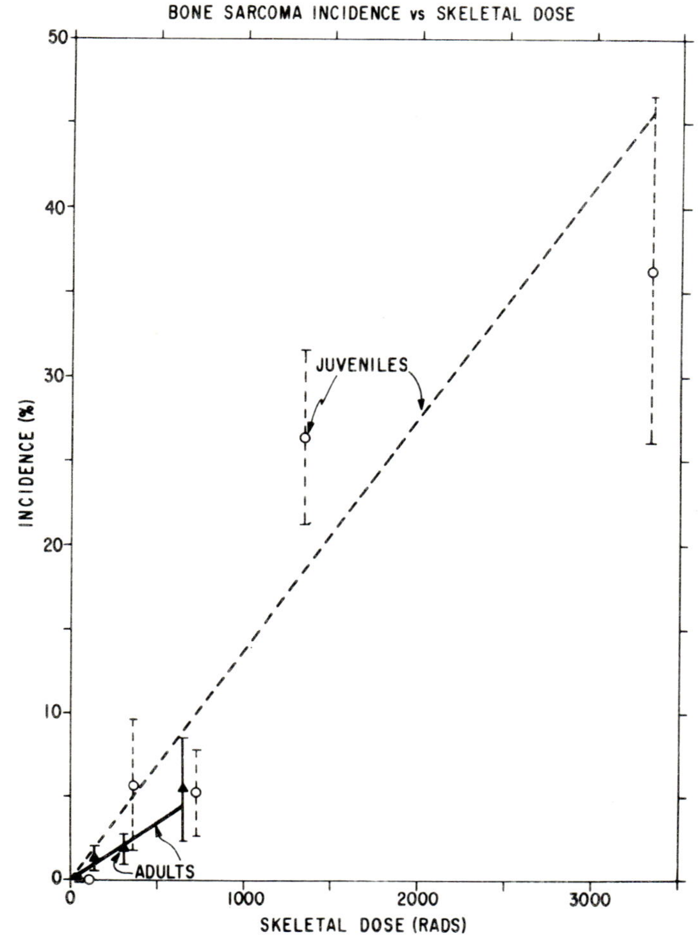

Fig. 2. Bone sarcoma incidence vs average skeletal dose in German patients injected with ^{224}Ra. The standard deviation in the incidence for each dosage group is shown by vertical lines. Incidence increases with dose. For the linear non-threshold lines shown, the cumulative risk from bone sarcomas during the first 14-21 years after the start of the exposure is 0.7% per 100 rads average skeletal dose for adults and 1.4% per 100 rads average skeletal dose for juveniles. Other dose-response relationships are possible, including a "practical threshold" at low doses. No bone sarcomas have been reported in the 210 adults in the 0-89 rads dose band, nor in the 12 juveniles in the 0-199 rads dose band. From our linear model, the predicted number of bone sarcoma cases is 0.8 for these 210 adults and 0.2 for the 12 juveniles. Thus, the lack of observed bone sarcomas in each of these respective low dose bands is not surprising, and neither rules out nor proves linearity at very low dosage.

^{224}Ra injections proved completely ineffective in the treatment of tuberculosis and the injection of ^{224}Ra into German children was stopped in 1951, due in large part to the efforts of Spiess who is indeed a German "Harrison Martland". (Martland's efforts were instrumental in stopping in 1925 the licking of radium paint brushes by the American dial painters and stopping in 1932 the injection and ingestion of ^{226}Ra for approved medical treatments in the U.S.A.)

About 200 adults with ankylosing spondylitis are still being injected with ^{224}Ra each year in Germany, but at lower doses (typically a total of about 280 μ Ci of ^{224}Ra for which the calculated average skeletal dose is 56 rads). This is indeed a most fascinating study in human radiobiology'.

Postscript: Several questions were raised at the colloquium as to the usefulness of the parameter, average skeletal dose. Therefore, I have computed the mean local dose to the soft-tissue layer which is 0-10 microns distant from the mineralized bone surfaces, since some persons believe that this may be the sensitive site for the induction of bone sarcomas. Assuming that half of the skeletal ^{224}Ra decays on bone surfaces and half within mineral bone, the mean local dose to this layer is about 9 times the average skeletal dose from ^{224}Ra, whereas for long-lived ^{226}Ra randomly distributed throughout the volume of mineral bone, the mean local dose to this layer is about 0.6 times the average skeletal dose from ^{226}Ra (details are in the manuscript by Spiess and Mays). Thus, the smallest mean local doses to the lining of the bone surface associated with induced bone cancer appear comparable thus far: about (9) (90 rads) $\simeq$ 800 rads for ^{224}Ra, and about (0.6) (1200 rads) $\simeq$ 700 rads for ^{226}Ra.

Dr. Brill: Were there any leukaemias in the German series?

Dr. Mays: Only 2 leukaemias are recorded, and it is uncertain whether or not these resulted from irradiation. The average skeletal dose was only 50 rads in the 1 case of paramyeloblastic leukaemia, whereas the case at the high dose (665 rads) was lymphatic leukaemia, a type not ordinarily associated with irradiation. A few cases of leukaemia could have occurred naturally in the injected population, although a random occurrence so soon after injection (2 and 3 years) might seem unlikely. It is interesting that no leukaemias have been diagnosed among the juveniles in this series, especially since these patients received the higher doses. Some of the 4 cases recorded as panmyelosis might have been mis-diagnosed leukaemias, but even if this were true the number of induced leukaemias would still be small compared to the 49 cases of induced bone sarcoma. Leukaemias have also been infrequent among the radium dial painters. The most likely explanation for the low incidence of leukaemia is the inability of the short-range α-particles from bone-deposited radium isotopes to reach deeply into the marrow.

References

Dougherty, T.F., and Mays, C.W. Bone cancer induced by internally deposited emitters in beagles. In: Radiation-Induced Cancer, edited by Anne Ericson, IAEA, Vienna, p. 361, 1969.

Mays, C.W., Dougherty, T.F., Taylor, G.N., Lloyd, R.D., Stover, Betsy J., Jee, W.S.S. Christensen, W.R., Dougherty, Jean H., and Atherton, D.R. Radiation-induced bone cancer in beagles. In: Delayed Effects of Bone-Seeking Radionuclides, edited by C.W. Mays, W.S.S. Jee, R.D. Lloyd, Betsy J. Stover, Jean H. Dougherty and G.N. Taylor, University of Utah Press, Salt Lake City, p. 387, 1969.

Spiess, H., and Mays, C.W. Bone cancers induced by ^{224}Ra (Th X) in children and adults; Health Physics, in press, 1970.

Dr. Goldman: At this late hour I shall attempt to summarize some of the salient features of Dr. Nelson's extensive review of beta- and gamma-emitting radionuclides and perhaps play the role of a provocateur in this regard. As a point of departure, I believe it would be useful to contrast the effects of internal and external emitters. In the former case the dose input time is usually protracted as compared to the acute or sum of acute doses used in most external radiation studies. Thus, in some instances of cellular response, the radionuclide effects may produce less "wasted radiation" for specific end-points. At lower dose rates, the period of continual stress may actually stimulate cellular renewal potential to some extent, making it more difficult to compare the two modes of irradiation on a rad for rad basis. Radionuclide dosimetry per se is complicated by both the temporal and spatial distribution of the ionization intensity. The absorbed tissue dose is dependent on the physical characteristics of the radiation — that is, the mean or peak energy, whether it is electromagnetic or particulate radiation in terms of range, its physical half-period and decay to possible additional radionuclide daughters. An example of the latter would be the yttrium-90 daughter which accounts for about 0.8 of the radiation energy from strontium-90 depositions, when in equilibrium.

Biologic factors, which are known with lesser certainty, must also enter into such an analysis. The route of administration, whether it is a surface contamination, an oral administration, intravenous, or an inhalation (which often is followed by an oral component), the chemical form of the radionuclide (soluble or insoluble), and the chemical and biological specicity and predilection for deposition site or mode of administration are all factors whose sum complicates the quantitation of radionuclide dosimetry. Even in the case of specific deposition, tissue metabolic factors of turnover and elimination must be factored into the dose equation. As if these complexities were not enough, the literature so elegantly summarized by Dr. Nelson includes the species-related variability of life-span, the differentially late effect end-points — that is, variation in the "signal-to-noise ratio" for these effects — and variations between species and sexes for the post-dose to effect appearance time. Finally, within a species given the same radionuclide at comparable doses, different kinds of end-points may be produced, indicating varying effectiveness depending on the age of the individual at the time of exposure. One must also include, I believe, some of the paradoxical synergistic and/or abscopal effects that have been reported.

This incomplete list of complexities tempts us to be "lumpers", rather than a "splitter". However, analysis of the late and subtle effects described may help us to play the role of the "splitter" to some degree. For example, a common condition exists among those radionuclides which, once in the body, distribute uniformly throughout most of the body cells. Such radionuclides are caesium-137, phosphorus-32, tritium-3 and carbon-14, and the common condition is that there is a continual decrease in the total body irradiation dose rate. If a radionuclide is administered at a sufficiently high level, the biologic effects may resemble the results of a chronic external penetrating radiation exposure. However, those radionuclides such as the alkaline earths, the halides, iron and cobalt, which concentrate in specific tissues by virtue of their special chemical affinity, represent a unique type of partial body irradiation which is necessarily tissue-specific and which is not usually feasible with partial body external radiation studies.

In evaluating these radionuclide effects, a target quality factor must also be considered. One should ask how the radioactivity is distributed in relation to the rads per cell lifetime for tissues that are at risk. If one wishes to consider carcinogenesis, for example, the rad dose must be minimally effective but not markedly lethal to the cells at risk. There appears to be a certain radionuclide dosage pattern in some of the reported cases in which there is a rather high "cell injury to cell killing" ratio. This pattern may be a model for other environmental hazards. Perhaps we should concentrate greater effort on some environmental radiation studies for which this model might be more applicable.

One example of the differential target concept is summarized in the work of Yuri Moskalev (Moskalev et al., 1969). He has noted in rats injected with ^{90}Sr that leukaemias are induced with about one tenth the injected dose (μCi/kg) required to produce osteosarcomas; in fact, at the highest incidence level of osteosarcomas there is actually reduction in the leukaemogenic potential of ^{90}Sr. On the other hand, cerium-144 injections produced pituitary tumours at fairly comparable incidence rates over a hundred-fold range of injected doses (approximately 5-10% over the 5 to 500 μCi/kg rate). The same nuclide induces liver tumours in substantial numbers of rats only at injection concentrations exceeding 200 or 300 μCi/kg.

He also has noted that rats appear to have a greater radiosensitivity for leukaemias than for osteosarcomas and the ^{90}Sr-induced leukaemias appear more quickly than ^{90}Sr-induced osteosarcomas.

A unique experiment concerned with the chronic administration of ^{90}Sr to our colony of beagles at Davis is currently under way (Goldman et al., 1969). Exposure is initiated during early foetal life and continues until young adulthood (1.5 years of age), by which time a uniformly labelled skeleton is produced in treatment levels covering almost a thousand-fold range of dosage. Beta radiation doses range from about 15 millirads per day to almost 20 rads per day. After the radionuclide administration period, the body burden develops a non-uniformity pattern which is in a mirror image to the radium deposition pattern noted following brief exposures; the strontium-labelled skeletons develop "cold spots" in regions that are usually associated with alpha-emitting "hot spots" from radium. These correlate well with the local rate of tissue turnover. That is, there is a sparing effect of dose rate on the highly cellular and sensitive cells in the trabecular portion of the skeleton. The continuingly decreasing radiation dose to associated marrow spaces is paralleled by a change in the radiogenic neutrophil depression, providing a model of continual stress on a rapidly renewing system which fairly accurately reflects the contemporary local dose rate. Thus, with increasing time and associated loss of body burden, there is an increase in the neutrophil recovery pattern (Bustad et al., 1969).

In some of the dogs at the highest dosage levels (greater than 1 rad per day) a dose-related incidence of myeloproliferative disease has been noted (Dungworth et al., 1969). At all effective levels the earliest cases have been noticed by 1-1.5 years of age. The incidence rate is related to the dose rate rather than to the cumulative radiation dose, which latter seems to correlate well with the appearance of ^{90}Sr-induced osteosarcomas (Goldman et al., 1969). These myeloproliferative disorders are similar in many respects to the splenic leukaemia following ^{226}Ra poisoning described by Martland (Martland, 1931), in which the acute cases very closely resemble granulocytic leukaemias, while the chronic cases are characteristic of myeloid metaplasia with myelofibrosis. In all cases a terminal progressive or precipitous anaemia is the premonitory sign of disease, the severity often correlating well with the degree of splenomegaly. The myeloproliferative disorders have been seen following 1,000 rads of cumulative skeletal irradiation, whereas the appearance of ^{90}Sr-induced osteosarcomas to date correlates well with a cumulative dose minima of approximately 10,000 rads.

In a parallel study done at our laboratory by Dr. J.F. Wright, three strains of mice were exposed to short-lived ^{89}Sr during their first half-year of life. Haemopoietic tumours were also induced with high frequency in the RF strain, but were not frequently seen in C57BL and BALB mice. A greater variation sensitivity was seen in the females than in the males. We feel this is, to some extent, related to the higher spontaneous incidence rate for tumours known to exist in the female mouse. The earliest tumours appeared by 5 months in the mice, as contrasted to the 1-1.5 years in the dog. We feel that these provide examples for the importance of considering both the age at exposure (juvenile vs adult) as well as the mode of exposure (acute vs chronic) in determining not only the sensitivity to radiation oncogenesis but the type of tumours which may be produced.

Dr. Nelson has ably pointed out that no tumours have been observed at low doses. This should not be surprising. Many studies have indicated that an efficient repair mechanism exists in tissues subjected to beta or gamma irradiation when the dose rate is sufficiently low. It may be quite difficult to determine if a fraction of the irradiation injury remains unrepaired. In most animal experiments, in addition, not enough animals have been used to definitively determine whether a non-threshold model or a curvilinear model truly exists; to me, the available evidence appears to fit best the non-linear or sigmoidal type response. In some instances a dose-time relationship may obtain in which the induction time may actually exceed the life expectancy of the experimental subject.

A subtle, late effect of bone-seeking radionuclides that we have noted when administration extends over the juvenile period is a change in the quality of bone. This change is characterized by a decrease in the size of the medullary cavity and by hypocellularity and an increase in cortical thickness. This "hyperostosis" is seen at all the higher levels of treatment in our beagle experiment (Goldman et al., 1969). Although the chronic radiation model for ^{90}Sr is potent in induction of haematopoietic deaths in the young, bone tumours are seen following the same cumulative rad dose (~10,000 rads) as was noted at Utah where adult dogs, following single acute administration, manifest bone cancers.

For extrapolation purposes I believe that it is useful to consider the number of rads per cell and/or tissue from the radionuclide in any comparison of effects in species. Such quantitation may be essential to fully utilize animal models in extrapolations to man.

Combinations of nuclides in different concentrations can be utilized to test some of the models which suggest synergism in inducing late effects. Such models may be important in planning studies for other environmental hazards that appear to be increasing exponentially with the technological complexities of our society. In addition, some of these radiation models may prove useful tools that may be combined with other environmental hazards such as chemical pollutants. This approach, for example, could be useful in studying cocarcinogenesis or the effects of an environmental pollutant on a tissue already under radiation stress.

What started out less than three decades ago as a need for radiation protection guides for the nuclear industry has evolved into perhaps one of the few documented models for the design of future toxicity studies of importance to our civilization's survival. The temporal and spatial distribution of ionizing radiation from beta- and gamma-emitting nuclides within specific tissues or cells at risk have produced little evidence of any unique potency of any particular radionuclide which does not appear to be a function of its physical characteristics. Since one of the missions of this colloquium is to address the subject not only of radiation and its late and subtle effects, but perhaps other environmental stresses, I thought this would be a good time to provoke further discussion.

Dr. Kohn: How would experimental design and interpretation be affected by the knowledge or suspicion that viruses may be associated with such tumours?

Dr. Goldman: While I cannot answer the virus aetiology question adequately, I do believe that properly designed low dose rate radionuclide studies can be performed which will address itself to this particular problem.

With regard to the virus model, I believe that the mouse material is essentially concerned with lymphoid tumours which also occur spontaneously. In the beagle work referred to here, the condition is myeloid and is normally exceedingly rare in the dog. Although it was not known beforehand, the spontaneous incidence of bone tumours in beagles used in the radionuclide studies is also normally low, whereas larger breeds of dogs do manifest significant incidences of spontaneous bone tumours. I am unaware of any data invoking a viral vector in the induction of myeloproliferative disorders.

Dr. Hasterlik: Have any central nervous system tumours been seen in the Davis or Salt Lake City animals?

Dr. Mays: No primary central nervous system tumours have been observed in our 262 radioactive toxicity beagles dying as of 1 March 1969 at the University of Utah, according to our Veterinary Pathologist, Dr. Glenn N. Taylor.

Dr. Goldman: Although a few instances of epilepsy have been observed which are unrelated to radiation treatment there have not been any central nervous system tumours seen to date in the radionuclide-treated dogs at Davis.

Some of the more recent work on the distribution of radium has shown that the body burden is not totally accounted for by the skeletal deposition. The dog work at Utah has shown that some of the pigmented cells have a particular affinity for the alkaline earths. In addition, there has been some work on intranuclear concentration of radiocalcium in which an autoradiograph of a karyotype has suggested a firm binding of calcium within nuclear structures (Herzog, 1966).

The studies about which I am aware, however, do not indicate any unique change in specific activity of strontium or calcium in any cellular substructure. Thus, for alkaline earth radioactivity I would not expect the radiation dose to extra skeletal cells to exceed one-thousandth that which is found in bone. The soft tissue dose from extra skeletal ^{90}Sr concentrations at levels below which we have seen bone and bone marrow effects would be quite small compared to the 300-400 microrads a day to which almost all tissues on this planet are subjected from natural background radiation sources.

I did not infer in my summarization of radionuclide complexities that the use of a critical organ in the study of a single radionuclide effect means that all other tissues are totally spared. Certainly, as Dr. Nelson has pointed out, about three-fourths of the ^{90}Sr dose to a mouse is outside of his skeleton, whereas perhaps only one-fourth of it is going to escape the skeleton of larger animals and man. Due to the beta energy range, the one-fourth of energy escaping the skeleton would certainly include cells for some millimetres away from bone and therefore they should not be entirely neglected. The effects summarized on haemopoietic disorders indicate that the cells at risk do not necessarily have to have high radionuclide concentrations.

References

Bustad, L.K., Goldman, M., Rosenblatt, L.S., McKelvie, D.H., and Hertzendorf, I.I. Hematopoietic changes in Beagles fed ^{90}Sr. In: Delayed Effects of Bone-Seeking

Radionuclides, edited by C.W. Mays et al., University of Utah Press, Salt Lake City, p. 279, 1969.

Dungworth, D.L., Goldman, M., Switzer, J.W., and McKelvie, D.H. Development of a myeloproliferative disorder in Beagles continuously exposed to ^{90}Sr. Blood, 34, 610, 1969.

Goldman, M., Della Rosa, R.J., and McKelvie, D.H. Metabolic dosimetric and pathological consequences in the skeletons of Beagles fed ^{90}Sr. In: Delayed Effects of Bone-Seeking Radionuclides, edited by C.W. Mays et al., University of Utah Press, p. 61, 1969.

Goldman, M., Dungworth, D.L., Bulgin, M.S., Rosenblatt, L.S., Richards, W.P.C., and Bustad, L.K. Radiation-induced neoplasms in Beagles after administration of ^{90}Sr and ^{226}Ra. In: Radiation-Induced Cancer. International Atomic Energy Agency, Vienna, 1969.

Herzog, R.K. Autoradiographic studies of DNA synthesis and alkaline earth incorporation in nuclear material of human white blood cells. Cornell University, Ph.D. Thesis, 1966.

Martland, H.S. The occurrence of malignancy in radioactive persons. Am. J. Cancer, 15, 2435, 1931.

Moskalev, Y.I., Streltsova, V.N., and Buldakov, L.A. Late effects of radionuclide damage. In: Delayed Effects of Bone-Seeking Radionuclides, edited by C.W. Mays et al., University of Utah Press, Salt Lake City, p. 489, 1969.

Dr. McClellan: Dr. Marvin Goldman, in his earlier comments, noted the complexity of the situation with regard to internally deposited radionuclides. I believe it is appropriate to extend this discussion to the complexity of what is considered by many to be the most significant route of accidental entry of radionuclides into the body — the inhalation route.

The complexity of the radiation dose pattern for the inhalation route of entry is illustrated in fig. 1 where the changing radiation dose rate for a constant amount (1 μCi) of inhaled and deposited (in lung) activity is related to time post-inhalation exposure for several significant radionuclides in different forms for the beagle dog. The curve for $^{239}PuO_2$ is taken from the work of W.J. Bair and associates (Park et al., 1968; Bair et al., 1966; Park et al., 1962) at Battelle-Northwest. The curves for $^{238}PuO_2$ and $^{242}CmO_2$ are extrapolated from that for $^{239}PuO_2$ taking into consideration the radiologic characteristics of each radionuclide. The curves for ^{90}Sr fused clay, ^{144}Ce fused clay, $^{144}CeCl_3$, $^{91}YCl_3$, $^{137}CsCl$, and ^{90}Y fused clay are from the AEC-sponsored Inhalation Research Program at the Lovelace Foundation (Annual Report, LF 39, 1967-1968). The differences in radiation dose rate patterns reflect differences in the radiologic characteristics of each radionuclide such as half-life and emission (alpha, beta and gamma) and the physical chemical form in which it was inhaled. These differences have a marked effect on the cumulative radiation dose to lung for equivalent lung deposition (fig. 2). For example, the infinite radiation dose to the lung associated with lung deposition of 1 μCi ^{90}Y fused clay in the dog is just over 1 rad, while 1 μCi of $^{239}PuO_2$ in the dog lung will yield an infinite radiation dose to the lung on the order of 10^3 rads. Clearly, these differences in radiation dose pattern will have a profound effect on the ultimate biological response.

An example of the type of data developed on effects when the cumulative radiation dose in rads is related to time post-inhalation exposure, is shown in fig. 3 for dogs that inhaled ^{144}Ce in fused clay. The experiment is now out to about 600 days post-exposure. To date, 9 dogs have died from 143 to 410 days after inhalation

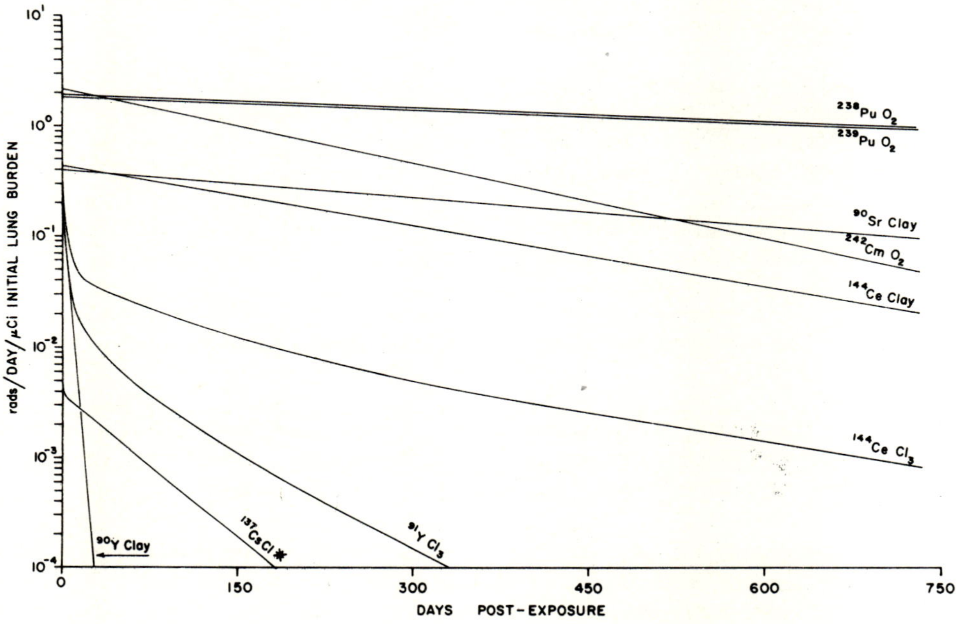

Fig. 1. Radiation dose rate to lung following inhalation of ^{90}Y, ^{90}Sr, and ^{144}Ce in fused clay, $^{91}YCl_3$, $^{137}CsCl$, and $^{144}CeCl$, and $^{238}PuO_2$, $^{239}PuO_2$, and $^{242}CmO_2$.

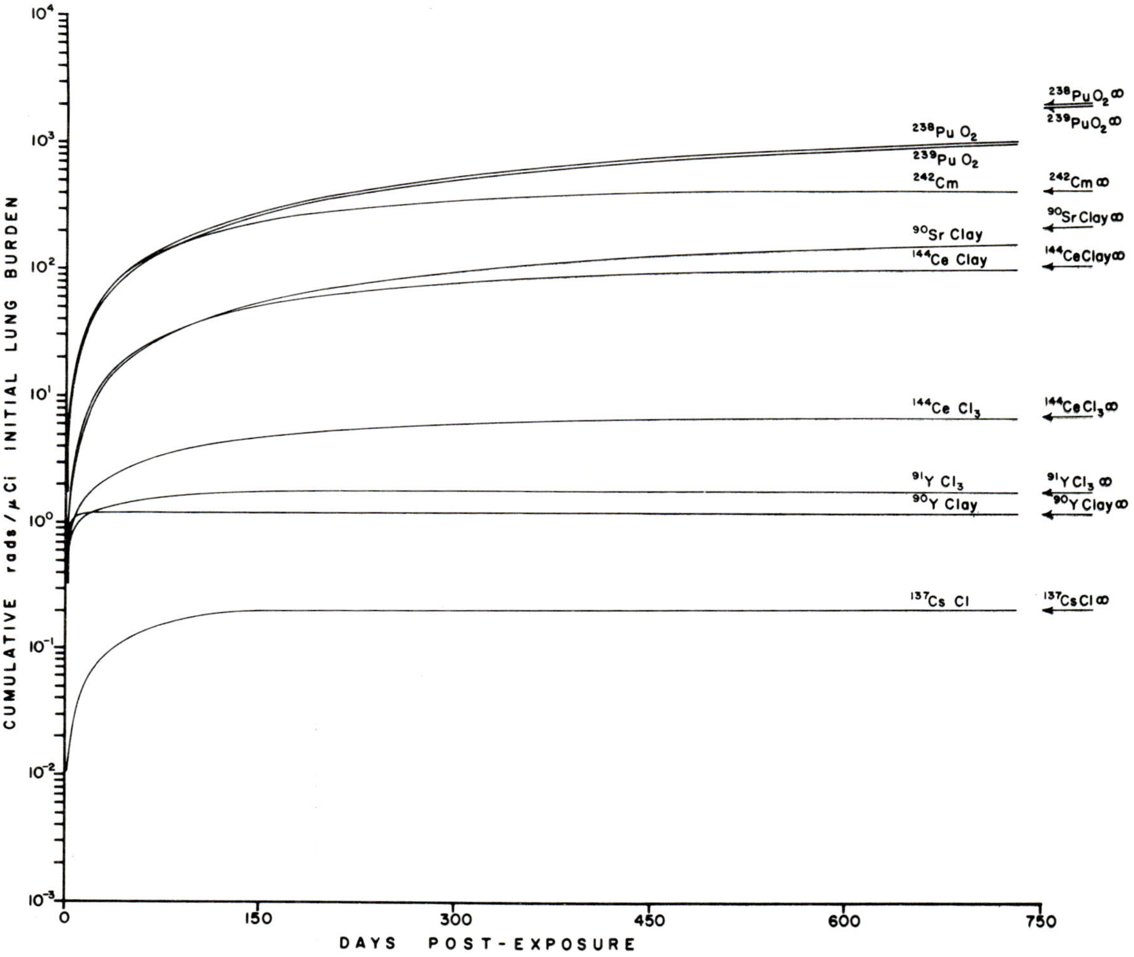

Fig. 2. Cumulative radiation dose to lung following inhalation of ^{90}Y, ^{90}Sr, and ^{144}Ce in fused clay, $^{91}YCl_3$, $^{137}CsCl$, and $^{144}CeCl_3$ and $^{238}PuO_2$, $^{239}PuO_2$ and $^{242}CmO_2$.

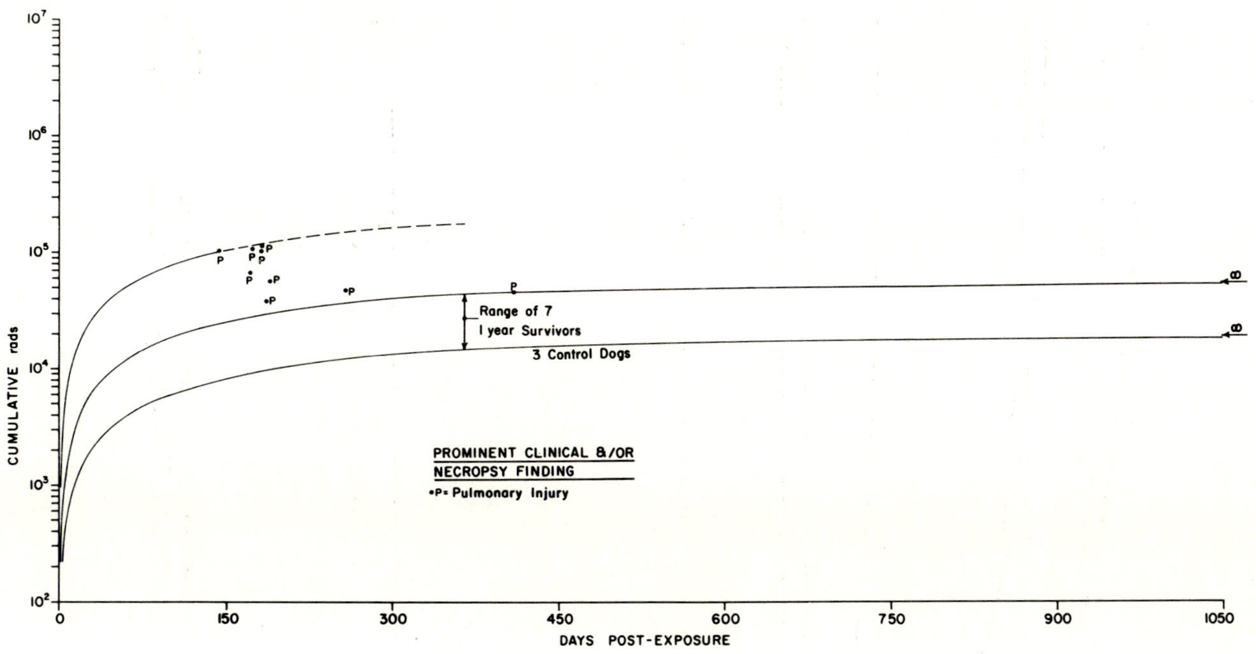

Fig. 3. ^{144}Ce fused clay longevity study — cumulative radiation dose to lung versus effect.

exposure with cumulative radiation doses to lung of 35,000 to over 100,000 rads. The first 8 deaths were all related to severe pulmonary fibrosis. The last death, at 410 days post-inhalation exposure, was also related to severe pulmonary fibrosis, however, it was noteworthy that marked metaplastic changes in the lungs were also noted. Six dogs are still surviving and are projected to have infinite radiation doses to lung of 18,000 to 40,000 rads. Undoubtedly, dogs surviving at this time are prime candidates for the development of neoplasia of the lung tissues as noted by W.J. Bair and associates at Battelle-Northwest with $^{239}PuO_2$ inhalation exposure of dogs.

Since the work of W.J. Bair and associates (Park et al., 1968) has not been described here, and recognizing its significance, I believe it appropriate to present a graphic presentation of some of their data as interpreted in our laboratory for the design of future studies (fig. 4). It may be noted that death prior to 1,000 days post-inhalation exposure was related to severe pulmonary fibrosis. Beyond 1,000 days post-inhalation exposure some deaths with pulmonary fibrosis alone were noted, however, in some cases lung tumours were noted in addition to the fibrosis. In a few cases lung tumours with minimal fibrosis was noted. Several dogs had both lung and lymphatic tissue tumours.

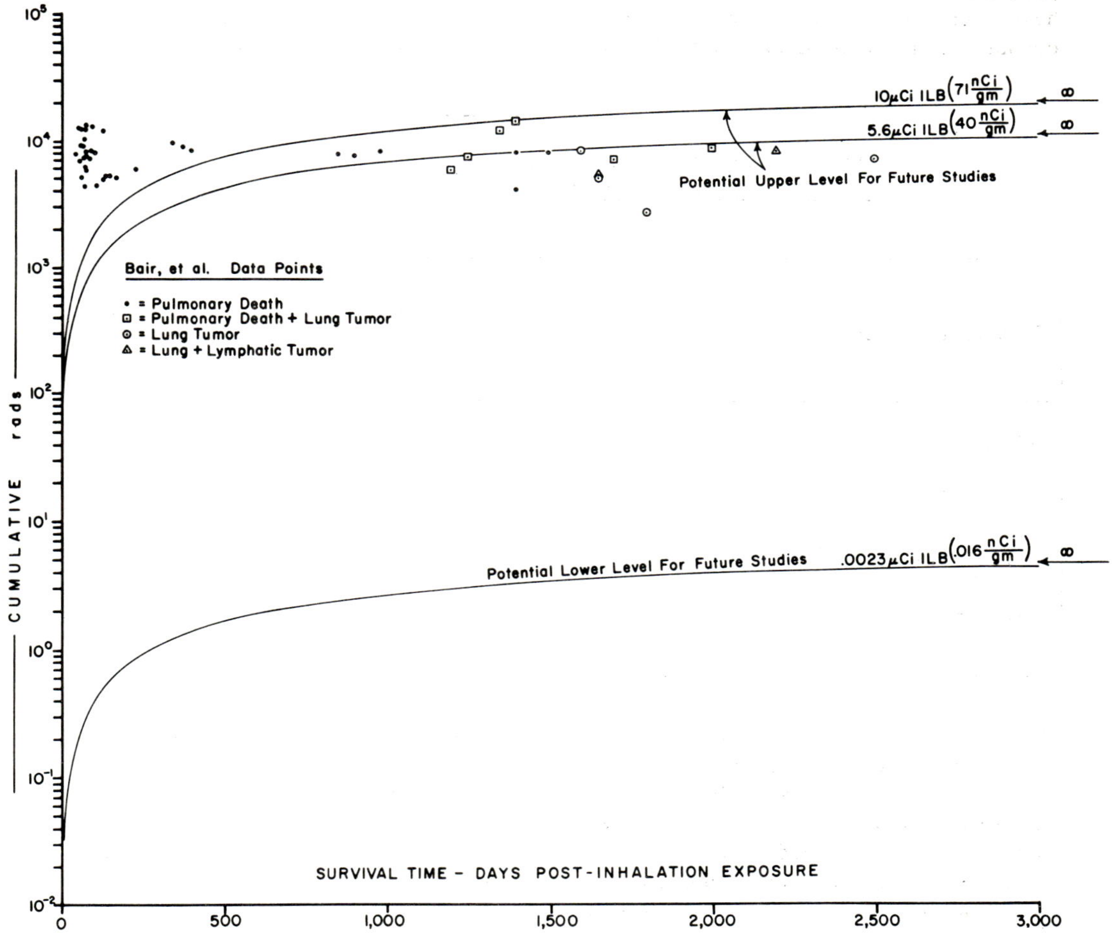

Fig. 4. Cumulative radiation dose to lung versus survival time for dogs that have inhaled $^{239}PuO_2$ (data of W.J. Bair and associates, Battelle-Northwest).

The cumulative radiation dose for the lungs of these dogs are substantial, in excess of 10^3 rads. Further, it may be noted that although these studies have been carried to approximately eight years post-inhalation exposure, there is still a considerable fraction of the dog's lifespan remaining, potential lifespan available for the development of neoplastic or other late effects at lower dose levels. Because of this, plans are being developed in our laboratory as well as at Battelle-Northwest for the inhalation exposure of additional dogs. Fig. 4 has several curves that represent the cumulative radiation dose projections for initial lung burdens that might be considered for use in future studies. The lower curve which represents an amount equivalent to a Maximum Permissible Lung Burden for man is several orders of magnitude below the levels where effects have been noted to date in dogs.

Both Drs. Nelson and Goldman noted the problem of assessing the effects of exposure to mixtures of radionuclides. This is certainly a very important problem, especially when viewed in relation to the practical use of radionuclide toxicity data; many potential real life hazard situations exist where man may be exposed not to just a single radionuclide but a mixture of radionuclides. I would like to note that studies are already in progress which are relevant to this problem and, more specifically, studies in which animals have been exposed to radionuclides that produce substantial radiation exposure of several organs. This is illustrated in table 1 for several radionuclides following inhalation by the dog

Table 1

Organs receiving significant radiation doses following inhalation of various radionuclides in several forms

Material inhaled	Lung				
	Lung	Tracheobronchial lymph nodes	Liver	Bone and bone marrow	Whole body
$^{90}SrCl_2$				+	
$^{144}CeCl_3$	+		+	+	
$^{91}YCl_3$	+		+	+	
^{144}Ce fused clay	+	+			
$^{137}CsCl$					+

For example, inhaled $^{90}SrCl_2$ is rapidly translocated to bone, so the radiation dose to lung is very small while the radiation dose to bone and contiguous bone marrow is high. With $^{144}CeCl_3$ and $^{91}YCl_3$ the radionuclide leaves the lung more slowly so significant radiation doses are delivered to lung, and following translocation to liver and bone significant radiation doses are delivered to these tissues. With ^{144}Ce fused clay the material has long-term retention in lung with small quantities translocated to tracheobronchial lymph nodes, liver, and skeleton. The radiation dose to lung is substantial and, because tracheobronchial lymph nodes have a small mass, they also accumulate a substantial radiation dose. Whether $^{137}CsCl$ is inhaled, ingested or injected, as an analogue of potassium, it distributes widely in the body so that whole body is the critical organ. Long-term studies using the beagle dog are now under way in our laboratory with each of the materials noted in table 1.

When several organs are at risk, the critical organ may shift with time. For example, following inhalation of $^{144}CeCl_3$, early deaths at about 30 days post-inhalation exposure are related to severe haematopoietic tissue damage from ^{144}Ce in bone, at about 140 days post-inhalation exposure deaths are related to pulmonary fibrosis from the early radiation exposure of this organ, and later deaths related to hepatocellular damage. Late neoplastic effects are anticipated in bone, bone marrow, liver and/or lung. At Argonne National Laboratory, Dr. Norris and associates (Fritz et al., 1967) have noted both late hepatic necrosis and bone tumours in beagle dogs following intravenous administration of ^{144}Ce.

The work I have noted provides an indication of research under way on the late effects of inhaled radionuclides. Further, it provides an indication of the type of data that are being developed which will be of value in planning future studies on the late effects of exposure to mixtures of radionuclides.

References

Bair, W.J., Park, J.F., and Clarke, W.J. Long-term study of inhaled plutonium in dogs. Report No. AFWL-TR-65-214, March 1966.

Fritz, T.E., Norris, W.P., Rehfeld, C.E., and Poole, C.M. Cerium-144 — toxic manifestations in beagle dogs. Report No. ANL-7409, 1967.

McClellan, R.O., and Rupprecht, F.C. (editors). Report No. LF-39, 1968.

Park, J.F., Willard, D.H., Marks, S., West, J.E., Vogt, G.S., and Bair, W.J. Acute and chronic toxicity of inhaled plutonium in dogs. Hlth Phys., 8, 651-657, 1962.

Park, J.C., Clarke, W.J., and Bair, W.J. Chronic effects of inhaled $^{239}PuO_2$ in beagles. Report No. BNWL-714, May 1968.

CHAPTER X

MODELS FROM RADIATION TOXICITY DATA

George A. Sacher

Last month, at the First European Symposium on Late Effects of Radiation, held in Casaccia, Italy, Dr. Mole gave a paper presenting his views on the subject of late effects (1970), and in the course of it delivered some uncompromising negative opinions about the utility of mathematical models in general, and of certain models in particular, for the description and prediction of late radiation effects in animal or human populations. I do not have the text of his remarks, so I cannot tell you precisely what he said, but I can speak authoritatively about what I think he said, which was that the subject of late radiation effects has as its subject-matter a large number of different causes of injury, disease or death, and the effort to reduce this infinite variety to simple mathematical order is foredoomed to failure.

This view, that there is an antinomy between pathological fact and mathematical model, is widely held, and indeed it was given expression here two days ago, when Dr. Lamerton appeared to us in the guise of a Hamlet-figure, torn between the ghostly stern voice of experimental complexity and the sweet song of theoretical simplicity, troubled by the necessity of deciding which voice to follow.

I share these feelings in some degree, for the problem of maintaining in one's thought a construct, or model, for the ordering of phenomena is difficult, unless the abstraction gets a great deal of reinforcement and support from the real world. What is the abstraction that is the source of this concern? It is time. Dr. Lamerton made this explicit when he said that he could not feel comfortable about life-shortening as a parameter, because the abstract representation of a deleterious radiation effect as a few days or percent reduction of life conceals the reality that some members of the population died untimely early deaths. Yet, virtually the whole thrust of modelling late effects is directed to formulating statements about the behaviour of populations in the time domain. The urgent question is, how can we close the gap between this abstract representation and the concrete presentations of animals and men who develop specific diseases and die thereof?

It is unfortunate that misunderstanding should arise on this point between experimentalists and clinicians on the one hand, and theoreticians and model builders on the other. For one thing, they need one another. The differences between them are not an unresolvable antinomy, but rather a dynamic and productive dialectic. For another thing, model-building is not a monopoly of a small corps of specialists. It is a proper activity of every good scientist. Insofar as there is a group of experts in model-building, their expertise lies not in the activity of discovering new hypotheses so much as in the more formal activity of finding for a new hypothesis that form of explicit statement that has the greatest generality and the greatest number of experimentally testable implications.

The word "testable" brings us to the heart of the matter. It is essential that the techniques of modelling and theory-building be highly developed and widely used, because with-

This work has been supported under the auspices of the U.S. Atomic Energy Commission.

out them a discipline can be stifled by an accumulation of unassailable, but basically vacuous, "laws".

Despite shortcomings which are quite apparent, mathematical research in the domain of late radiation effects has shown a consistent pattern of development, and has built up a reasonably (but far from completely) coherent system of interrelated theories and models of many types, ranging from the empirical and phenomenological to the mechanistic and speculative. Let us briefly examine some of these developments in their historical sequence.

During the early post-war period, the modelling of late radiation effects was mostly confined to the characterization of the reduction in mean after-survival time. This domain of modelling is associated with the names of Blair (1952), Boche (1954) and Sacher (1956).

Within a decade, the appearance of more extensive and accurate data caused interest to shift toward the characterization of radiation effects in terms of life-tables, and a formulation of radiation lethality was evolved in terms of a particular life-table function, the Gompertz function, which you get by plotting the logarithm of the age-specific rate of mortality against age (Sacher, 1956; Jones, 1956; Berlin and DiMaggio, 1956). The Gompertz function plots for most metazoan species are approximately linear, meaning that the death rates go up geometrically with age, or, alternatively, that the log death rates rise as a linear function of age.

Against that background, it seemed to me then, as it still does today, that a significant new level of simplicity and order was achieved by the observation that the perturbation of the life-table produced by a single burst of ionizing radiation given early in life can be described as a displacement of the Gompertz line parallel to itself (Sacher, 1956). In other words, one can describe the effects of a single dose of radiation by saying that, in terms of the actuarial function which accumulates proportional to age, the radiation exposure introduces a permanent increment of some kind of morbific injury*, which then summates with the ageing injury.

Dr. Grahn earlier gave you another aspect of this story (Grahn, 1970) in regard to the administration of duration of life exposure, showing that the data for lifetime irradiation of mice agree with the Gompertz model, which predicts an increase in the Gompertz function slope with increase in dose rate.

The next stage of experimental inquiry was directed to the development of data about the interspecies pattern of radiation life-shortening. Out of this came evidence for an important generalization, based on the observation that the upward displacement of the Gompertz function, ΔG, is in proportion to dose, D, so that the displacement per unit dose, $\Delta G/D$ is approximately constant for a species (Sacher, 1966). The interspecies comparison of $\Delta G/D$ values for experimental species showed that $\Delta G/D$ is nearly constant for all the species that have been adequately studied: mouse, rat, guinea-pig and dog. The species estimates range from 0.0030 to 0.0038 R^{-1} with an unweighted average of 0.0034 R^{-1}.

When the same quantitative approach is applied to human populations, and specifically to the mortality experience obtained from the Japanese atom bomb survivors

---

* This is introduced as a technical term, to signify injury of a kind that leads to morbidity and death, without the semantic contradictions that attach to the terms "lethal" or "sublethal" in this context.

(Jablon et al., 1965), the excess mortality per rad, $\Delta G/D$, for all causes of death is apparently smaller, by a factor of 2 or more, than it is for the animal populations. We are thus made aware that even when there is a high degree of consistency between experimental species, there can still be a large discrepancy in the contrast between man and the other animals. Fortunately, the discrepancy is in our favour, but it means that the theory of radiation life-shortening is still deficient in some important respects.

An unexpected area of agreement between mouse and man is the concordance of these two species in susceptibility to radiation leukaemia on a rate-of-incidence basis. A single X-ray dose can produce up to 90% incidence of lymphoid leukaemia in mice irradiated at young ages. This corresponds to approximately a 30-fold factor of increase in the instantaneous rate of occurrence of leukaemias (Sacher, 1956).

Human leukaemia has on the order of a thousand-fold lower absolute incidence than murine leukaemia, and the statement has been made quite often that there is therefore no value in the use of a murine model for human leukaemia. Yet, if we express human leukaemia incidence in terms of the factor of increase over the spontaneous, the increase per unit dose is about the same for man as it is for the mouse. This is an illuminating instance of an empirical relationship which was found as a consequence of studies on the Gompertz model, but which is not explained by that model, and, in addition, raises fundamental questions about the validity of the whole class of mutation-related models of carcinogenesis.

I shall now consider the modelling process in greater detail, and take up some of the questions and doubts that I mentioned at the beginning.

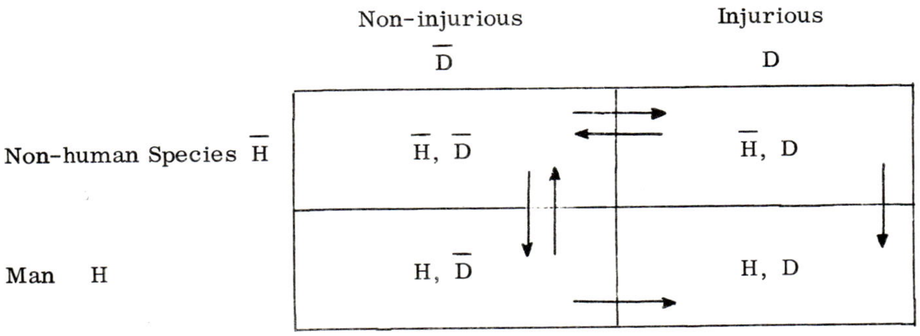

Paradigm for the modelling of destructive effects in man. Information about the cell "injurious/human", (H, D), cannot be generated within the cell, so it must be obtained by appropriate models based on two kinds of correspondence: (1) correspondence of the injury, recovery and death processes in man and animals, and (2) correspondence of constitution between man and animals at the tissue and cell level.

The diagram above presents a paradigm that I have found quite valuable for my own thought. It is a 2 x 2 matrix, which dichotomizes all living creatures into "human" and "non-human", and all experimental procedures into "injurious" and "non-injurious". Our problem is to fill in the cell "injurious/human". There are various strategies for doing so, according to the different kinds of information available to the clinician, epidemiologist or biologist. My model-making activities, as an experimental biologist, are built on the premise that the game is to fill in that cell solely on the basis of the information attainable from the other three cells. This can be done to the extent that man has cellular and physiological characteristics in common with some of the experimental objects we are free to study. The determination of these homologies, and degrees of relationship, are therefore a necessary part of the synthesis that must be achieved before experimental radiobiology can attain the goal of understanding late radiation effects in man.

The rigorous characterization of those system-properties requires that we detach ourselves from the obvious, concrete attributes of the various species and seek to give an abstract representation of each species in terms of a set of quantitative parameters. Such a reduction is a model. It can be tested, by making predictions which can be compared with experiment. By this process, we shall eventually learn how many parameters are required to determine the effects of radiation exposure on a specified function for a specific mammal. From this standpoint, I shall take up again the question of survival time as an end-point, taking as an illustration some data which came from the duration-of-life experiments that we have been doing at Argonne over the past decade.

We gave mice lifetime irradiation at a number of daily doses, running from 5 R/day up to 1650 R/day, starting at age 100 days. In fig. 1, the average survival time at each daily dose level is given on the abscissa, and the corresponding mean accumulated dose is shown on the ordinate (Sacher and Grahn, 1964). This is a rather complex functional

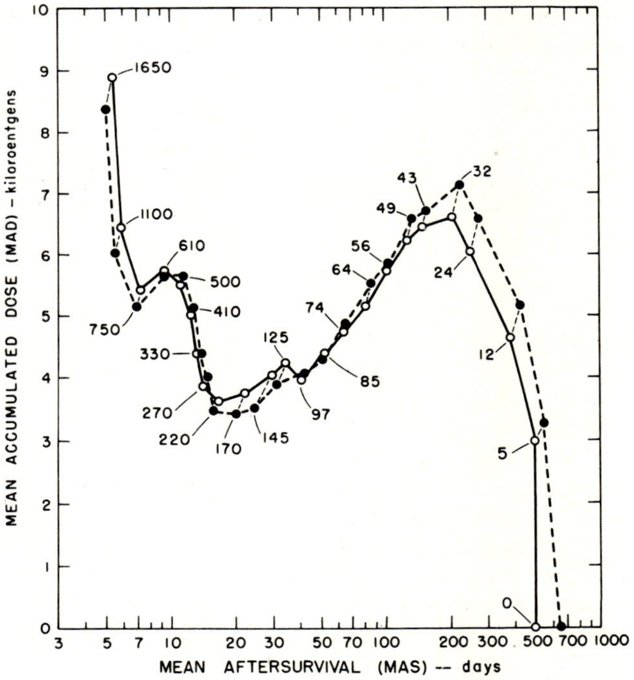

Fig. 1. Mean accumulated dose (MAD) as a function of mean after-survival time (MAS) for male and female LAF_1 mice exposed to ^{60}Co gamma rays for the duration of life, beginning at 100 days of age. The daily doses given are recorded in the chart. Open circles - males; closed circles - females. From J. natn. Cancer Inst., 32, 288, 1964.

relationship, even though all the numbers on it are the direct experimental observables of dose rate, mean accumulated dose, and mean after-survival time. It is necessary that we give to these data a more readily comprehended representation, that will enable us to say what is the quantitative course of lethal radiation injury in the mouse. This was done by a model-making process which is based on three simple assumptions; first, that lethality occurs at a constant determinate end-point; second, that all kinds of physiological injury combine additively to produce the summated morbific injury which, when it reaches the lethal end-point, leads to death; third, that the amount of injury produced is proportional to dose.

Although we make no assumption about how many injury processes there are, or the nature of the recovery processes, we can deduce a response function which is theoretically what would happen if we gave animals of this strain a dose of 1 R instantaneously, and then observed the process of injury as it proceeded. The outcome is shown in fig. 2. This is an empirical function, smoothed by numerical interpolation, which describes the sequence of injury produced by an impulse exposure in a linear model of the mouse, that obeys a dosage-survival relationship exactly as given by the real mice in fig. 1, and conforms to the three assumptions listed above.

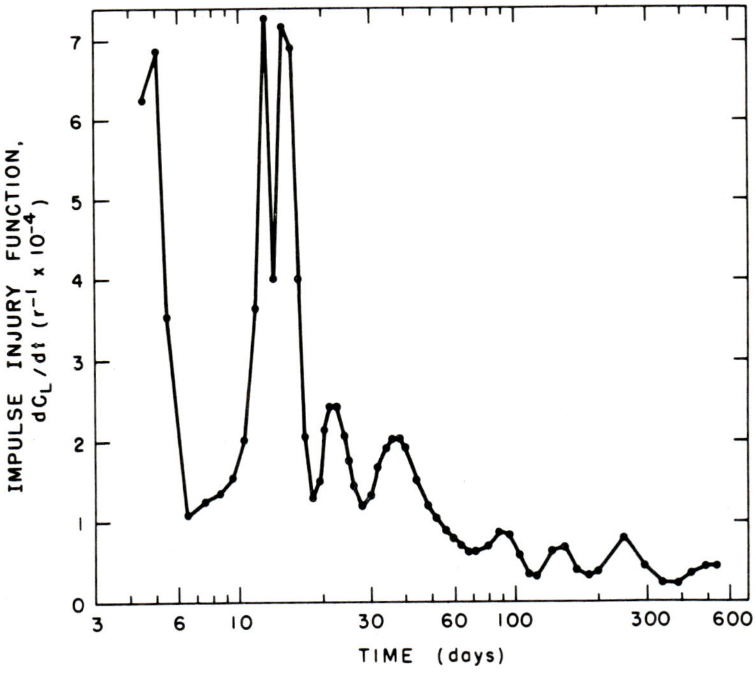

Fig. 2. The intensity of morbific injury in LAF_1 female mice as a function of time after the administration of a single brief exposure of 1 R at time zero. This curve was computed, without loss of information, from the dosage/survival data for female mice in fig. 1. The points are not data points, but rather the points at which the interpolation polynomial was evaluated. Time is plotted on a logarithmic scale so that the initial phasic components can be seen more clearly. Each peak is a separate component of injury, and the rate of decline is a measure of the recovery rate for that component (Sacher and Grahn, 1964).

These empirical response functions must, if they are to be useful, allow one to compute what happens when several doses are delivered in sequence. We have investigated this for the radiation lethality function.

If each dose fraction produces the impulse response function of fig. 2, then we can find out what happens when we give exposure as a specified function of time by carrying out a mathematical process called <u>convolution</u>. This is a procedure to compute, for each time, t, after the beginning of exposure, the integrated amount of injury arising from each increment of exposure, $A(\tau)d\tau$, for all times of exposure, τ, from $\tau = 0$ to $\tau = t$. If we call the integrated injury $J_1(\tau)$, and if the impulse injury function at time t arising from unit dose given at time $\tau < t$ is $S(t-\tau)$, then the amount of injury produced by dose $A(\tau)d\tau$ at time τ is $A(\tau)S(t-\tau)d\tau$, and the accumulated injury at time t is

$$J_1(t) = \int_0^t A(\tau)S(t-\tau)d\tau$$

This function can be computed numerically when $A(\tau)$ and $S(t-\tau)$ are known. We have carried out these computations for some illustrative exposure patterns (Sacher, 1965).

Figure 3 shows what happens if we convolute the impulse function with a "square-wave" exposure pattern, in which exposure is given at a constant rate for a time period of H days. This is also an adequate representation of highly fractionated exposure. Morbific injury builds up on a complex curve until exposure is terminated at time H, and then dies away, again as a complex function of time.

Given the quantitative nature of this response function, the convolution indicates that the last increments of dose, from the exposures received in the last days or weeks before the end-point is reached, make a comparatively small contribution to the lethality. This phenomenon was also noted by Mole, and he coined the phrase "wasted radiation" to characterize the observation that the dose needed to reach a given end-point is smaller if exposure is terminated before the end-point is reached than it is if exposure is continued up to the end-point (Mole, 1955).

The phrase "wasted radiation" is, or implies, a qualitative model of radiation effect, but it has the serious shortcoming that it has by itself no testable implications, and it does not give rise to a procedure for estimating the effectiveness of any specified dose-time pattern of exposure. This is an instance of the important principle that there are kinds of explanation which are true, in a tautological sense, and nevertheless are not proper scientific explanations, because they terminate the process of inquiry instead of advancing it (Popper, 1959). The real problem of the wasted radiation is still very much with us 15 years later, but the decision as to whether this is due to the tranquilizing effect of the phrase "wasted radiation" must be left as a problem in the psychology and sociology of the research process.

The real need is to know <u>why</u> there is a phenomenon of wasted radiation. This is not a simple matter, as I have learned since I first took up the problem a number of years ago. At least four mechanistic factors can be shown to be involved, and we will not be able to make accurate estimates of the effects of different time-patterns of exposure (the general problem that subsumes the wasted radiation problem) until these factors can be taken into account. This cannot be accomplished in one step, however, so my colleagues and I have found it desirable to introduce three diverse mathematical models which characterize the

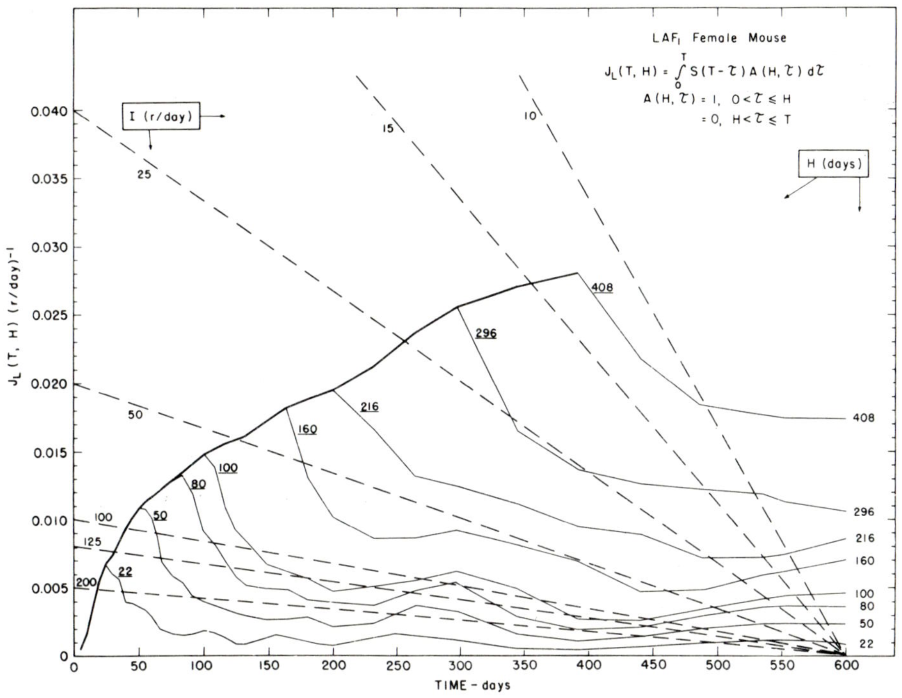

Fig. 3. The course of morbific injury in LAF_1 female mice given terminated exposure to ^{60}Co gamma rays, computed by the convolution equation given in the figure, using the data for female mice in fig. 1. The impulse function, $S(t-\tau)$, is the empirical function graphed in fig. 2, and $A(H, \tau)$ is the exposure function. The dashed lines are the daily dosages. By the linear hypothesis, a terminated exposure at length H at a given daily dosage, I, will lead to death at the time that the injury curve for exposure duration H first intersects with the slanting line which intercepts the ordinate at 1/I.

factors separately in a simpler, more manageable fashion.

One factor is latency in the appearance of functional, morbific injury. This was first evaluated quantitatively by means of the linear cumulant function model (Sacher, 1955; Sacher and Grahn, 1964), which is discussed briefly above. The cumulant function is an example of an empirical model, which enables us to compute, from the data themselves, everything that can be learned about the additive properties of the lethal response to repeated exposures (Sacher, 1965). It should be remarked in passing that this model embodies the minimum number of assumptions. Blair (1952) also developed a linear model, but he violated Occam's Rule by introducing two gratuitous, and incorrect, further assumptions about the number of injury processes and the form of the injury function. This denied him, *inter alia*, the opportunity to discover the latency property, for he had already assumed it not to exist.

A good model serves when it fails, as well as when it succeeds. The linear model can be tested by means of the convolution procedure referred to above, and the discrepancies that appear between prediction and observation can be used, together with other information, to guide further development. The linear convolution process does not predict correctly the relation between the total dose and number of daily fractions to yield 50% lethality within 30 days from the end of exposure (Sacher, 1965). A different kind of model is required for this purpose, which is non-linear, and therefore must be mechanistic and parametric, whereas the linear model can be formal and non-parametric (Sacher and Trucco, 1966). The non-linear model gives rise to a logistic equation as a simplified picture of damage and recovery in two cell demes, of dividing and post-mitotic cells respectively. This model shows how latency of morbific injury can arise from the population age structure in renewal tissues, such as the erythron. It predicts correctly the linear relation between dose and number of daily fractions for 50% lethality, and it also predicts that there is a shoulder in the split-dose recovery function. The existence of such a shoulder, in fair numerical agreement with prediction, has been demonstrated (Phillips and Ainsworth, 1969).

The logistic cell population model ignored certain properties of radiation damage in cells. One of these properties, that of division delay after irradiation, was examined separately (Sacher, 1968). Division delay is proportional to dose for a variety of cellular systems, and a simple mathematical model demonstrates that this property can be partly explained by means of second-order kinetics for an intracellular repair process.

The linear and logistic models for morbific injury are alike in being deterministic, i.e. they postulate that there is an exact functional dependence of injury on dose, and that the end-point is a determinate, constant value. These postulates are inconsistent with the observed properties of the lethal response in several ways. Consideration of these discrepancies, and of the general nature of homeostatic, life-sustaining processes in metazoans, led to the development of a probabilistic theory of failure and death in physiological systems. Mathematical models of stochastic mortality processes were derived and applied to various problems in late radiation mortality (Sacher, 1956; Sacher and Trucco, 1962). This theory accounts for some properties of lethal processes that cannot be explained by deterministic models (Sacher, 1965).

It should be particularly noted that these various models are intentionally simple and fragmentary, but because of that simplicity, they have served, and continue to serve, their purposes. One can use a model, knowing that it is "wrong", if one is careful to confine the applications to the limited domain within which the model is accurate in the required degree.

I do not want to leave the impression that we are anywhere near our goal. We have concentrated our efforts up to now on finding out what factors are involved: the construction of a good prediction model requires in addition procedures for statistical parameter estimation. Also, the above discussion has neglected some important radiobiological factors, in particular the details of the kinetics of intracellular damage and repair which have been revealed by the past decade of research in cellular radiobiology.

The best test of the model-building approach is to apply it to an exigent problem, such as radiation tumour therapy or immunosuppression by radiations or chemicals. Cohen and Scott (1968) adapted the non-linear population recovery model of Sacher and Trucco (1966) to the evaluation of the effectiveness of fractionation schedules, and it is to be hoped that more work can be started on the critical evaluation of mathematical models in relation to specific problems of therapy.

The models discussed thus far are diverse in kind, but alike in that each has as its referent the individual system (organism) or homogeneous group of systems (population). These models derive their value from the assumption that the specific system being modelled is typical of a class of "similar" systems, all amenable to application of the model. In the usual course of events, such an assumption is adequately tested by the accumulation of independent trials on other systems, but in regard to the lifetime effects that concern us here, this procedure is entirely inadequate. We do not yet have the information needed for valid extrapolation of long-term morbid effects from animals to man. The only hypothesis that has been seriously examined up to now is the hypothesis that the increase in age-specific mortality rate per rad is a constant independent of species lifespan (Sacher, 1966). We saw that the data for mice, rats, guinea-pigs and dogs are in good accord with the hypothesis, but that the predicted effect for man, expressed as the factor of increase of mortality rate, is considerably in excess of the observed increase. It is clear that other factors will need to be taken into account before we have an adequate understanding of radiation life-shortening in mammals.

An appropriate strategy for this situation is conveyed by the precept <u>reculer pour mieux sauter</u>. It became necessary for me to step back from the problem of radiation life-shortening to examine the broader question of vertebrate longevity and its determiners. This is an absorbing problem, which raises fundamental questions about the stability (longevity) of organisms and the systemic (organizational) factors on which it depends (Sacher, 1959, 1965). The search for systemic factors led to the discovery that two anatomical dimensions, body weight and brain weight, accurately predict the life-spans of mammalian species (Sacher, 1959), and to the recent observation that the metabolic rate has a negative correlation with longevity independent of body and brain weight (Sacher, 1969). Now that these important longevity factors have been identified, it is possible to design rational experiments to account for species differences in the life-shortening effects of radiations.

The analysis of the comparative physiology of longevity and its relation to radiation life-shortening is, therefore, like the cumulant function analysis discussed earlier, an instance of the general principle that good scientific method in theory construction requires the development of systematic procedures for the discovery of phenomena as well as for their explanation. Mathematical and statistical models are tools that can contribute to both of these processes, and to the effectiveness and economy of experimental procedures.

Conclusion

The use of mathematical models to assist the process of explanation of biological systems is still in its infancy. Much needs to be learned about new mathematical tools, but even more urgent is the need to develop sound methodologies of abstraction and generalization at the verbal and logical, as well as at the mathematical level.

The most important property of a scientific explanation is that it be falsifiable, i.e. have testable consequences (Popper, 1959). Mathematical models, if they are explicit, usually satisfy this requirement, but the virtue of the method is sometimes lost because of the all-too-human tendency of the author to devote his energies to defending his model, rather than to looking for the evidence needed to transcend it. However, some verbal explanations, precisely because they are true in an empty sense, can be insidiously harmful to the scientific process.

Another lesson to be learned is that Occam's razor can wound the unwary user. In the case of linear models of radiation injury, for example, the assumption that there is just one recovery constant was unparsimonious, because it was gratuitous. This unwarranted assumption gave rise to misconceptions, some of which are still with us.

Other considerations being equal, simplicity is a more important virtue than veridicality. The mathematical studies of radiation injury and lethality establish that the underlying processes are multifactorial, non-linear, and probabilistic. These properties were established by means of three relatively simple models: a multifactor model that is linear and deterministic (Sacher, 1956; Sacher and Grahn, 1964), a non-linear model that is single-factor and deterministic (Sacher and Trucco, 1966), and a probabilistic model that is single-factor, and either linear or non-linear (Sacher, 1956; Sacher and Trucco, 1962). These partial models are still useful. A satisfactory unified model, incorporating all the established kinetic properties, has not yet been produced, but it is not for want of effort. The important requirement for the development of such a model is the recognition of an urgent need in relation to some important, but circumscribed, problem, such as those arising from tumour therapy, or immunosuppressive therapy, or environmental pollution. If the need is recognized, and adequate support is forthcoming, the problems can be solved.

References

Berlin, N.I., and DiMaggio, F.L. A survey of theories and experiments on the shortening of life span by ionizing radiation. Report AFSWP-608, Department of Defense, Washington, D.C., 1956.

Blair, H. A formulation of the injury, life span, dose relations for ionizing radiations. I. Application to the mouse. USAEC Report UR-206, Univ. of Rochester, 1952.

Boche, R.D. Effects of chronic exposure to X-radiation on growth and survival. In Biological Effects of External Radiation. edited by H. Blair, New York, McGraw-Hill (first issued as USAEC Report MDDC-204, Univ. of Rochester, 1946), 1954.

Cohen, L., and Scott, M.J. Fractionation procedures in radiation therapy: a computerized approach to evaluation. Br. J. Radiol., 42, 529-533, 1968.

Grahn, D. Biological effects of protracted low dose radiation exposure of man and animals. These Proceedings, pp. 101-36 1970.

Jablon, S., Ishida, M., and Yamasaki, M. Studies on the mortality of A-bomb survivors. 3. Description of the samples and mortality, 1950-1960. Radiat. Res., 25, 25-5 1965.

Jones, H.B. A special consideration of the aging process, disease and life expectancy. In Adv. Biol. Med. Physics, 4, 281-337, 1956.

Mole, R.H. On wasted radiation and the interpretation of experiments with chronic irradiation. J. natn. Cancer Inst., 15, 907-914, 1955.

Mole, R.H. Late effects of exposure to ionizing radiation: animal experimentation and human protection. Proc. First European Symposium on Late Effects of Radiation, edited by G. Silini and P. Metalli, Casaccia, Italy (in press).

Phillips, T.L., and Ainsworth, E.J. Altered split-dose recovery in mice irradiated under hypoxic conditions. Radiat. Res., 39, 317-331, 1969.

Popper, K. The logic of scientific discovery. New York, Basic Books, 1959.

Sacher, G.A. Survival of mice under duration-of-life exposure to X-rays at various rates. In Biological Effects of External X and Gamma Radiation, Part 2, TID-5220, edited by R.E. Zirkle, Dept. of Commerce, Office of Technical Services, Washington, D.C. First issued as USAEC Report CH3900, Univ. of Chicago Metallurgical Laboratory, 1956a.

Sacher, G.A. On the statistical nature of mortality, with special reference to chronic radiation mortality. Radiology, 67, 250-257, 1956b.

Sacher, G.A. Relation of lifespan to brain and body weight in mammals. In Ciba Foundation Colloquium on the Lifespan of Animals. edited by G.E.W. Wolstenholme and M. O'Connor, Boston, Little, Brown & Co., pp. 115-133, 1959.

Sacher, G.A. Lethal effects of whole-body irradiation in mice. The dose-time relation for terminated and time-dependent exposure. Radiol. Clin. N. Am., 3, 227-241, 1965a.

Sacher, G.A. On longevity as an organized behavior: the role of brain structure. In Contributions to the Psychobiology of Aging, edited by R. Kastenbaum, New York, Springer Publ. Co., pp. 99-110, 1965b.

Sacher, G.A. The Gompertz transformation in the study of the injury-mortality relationship. Application to late radiation effects and ageing. In Radiation and Ageing, edited by P.J. Lindop and G.A. Sacher, London, Taylor & Francis Ltd., pp. 411-441, 1966.

Sacher, G.A. Mathematical analysis of the division delay produced by ionizing radiation. Radiat. Res., 33, 644-658, 1968.

Sacher, G.A. Unpublished observations, 1969.

Sacher, G.A., and Grahn, D. Survival of mice under duration-of-life exposure to gamma rays. I. The dosage-survival relation and the lethality function. J. natn. Cancer Inst., 32, 277-321, 1964.

Sacher, G.A., and Trucco, E. The stochastic theory of mortality. Ann. N.Y. Acad. Sci., 96, 985-1007, 1962.

Sacher, G.A., and Trucco, E. Theory of radiation injury and recovery in self-renewing cell populations. Radiat. Res., 29, 236-256, 1966.

CHAPTER XI

EPIDEMIOLOGICAL CONCLUSIONS FROM RADIATION TOXICITY STUDIES

Robert W. Miller

Epidemiology is in general observational rather than experimental. The epidemiologist must make the most of natural circumstances in seeking new information about disease. Unlike the laboratory investigator, he must take things as they are, rather than as he might ideally want them to be.

In the establishment of a causal relationship, statistics alone are usually not enough. Implications of causality will be greatly aided by demonstrating:

1. A specificity of effect (e.g. for certain rather than for all causes of morbidity).
2. A response that is proportionate to dose.
3. Absence of an influence of concomitant variables.
4. Results that are consistent with other information available from laboratory, clinical, and epidemiological studies.

My purpose, however, is not to speak of epidemiologic principles in the abstract, but to apply them in interpreting radiation effects in man. In particular, I will examine certain findings of the Atomic Bomb Casualty Commission (ABCC) in relation to one another and in relation to observations from other sources.

Effects on the Embryo

Only one congenital malformation has been described to date as a result of exposure to the atomic bomb; namely, small head circumference with mental retardation. Each of the four indications of causality listed above has been demonstrated. Yet, in describing radiation-induced diseases among the survivors of Hiroshima and Nagasaki, this one is often omitted.

The most recent report on the effects of intrauterine exposure (Wood et al., 1967a) confirms those previously published (Plummer, 1952; Miller, 1956). The effect was primarily among children of women who were exposed to the atomic bomb within 15 weeks of their last menstrual period (table 1). Among the 56 in this category who were within 1800 metres of the hypocentre, a head circumference two or more standard deviations (S.D.) below the mean for age and sex was expected in 1.4 persons (2.5%), as compared with 23 observed, 9 of them mentally retarded. Among the 105 exposed more than 15 weeks after the mother's last menstrual period, small head circumference was expected in 2.6 as compared with 6 observed, 2 of whom were mentally retarded. The usual frequency of comparable retarded intelligence among the non-exposed of the same age in Hiroshima and Nagasaki was about 1% (Wood et al.,

Table 1

Effects of intrauterine exposure to the Hiroshima atomic bomb; head circumference 2 or more S.D. below average; exposure within 1800 metres of the hypocentre (from Wood et al., 1967)

	Gestational Age	
	≤15 weeks	>15 weeks
Total exposed	57[a]	109
Total examined	56[a]	105
Small head circumference		
with mental retardation	9	2[b]
with normal intelligence	14	4[c]

[a]Excludes 2 with pre-existent Down's syndrome.
[b]Exposed at 21 and 24-25 weeks.
[c]Exposed at 16, 32, 32, and 36-40 weeks

1967b). Table 2 reveals a dose-response relationship, i.e. the effect diminished in frequency and severity as the distance from the hypocentre increased. These findings are in accord with the results of animal experimentation and with a series of cases collected in the late 1920's concerning the excess of this anomaly among children born of mothers who received pelvic radiotherapy during early pregnancy (Murphy, 1928; Goldstein and Murphy, 1929). In Hiroshima the malformation occurred excessively within the range of high radiation dosage and not in relation to heavy destruction and economic loss, which extended far beyond. Estimates of the teratogenic dose-range in man have not as yet been published, but about half of the mothers of affected children reported that they had signs of severe acute radiation sickness (Miller, 1956). No other anomalies occurred excessively among the survivors (Plummer, 1952; Miller, 1956), although many others have been observed in animals exposed experimentally to X irradiation (Rugh, 1959).

Genetic Effects

In preparation for comments later about leukaemogenesis, we turn our attention now to genetic effects of irradiation, as evaluated in the F_1 generation.

It is commonly thought that congenital anomalies are the only measure of the submicroscopic genetic effects of ionizing radiation. The studies conducted at the ABCC, however, concerned six indicators of genetic damage (Neel and Schull, 1956; Neel, 1963; Schull et al., 1966; Kato et al., 1966). No influence of radiation was demonstrable in the study, which involved about 70,000 pregnancies and was likely to have detected a two-fold increase

Table 2

Radiation effect on head circumference and intelligence following intrauterine exposure to the Hiroshima atomic bomb within 15 weeks of the mother's last menstrual period (from Wood et al., 1967)

Intelligence	Head circumference	Distance from hypocentre (metres)			
		≤1200	1200-1500	1501-1800	1801-2200
Retarded	>3 S.D. below mean	6	0[a]	0	0
Retarded	-2 to -3 S.D.	2	0	1	0
Normal	>3 S.D. below mean	1	2	0	0
Normal	-2 to -3 S.D.	1	6	5	0
Total exposed		11	23[a]	23[b]	21[b]

[a]Excludes 2 with pre-existent Down's syndrome.
[b]One not examined.

in malformation rates or a 1.8-fold increase in stillbirth and neonatal death rates; there was no effect attributable to radiation on birth weight, on anthropometric values at 8 to 10 months of age or on mortality. The sex ratio following preconception radiation in theory would be diminished if the mother was irradiated and increased if the father was (Neel, 1963). In a study of about 120,000 births, such shifts did occur in the first 10 years following exposure to the atomic bombs, but not thereafter (Kato et al., 1966). Thus, though laboratory experimentation leaves no doubt that radiation is mutagenic, the effect could not be demonstrated in the F_1 generation studied at ABCC.

Cytogenetic Abnormalities

Table 3 summarizes the results obtained in a series of studies of chromosomal abnormalities among various age-groups exposed to the Japanese atomic bombs. It will be noted that among those 30 years of age or younger at the time of the bomb (ATB) who received at least 200 rads, 34% had complex cytogenetic abnormalities 20 years later as compared with 1% of the controls (Bloom et al., 1966). The percentage so affected who were over 30 years of age ATB was almost double that of the younger group, and 4 of the 77 in the older group had clones of genetically abnormal cells (Bloom et al., 1967). The frequency of complex cytogenetic abnormalities apparently increases naturally with age, from 1% in the younger group to 16% in the older group (table 3). Among persons who were in utero ATB and whose mothers received at least 100 rads, 39% displayed complex chromosomal abnormalities as compared with 4% of the controls (Bloom et al., 1968). Finding these abnormalities even among persons exposed during the first trimester indicates that radiation can induce

Table 3

Frequencies by age group of complex cytogenetic abnormalities among Japanese survivors of the atomic bombs

Age group	Exposed		Controls	Reference
	Min. dose (rads)	Affected		
≤ 30 yrs ATB	200	34% of 94	1% of 94	Bloom et al., 1966
Over 30 yrs ATB	200	61% of 77	16% of 80	Bloom et al., 1967
In utero ATB	100[a]	39% of 38	4% of 48	Bloom et al., 1968
Preconception	150[a]	0% of 103	....	Awa et al., 1968
Preconception	100[b]	0% of 25	....	Awa et al., 1968

[a]Maternal dose.
[b]Dose received by at least one parent.

long-persisting changes in the lymphocyte precursors. In contrast to the cytogenetic defects observed following intrauterine (post-conception) exposure, none were found following preconception irradiation (Awa et al., 1968). These observations revealed that in man chromosomal damage was induced even though an effect on the F_1 generation was not demonstrable. The results are consistent with other observations pertaining to therapeutic and other radiation exposures (Evans et al., 1967). A dose-response relationship was not sought because of the burden of work involved, but the other evidence of causality in the absence of known concomitant variables with the same effect, leaves no doubt that the increase in complex cytogenetic aberrations was radiation-induced.

Leukaemogenesis

Whole-body exposure

The leukaemogenic effect of radiation in man was suspected at about the same time and in the same way that teratogenic effects were, that is, through case-reports (Dunlap, 1942). Lymphoma was experimentally induced in mice in 1930 (Krebs et al., 1930). Then, by simply reviewing the death notices published weekly in the *Journal of the American Medical Association*, March (1946) and Ulrich (1946) independently found that U.S. radiologist died significantly more often of leukaemia than did other physicians. In consequence, a leukaemogenic effect of exposure to atomic radiation was expected and found among the survivors in Hiroshima and Nagasaki (Folley et al., 1952; Brill et al., 1962; Bizzozero et al., 1966). A dose-response relationship was observed which can be attributed to no variable except radiation. A peak in occurrence was reached in 1951, more marked for the acute leukaemias than for chronic granulocytic leukaemia (fig. 1). Chronic lymphocytic leukaemia, rare

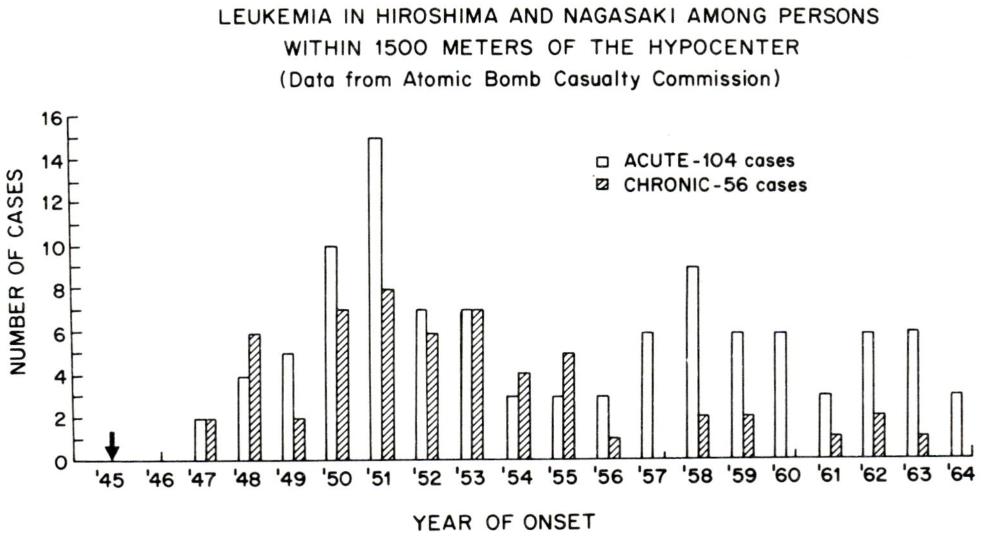

Fig. 1. Number of cases of leukaemia by type and year of onset among survivors of Hiroshima and Nagasaki who had been within 1500 metres of the hypocentre. (Reprinted from J.F. Fraumeni, Jr., and R.W. Miller, J. natn. Cancer Inst., 38, 593-605, 1967.)

among the Japanese (Finch et al., 1969), was not increased in frequency. In children, leukaemia was generally acute, as usual, the lymphocytic form being as common as granulocytic (Brill et al., 1962). In all age-groups, acute leukaemia continued to occur at higher than usual rates through 1966, whereas chronic granulocytic leukaemia had fallen to near normal rates (Bizzozero et al., 1966). The ABCC study leaves no doubt that whole-body exposure to ionizing radiation in sufficient dose can induce leukaemia in man.

Partial-body exposure

Human leukaemia may also be induced by partial-body radiation, as indicated by the dose-response effect observed in British men given radiotherapy for ankylosing spondylitis (Court Brown and Doll, 1957, 1965). Again the peak was reached about 5 years after first exposure (course of therapy), the predominant form in adults was granulocytic, and no increase occurred in the frequency of chronic lymphocytic leukaemia. In all, 52 cases of leukaemia were observed as compared with 5.48 expected, and 15 persons developed aplastic anaemia (perhaps subclinical leukaemia) as compared with 0.51 expected. This study in conjunction with that of ABCC revealed that ionizing radiation can induce more than one form of leukaemia in man, but not all forms, the notable exception being chronic lymphocytic leukaemia.

Other leukaemogenic circumstances

Epidemiology is largely a study of the origins of disease. Through this approach, a foothold to aetiology may be gained by recognition of attributes or exposures that carry high risk of a disease. When several such high-risk groups have been defined, one may look for a factor in common. With regard to leukaemia, radiation exposure is but one circumstance with an increased frequency of this neoplasm (table 4). At much higher risk are (1) the child whose identical twin develops leukaemia before 6 years of age, (2) adults with polycythaemia vera treated with X ray and/or ^{32}P, and (3) persons with Bloom's syndrome or Fanconi's aplastic anaemia (Miller, 1967). Their probability of developing leukaemia is about 1 in 6; that is, about ten times greater than that of Hiroshima survivors who were within 1,000 metres of the hypocentre. At lower risk of leukaemia are children with Down's syndrome (1:95 under 10 years of age) and radiation-treated patients with ankylosing spondylitis (1:270 over an interval of 15 years). These high-risk groups have in common a distinctive genetic feature, though not of uniform nature. Identical twins have identical genes; Bloom's and Fanconi's syndromes are genetically induced disorders with chromosomal fragility*; polycythaemia vera often exhibits aneuploidy before radiation and chromosomal breaks subsequently; exposure to ionizing radiation or to benzene produces long-lasting chromosomal breaks; and Down's syndrome is characterized by congenital aneuploidy.

Table 4

Groups at exceptionally high risk of leukaemia[a]

Group	Approximate risk	Time interval
Identical twins of children with leukaemia	1 in 5	Weeks or months
Radiation-treated polycythaemia vera	1 in 6	10-15 years
Bloom's syndrome	1 in 8	< 30 years of age
Hiroshima survivors who were within 1000 metres of the hypocentre	1 in 60	12 years
Down's syndrome	1 in 95	< 10 years of age
Radiation-treated patients with ankylosing spondylitis	1 in 270	15 years
Siblings of leukaemic children	1 in 720	10 years
U.S. white children <15 years of age	1 in 2880	10 years

[a]from Miller (1967).

Leukaemia in patients with polycythaemia vera has been attributed to radiotherapy (Modan and Lilienfeld, 1965). In table 4, however, it will be noted that the risk of the neoplasm in polycythaemia vera was ten times higher than it was among heavily exposed Hiroshima survivors and 45 times higher than in radiation-treated ankylosing spondylitis. One must conclude that in polycythaemia vera, radiation exposure or damage is greater than in the other two instances or that polycythaemia vera predisposes to leukaemia in the absence of radiation exposure. Further studies must be made to distinguish between these two possibilities.

---

* Chromosomal fragility is used in the sense that there is a greater incidence of chromosome breaks and rearrangement in cells in culture than normal.

A recently developed laboratory procedure may help to clarify the role of irradiation in human leukaemia. Todaro et al. (1966) have developed a quantitative procedure to measure susceptibility of human skin fibroblasts to transformation in vitro following infection with SV40, a virus which produces neoplasms in experimental animals. Normally, skin fibroblasts grow in a monolayer. When SV40 is added, the fibroblasts are transformed into epitheloid cells, which through loss of contact inhibition pile up into easily visualized colonies ("microtumours"). A marked increase in the number of transformed colonies is observed when fibroblasts from patients with Fanconi's anaemia are infected with SV40, and to a lesser extent in Down's syndrome. In both disorders, there are chromosomal abnormalities and a predisposition to leukaemia. When normal human fibroblasts are irradiated in vitro, no increase in susceptibility to transformation is observed, but when the cells are infected with SV40 before or after irradiation, the transforming capacity of the virus is enhanced, the response being proportionate to the radiation dose (Pollock and Todaro, 1968). In view of these laboratory findings, it would be of interest to determine if skin fibroblasts from atomic bomb survivors or other persons heavily irradiated decades ago display increased susceptibility to transformation by SV40 in vitro.

Childhood cancer following intrauterine or preconception irradiation

Several studies, taken individually, suggest that very small radiation exposures before conception or during pregnancy may as much as double the child's risk of leukaemia. When these studies are taken collectively, however, there is reason to suspect that some fault in the methods, difficult or impossible to escape, may be implicating radiation spuriously.

The individual results are as follows. In 1958, Stewart and her associates described a study in which mothers of 677 leukaemic children in England and Wales reported about twice the frequency of abdominal exposure to diagnostic radiation during the relevant pregnancy as compared with mothers of normal children living in the same locale. A similar difference was found among mothers of 739 children with all other neoplasms as compared with the control series. The possibility exists that mothers of children with cancer reported or remembered their radiologic exposures differently than did mothers of healthy children. MacMahon (1962) avoided this potential bias in interview histories by studying obstetric records for irradiation during pregnancy among mothers of 304 leukaemic children and 252 children with other cancer as compared with a 1% sample of all other births in the area (New England). He found a 40% excess of (1) leukaemia and (2) all other neoplasia among children whose mothers' records showed diagnostic radiation of the abdomen during pregnancy. Similar results were obtained by Graham et al. (1966) with respect to leukaemia, and by Stewart and Kneale (1968) for each of six categories of childhood cancer. A causal relationship would be indicated if a dose-response effect could be demonstrated, if the results were consistent with those from animal experimentation, and if concomitant variables could be excluded. The exposures involved were too small to permit evaluation of a dose-response effect, and there are no data from animal studies which support the observations in man.

Recently, Graham and his associates (1966) described an excess of leukaemia among children whose mothers or fathers gave histories of diagnostic radiation exposure up to a decade before the children were conceived. Again, there is no support for this observation from animal experimentation, and in a prospective study (Hoshino et al., 1967) of 22,400 children conceived after their parents were heavily exposed to the atomic bomb in Hiroshima or Nagasaki, no excess of leukaemia was found.

Table 5 summarizes the results following minimal doses of X ray, and indicates that such irradiation was equally oncogenic whether exposure occurred before conception or

Table 5

Relative risk of various childhood cancers following intrauterine or preconception diagnostic radiation exposure

Neoplasm	Relative risk[a]
Intrauterine exposure	
Stewart and Kneale (1968)	
Leukaemia	1.5
Lymphosarcoma	1.5
Cerebral tumours	1.5
Neuroblastoma	1.5
Wilms' tumour	1.6
Other cancer	1.5
MacMahon (1962)	
Leukaemia	1.5
Central-nervous system tumours	1.6
Other cancer	1.4
Graham et al. (1966)	
Leukaemia	1.4
Preconception exposure	
Graham et al. (1966)	
Leukaemia	
Mother exposed	1.6
Father exposed	1.3

[a] Relative risk in controls = 1.0.

during pregnancy, whether the neoplasm studied was leukaemia or any other major cancer of childhood, and whether the study was based on interviews, which may be biased, or on hospital records. Taken in the aggregate, the similarity of results in the absence of a dose-response effect or of supporting data from animal experimentation raises a question about the biologic plausibility of a causal relationship. In particular, one must ask if preconception irradiation is likely to induce leukaemia in the absence of demonstrable mutagenic or cytogenetic abnormalities in the F_1 generation.

Cancer Other than Leukaemia

Lung cancer

Wanebo et al. (1968a) have recently reported that "the accumulated information on lung cancer strongly suggests that exposure to ionizing radiation has increased the risk of lung cancer among atomic bomb survivors." These investigators observed 17 such cases as compared with 9 expected (dose = 90 or more rads). An immense weakness in the report was the finding that the lung cancers induced were non-specific as to histologic type, rather than of the undifferentiated or small-cell type, as in U.S. uranium miners (Wagoner et al., 1965) and workers heavily exposed to mustard gas, a radiomimetic chemical (Wada et al., 1968).

Breast cancer

Wanebo et al. (1968b) have reported that "information on breast cancer among survivors of the atomic bombings of Hiroshima and Nagasaki has now accumulated to the point where a fairly definite carcinogenic effect seems established." Six cases were observed among women who were exposed to 90 rads or more, as compared with 1.53 expected, an excess of only 4.5 cases. There was no specificity as to histologic type.

It may be difficult or impossible to avoid certain biases that could produce such a small excess; e.g. unequal ascertainment of cases with respect to exposure category, or dissimilar cancer risks in relation to some variable other than radiation which distinguished the heavily exposed from others in the study. The authors considered these biases, and believed that they were not present. The absence of a dose-response relationship handicaps interpretations of the results, as does the small or uncertain increase in breast cancer observed in studies of other radiation-exposed persons (cited by Wanebo et al., 1968b).

Thyroid cancer

Wood et al. (1969) have recently described an excess of thyroid cancer among Japanese atomic-bomb survivors. The increase was greater in women than in men, with the effect proportionate to the radiation dose, but no specificity as to cell type. These observations are in accord with the results of animal experimentation (Lindsey and Cheikoff, 1964) and with the increase in frequency of thyroid cancer following therapeutic radiation early in childhood (Hempelmann, 1968).

On the basis of the indicators of a causal relationship described at the outset of this presentation, one may conclude that among the Japanese atomic-bomb survivors only leukaemia and thyroid cancer have been shown to be radiation-induced. The evidence pertaining to cancer of the breast or lung is still very much in doubt.

Conclusion

The delineation of delayed effects of radiation in man is epidemiologic in nature. Observations from ABCC have been cited to illustrate (1) factors involved in establishing causality and (2) the importance of relating individual findings in the same study to one another and to those from other studies.

References

Awa, A.A., Bloom, A.D., Yoshida, M.C., Neriishi, S., and Archer, P.G. Cytogenetic study of the offspring of atom bomb survivors. Nature, Lond., 218, 367-368, 1968.

Bizzozero, O.J., Jr., Johnson, K.G., and Ciocco, A. Radiation-related leukemia in

Hiroshima and Nagasaki, 1946-1964. New Engl. J. Med., 274, 1095-1101, 1966

Bloom, A.D. Neriishi, S., Kamada, N., Iseki, T., and Keehn, R.J. Cytogenetic investigation of survivors of the atomic bombings of Hiroshima and Nagasaki. Lancet, 2, 672-674, 1966.

Bloom, A.D. Neriishi, S., Awa, A.A., Honda, T., and Archer, P.G. Chromosome aberrations in leucocytes of older survivors of the atomic bombings of Hiroshima and Nagasaki. Lancet, 2, 802-805, 1967.

Bloom, A.D., Neriishi, S., and Archer, P.G. Cytogenetics of the in-utero exposed of Hiroshima and Nagasaki. Lancet, 2, 10-12, 1968.

Brill, A.B., Tomonaga, M., and Heyssel, R.M. Leukemia in man following exposure to ionizing radiation: Summary of findings in Hiroshima and Nagasaki, and comparison with other human experience. Ann. Intern. Med., 56, 590-609, 1962.

Court Brown, W.M., and Doll, R. Leukaemia and aplastic anaemia in patients irradiated for ankylosing spondylitis. Med. Res. Council, Spec. Rep. Series No. 295, Her Majesty's Stationery Office, London, 1957.

Court Brown, W.M., and Doll, R. Mortality from cancer and other causes after radiotherapy for ankylosing spondylitis. Br. Med. J., 2, 1327-1332, 1965.

Dunlap, C.E. Effects of radiation on blood and hemopoietic tissues, including spleen, thymus and lymph nodes. Arch. Path., 34, 562-608, 1942.

Evans, H.J., Court Brown, W., and McLean, A.S. Human Radiation Cytogenetics. North-Holland Publishing Co., Amsterdam, 1967.

Finch, S.C., Hoshino, T., Itoga, T., Ichimaru, M., and Ingram, R.H., Jr. Chronic lymphocytic leukemia in Hiroshima and Nagasaki, Japan. Blood, 33, 79-86, 1969.

Folley, J.H., Borges, W., and Yamawaki, T. Incidence of leukemia in survivors of atomic bomb in Hiroshima and Nagasaki, Japan. Am. J. Med., 13, 311-321, 1952.

Goldstein, L., and Murphy, D.P. Etiology of the ill-health in children born after maternal pelvic irradiation. Part II. Defective children born after post-conception pelvic irradiation. Am. J. Roentg., 22, 322-331, 1929.

Graham, S., Levin, M.L., Lilienfeld, A.M., Schuman, L.M., Gibson, R., Dowd, J.E., and Hempelmann, L. Preconception intrauterine and postnatal radiation as related to leukemia. Natn. Cancer Inst. Monogr., 19, 347-371, 1966.

Hempelmann, L.H. Risk of thyroid neoplasms after irradiation in childhood. Science, N.Y 160, 159-163, 1968.

Hoshino, T., Kato, H., Finch, S.C., and Hrubec, Z. Leukemia in offspring of atomic bom survivors. Blood, 30, 719-730, 1967.

Kato, H., Schull, W.J., and Neel, J.V. A cohort-type study of survival in the children of parents exposed to atomic bombings. Am. J. hum. Genet., 18, 339-373, 1966.

Krebs, C., Rask-Nielsen, H.C., and Wagner, A. Origins of lymphosarcomatosis and its relation to other forms of leukosis in white mice. Acta radiol., Suppl., 10, 1-53, 1930.

Lindsey, S., and Cheikoff, I.L. The effects of irradiation on the thyroid gland with particular reference to the induction of thyroid neoplasms: a review. Cancer Res., 24, 1099-1107, 1964.

MacMahon, B. Prenatal X-ray exposure and childhood cancer. J. natn. Cancer Inst., 28, 1173-1191, 1962.

March, H.C. Leukemia in radiologists. Radiology, 43, 275-278, 1946.

Miller, R.W. Delayed effects occurring within the first decade after exposure of young individuals to the Hiroshima atomic bomb. Pediatrics, 18, 1-18, 1956.

Miller, R.W. Persons with exceptionally high risk of leukemia. Cancer Res., 27, 2420-2423, 1967.

Modan, B., and Lilienfeld, A.M. Polycythemia vera and leukemia - the role of radiation treatment. A study of 1222 patients. Medicine, 44, 305-344, 1965.

Murphy, D.P. Ovarian irradiation; its effect on the health of subsequent children: review of the literature, experimental and clinical, with a report of 320 human pregnancies. Surgery Gynec. Obstet., 47, 201-215, 1928.

Neel, J.V. Changing Perspectives on the Genetic Effects of Radiation. Thomas Publishing Co., Springfield, 1963.

Neel, J.V., and Schull, W.J. The effect of exposure to the atomic bombs on pregnancy termination in Hiroshima and Nagasaki. National Academy of Sciences-National Research Council, Publ. No. 461, Washington, D.C., 1956.

Plummer, G. Anomalies occurring in children exposed in utero to the atomic bomb in Hiroshima. Pediatrics, 10, 687-693, 1952.

Pollock, E.J., and Todaro, G.J. Radiation enhancement of SV40 transformation in 3T3 and human cells. Nature, Lond., 219, 520-521, 1968.

Rugh, R. Vertebrate radiobiology (embryology). A. Rev. nucl. Sci., 9, 493-522, 1959.

Schull, W.J., Neel, J.V., and Hashizume, A. Some further observations on the sex ratio among infants born to survivors of the atomic bombings of Hiroshima and Nagasaki. Am. J. hum. Genet., 18, 328-338, 1966.

Stewart, A., Webb, J., and Hewitt, D. A survey of childhood malignancies. Br. Med. J., 1, 1495-1508, 1958.

Stewart, A., and Kneale, G.W. Changes in the cancer risk associated with obstetric radiography, Lancet, 1, 104-107, 1968.

Todaro, G.J., Green, H., and Swift, M.R. Susceptibility of human diploid fibroblast strains to transformation by SV40 virus. Science, N.Y., 153, 1252-1254, 1966.

Ulrich, H. Incidence of leukemia in radiologists. New Engl. J. Med., 234, 45-46, 1946.

Wada, S., Nishimoto, Y., Miyanishi, M., Kambe, S., and Miller, R.W. Mustard gas as a cause of respiratory neoplasia in man. Lancet, 1, 1161-1163, 1968.

Wagoner, J.K., Archer, V.E., Lundin, F.E., Jr., Holaday, D.A., and Lloyd, J.W. Radiation as the cause of lung cancer among uranium miners. New Engl. J.Med., 273, 181-188, 1965.

Wanebo, C.K., Johnson, K.G., Sato, K., and Thorslund, T.W. Lung cancer following atomic radiation. Am. Rev. resp. Dis., 98, 778-787, 1968a.

Wanebo, C.K., Johnson, K.G., Sato, K., and Thorslund, T.W. Breast cancer after exposure to the atomic bombings of Hiroshima and Nagasaki. New Engl. J. Med., 279, 667-671, 1968b.

Wood, J.W., Johnson, K.G., and Omori, Y. In utero exposure to the Hiroshima atomic bomb, an evaluation of head size and mental retardation: twenty years later. Pediatrics, 39, 385-392, 1967a.

Wood, J.W., Johnson, K.G., Omori, Y., Kawamoto, S., and Keehn, R.J. Mental retardation in children exposed in utero to the atomic bombs in Hiroshima and Nagasaki. Am. J. Publ. Hlth, 57, 1381-1390, 1967b.

Wood, J.W., Tamagaki, H. Neriishi, S., Sato, T., Sheldon, W.F., Archer, P.G., Hamilton, H.B., and Johnson, K.G. Thyroid carcinoma in atomic bomb survivors Hiroshima and Nagasaki. Am. J. Epid., 89, 4-14, 1969.

DISCUSSION OF CHAPTERS X AND XI

Dr. Bond: Both Drs. Sacher and Miller in their excellent papers pointed out admirably the purposes, value and limitations of models. They dealt mainly with irradiation of the whole mammal, and the end-points of visible long-term effects were studied. I cannot add to these models, nor subtract. It is a truism to state that the models provide a framework upon which one can build, and to provide a means for extrapolation, however empirical, to other situations such as different species, age, range of dose, dose rate, etc.

I should like to deal with a rather small portion of the overall problem of models and extrapolation, and shall confine my remarks to possible effects at very low doses and dose rates. The importance of assessing the degree of effect at low doses is obvious. With increasing uses of radiation, more individuals in the population are becoming exposed to small doses of radiation. Thus, in addition to background, exposure results from medical diagnostic procedures, fall-out radiation, radiation from nuclear power plants, X radiation from TV sets, etc. The doses are small, of the order of millirads per year and at most a few rads per generation. It is important that possible effects at low doses not be underestimated. On the other hand, overestimation of the degree of possible effects can be quite costly to society in terms of dollars, effort, apprehension, and denial of real benefits. It would be preferable to deal with actual data on effects at very low doses. In the absence of such data, every effort should be made to ensure that extrapolations are realistic.

There are very few direct measurements of the biological effects of low doses of radiation (of the order of 5 R or less). If one looks at so-called simpler systems, and deals with cell survival or the type of studies that Dr. Bender reported on here there are few data at lower doses. However, one can obtain rather complete dose-effect curves, and can perhaps feel comfortable in extrapolating to the degree of effect at low doses. Empirical curve fitting is resorted to, but we do not really know the shape of the curve at very low dose levels.

In more complex systems, the situation is of course much more complicated. What one is interested in practically are the effects on the mammal, such as those dealt with by Dr. Sacher. These include a host of possible long-term effects, such as longevity, leukaemia, other malignancies, cataract formation, and genetic effects. Data at very low doses are non-existent. Dose-effect curves can be constructed, but they are empirical indeed. One does not know mechanisms even at the cellular level, let alone at finer levels of organization. Frequently one does not even know what cell system is responsible for the gross effect noted. There is a greater chance for complicating factors such as abscopal effects, hormone influences, interaction with viruses, etc. to play a role. The main point is that, with mammals, it is unusually difficult to obtain meaningful data at low doses. Dose-effect curves are quite empirical and consequently extrapolation is fraught with considerably more difficulties than encountered with simple cell systems, and is commensurately less satisfactory. Even in studies on the genetic effects of radiation in the mammal, it is not possible to work directly with very low doses of radiation. The difficulties of extrapolating to low doses are at least as difficult as those encountered in simple cell systems.

One approach to fill the voids would appear to lie in dealing with a given long-term effect in a mammal, which can be attributed definitely to a particular cell system. If one could develop dose-effect curves for pertinent changes in the cell system involved, and relate these to dose-effect curves for a given late effect in the mammal, one might be in a better position to bridge the gaps and extrapolate more competently to lower dose levels for effects in the mammal.

What would be the attributes of such a system? The system of course would have to be in a mammal. Damage to the system must produce a late effect that is clinically discernible. Preferably one should be able to study the effects at very low, intermediate and high doses. With high and intermediate dose levels one should be able to develop dose-effect relationships in the mammal, and extrapolate to effects at low dose levels. With intermediate to low dose levels, cell death and abscopal effects should be minimal, allowing perhaps more confident extrapolation. If one were able actually to study the effect at very low dose levels, one could then determine whether or not extrapolation from high dose levels is adequate for prediction purposes.

With all late effects at relatively low doses in the mammal one is presumably dealing with cell injury and not cell death. One should be able to study events at the cellular or subcellular level, and to correlate these with clinical manifestations resulting from damage to that cell system. Ideally it should be possible to study cell kinetics in the cell system involved.

There are a number of systems in the mammal that have some of these attribute Neoplasia of the breast in the rat is one example, in which one at least knows the location of the cells of interest. One does not, however, know the actual cell population responsible for the neoplasia. Leukaemia represents an obvious gross end-point of importance; however, one has little knowledge of the actual cells responsible, nor of the location of these cells within the body. Thus these systems, while they are attractive in some respects, have serious drawbacks with respect to attempting to correlate effects at the subcellular, cellular and mammalian level.

There is one system that in my estimation has distinct possibilities, and this is the lens of the eye and lens opacification following exposure to radiation. The system has a number of characteristics that make it desirable. Certainly one knows which are the cells that lead to the clinical manifestation, lens opacification or cataract formation. The late effect can be dealt with "clinically", and the response can be quantified. The clinical end-point, lens opacification, is seen throughout a wide range of doses, and down to very low dose levels. One can study the effects of fractionation, radiation quality, dose rate, etc. The possibility exists to study the cell populations involved in some detail, and to actually do studies at the subcellular or biochemical level.

The system is extremely sensitive, and very small doses lead to readily discern ible effects. The lens of the eye is of course normally transparent. The effect results apparently mainly from cell injury. As opposed to cell injury in other systems, the damaged cells are not lost and are therefore susceptible to observation. The damaged cells remain wi in the lens, and even very small degrees of injury change the degree of transparency of the lens. Thus very small degrees of damage can be detected. The clinical effect, cataract, appears to result directly and only from damage to the cells involved, i.e. there is no abscop effect. In addition, lens opacification represents a late effect that has many of the aspects of normal ageing. In the mouse, irradiation appears to displace forward in time, a process that occurs later in the normal animal.

This system is now being studied extensively by Dr. Bateman, Dr. Rossi and myself at Brookhaven. I do not intend to give detailed results, but I shall outline briefly the types of studies that can be done. Complete dose-effect curves have been obtained for X radiation and neutrons of different qualities. Effects have been quantified with X rays at doses of 10 R, or lower and with neutrons at doses well below 0.5 rads. Dose rate effects are under study for both X rays and neutrons. The RBE has been determined for a number of neutron spectra. Studies on the detailed cytological and pathological changes in the lens are being undertaken, principally by Dr. Horton Johnson. The types of cellular lesions involved have been characterized.

A defect in the system lies in the inability to establish dose-effect curves, in the usual meaning of the term. The scoring system used to indicate the degree of opacification, while quite reproducible in the hands of a single observer, is nonetheless arbitrary. Thus a given degree of biological effect cannot be expressed accurately in terms of another degree or level of effect, i.e. if one arbitrarily scores lesion B as being twice as extensive as lesion A, and lesion C as being twice as extensive as lesion B, it cannot be stated that lesion B is in fact two times as extensive as lesion A, or that lesion C is four times as extensive as lesion A. Nonetheless, it is possible to derive "dose-effect" relationships. By arbitrarily fitting the response with high LET radiation to an exponential curve, one can construct a curve for low LET radiation by means of the RBE. Such a curve for low LET radiation has a very "broad shoulder". As would be expected, the RBE is a strong function of dose, and increases with decreasing dose. The RBE rises from a value of less than 10 at high doses, to values well in excess of 100 at extremely low doses (of the order of 25 R of X rays and 0.25 rads of neutrons).

The studies are not far enough along to deal adequately with the degree to which extrapolation from high dose levels will satisfactorily describe the degree of effect actually observed at low dose levels. It is clear, however, that the exact shape of the curve at low dose levels, for low LET radiation, could not be accurately predicted from effects at high dose levels only. I shall not attempt to give additional data in the short time available.

In summary then, models of all kinds are necessary, useful and desirable. If nothing else, models provide incentive for individuals to do work to disprove them. Models at the cellular or subcellular level are quite important, as are models based on observation of "clinical" effects in the intact mammal. Each is valuable and desirable. However, what is badly needed, in my estimation, is further concentrated work on systems and models in which one can deal with damage at both the cellular and subcellular level, and at the same time with clinical manifestations resulting from such damage. It is the wedding of these approaches, in systems in which it is possible to do so, that gives the most promise of getting at actual mechanisms, and the relationship between events at the various levels of biological organization. Thus such studies are important from a mechanistic viewpoint; however, they are also vital in a more pragmatic sense. It is increasingly necessary to obtain information on, or to estimate accurately the degree of effect of radiation in man exposed at low dose levels. Underestimation of the degree of effect is of course undesirable, serious overestimation of the degree of effect can be restrictive and quite costly. Thus in my estimation considerable work is justified in efforts towards improving our ability to predict accurately the degree of biological effect from irradiation at low dose levels.

<u>Dr. Stewart:</u> In 1961, on the basis of circumstantial evidence, it was suggested that the increased risk of dying from leukaemia (which only became a subject of anxiety after the discovery of antibiotics) was due to the effect of these drugs on a hidden association between infection hazards and pre-leukaemia (Stewart, 1961). According to this "special relationship" theory, there was probably an interval of several years between the initiation of a leukaemic process and the onset of symptoms (Wise, 1961), during which the effectiveness of the reticulo-endothelial system was being progressively undermined by an

ever-increasing number of neoplastic cells. As a result of this corrosive action, resistance to infections was first slowly and then rapidly being reduced to the point where even a minor infection was likely to prove fatal.

This theory offered great scope for antibiotics and improved standards of hygiene to reduce the probability of an individual who would otherwise have died from leukaemia dying from pneumonia or other complications of minor infections. There was, however, no direct evidence of the process described, nor was it envisaged in the Multiple Hit theory of cancer causation, which implies late grafting of invasive or malignant properties on to small clones of non-invasive or pre-malignant cells (Burch, 1965).

Following the discovery of how to use radiogenic cases to measure cancer incubation periods (Stewart and Kneale, 1968), a crucial test of the special relationship theory has been devised which demands an understanding of the early peak of leukaemia mortality (Hewitt, 1955) and of the secular trend of leukaemia and pneumonia mortality (Stewart, 1961) (see figs. 1 and 2). The early peak of leukaemia mortality is important for two reasons. In the first place, no-one has been able to understand why children between 2 and 4 years of age should have been so much more affected by the increased risk of dying from leukaemia than younger children, who have sometimes shown a declining incidence (Hewitt, 1964). Secondly, the fact that children under 2 years of age had failed to respond to a presumed backlash effect of antibiotics was regarded as a reason for rejecting the special relationship theory because infection sensitivity rapidly decreases with advancing age during childhood (Doll, 1965). Given the length of incubation period postulated in the special relationship theory, this was not a valid objection. For it clearly requires a post-natal setting to express an unusual degree of infection sensitivity. It was, however, allowed to stand until it became possible to show that incubation periods of 3 to 5 years are typical for juvenile leukaemias (see fig. 3). This figure is based on cases caused by obstetric X rays and, therefore, initiated during the third trimester of prenatal life. It does, however, indicate that when death from leukaemia occurs before the age of 2 years, it is probably the result of a lesion which has either pre-dated conception or happened during the first trimester of prenatal life. In which case, leukaemia in this age group cannot be affected by antibiotics to anything like the same extent as older cases because all but a fraction of their incubation periods are spent in a setting which precludes pneumonia being a cause of death during pre-leukaemia (i.e. in utero).

The secular trends of leukaemia and pneumonia mortality are depicted in fig. 2 and show the nature of the relationship which was being tested and the basic data. For the tests involved detailed comparisons between contemporary death rates for both diseases in two age groups (under 2 years and 2 to 4 years) over many years (Registrar-General, 1911-1965). The first test necessitated dividing the period 1911-1955 into nine quinquennia, preparatory to applying Spearman's Rank Correlation test to the null hypothesis that the two causes of death were occurring independently of one another in consecutive five-year periods (see table 1). This test revealed a zero correlation for the younger age group and a negative correlation for the older age group - that is to say, in the older age group pneumonia deaths showed signs of blocking leukaemia deaths, but this was not the case for younger deaths.

The strength of this presumed blocking effect was measured by applying the following formula to the annual death rates for the two diseases in two age groups:

$$L = (1 - kP) \,/\, (1 - P)\, I$$

where L = observed leukaemia death rate

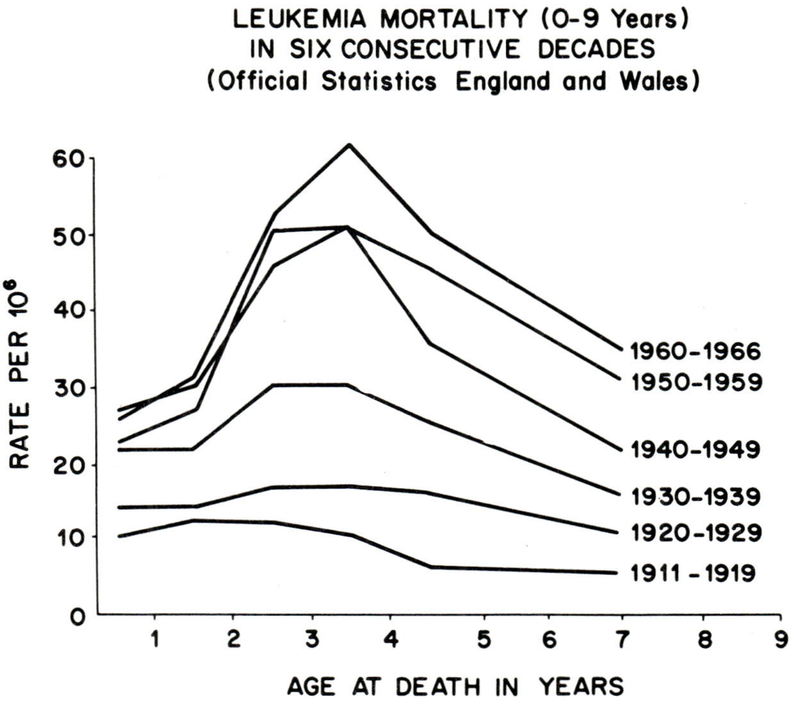
LEUKEMIA MORTALITY (0-9 Years)
IN SIX CONSECUTIVE DECADES
(Official Statistics England and Wales)
RATE PER 10^6
60
50
40
30
20
10
0
1960-1966
1950-1959
1940-1949
1930-1939
1920-1929
1911-1919
1
2
3
4
5
6
7
8
9
AGE AT DEATH IN YEARS

Fig. 1.

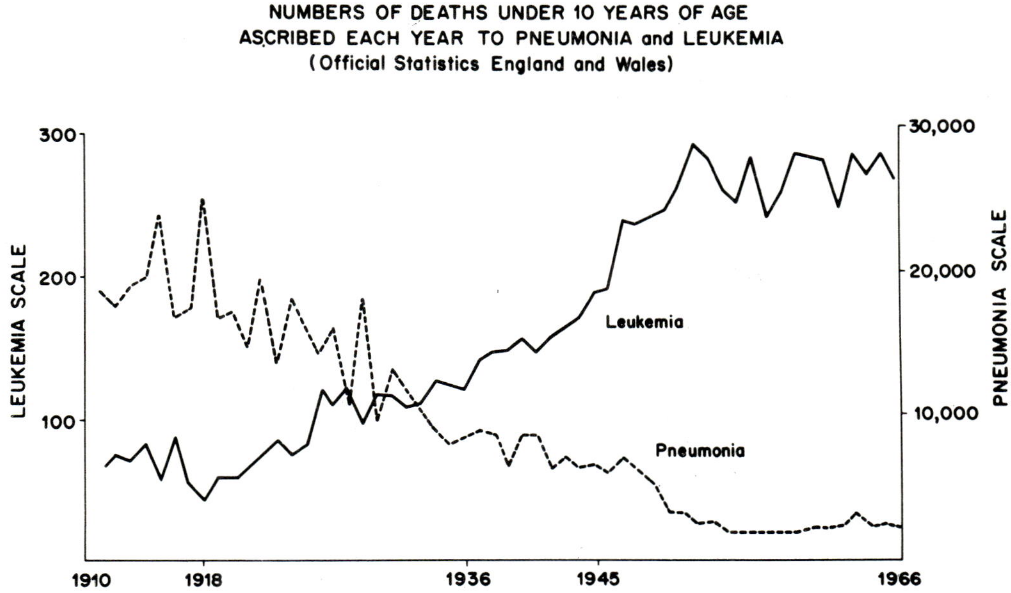
NUMBERS OF DEATHS UNDER 10 YEARS OF AGE
ASCRIBED EACH YEAR TO PNEUMONIA and LEUKEMIA
(Official Statistics England and Wales)
LEUKEMIA SCALE
300
200
100
PNEUMONIA SCALE
30,000
20,000
10,000
Leukemia
Pneumonia
1910
1918
1936
1945
1966

Fig. 2.

AGE DISTRIBUTIONS OF 190 JUVENILE LEUKEMIAS INITIATED BY OBSTETRIC X-RAYS SHORTLY BEFORE BIRTH (KNEALE Analysis of O.S.C.C. Data)

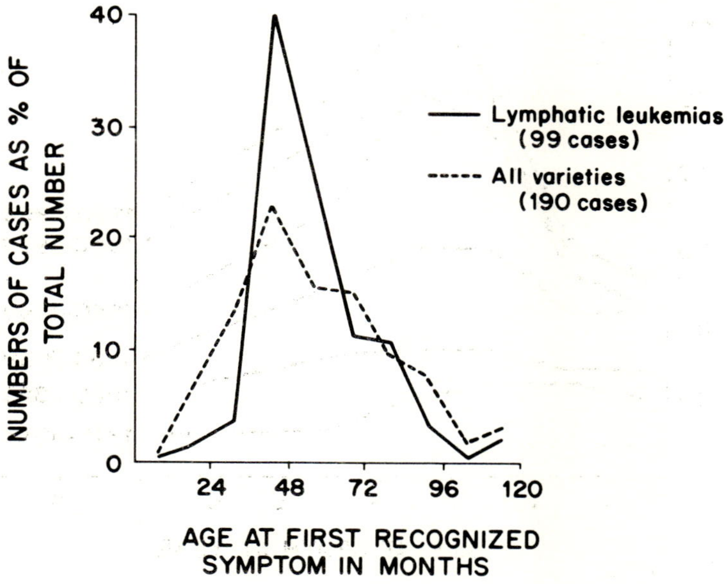

Fig. 3.

Table 1

Spearman's Rank correlation coefficients for leukaemia and pneumonia deaths in stated periods and age groups

Quinquennium	Rank Correlation Coefficients	
	0-1 years	2-4 years
1911-1915	0.0	0.0
1916-1920	- 0.5	- 0.5
1921-1925	- 0.9	+ 0.6
1926-1930	+ 0.3	- 0.5
1931-1935	+ 0.2	- 0.8
1936-1940	+ 1.0	- 0.8
1941-1945	+ 0.1	- 0.9
1946-1950	- 0.2	- 0.6
1951-1955	0.0	+ 0.7
Mean values	0.000	- 0.311
Standard errors	0.167	0.167

P = observed pneumonia death rate
I = initiation rate of pre-leukaemias
k = ratio of death rates from pneumonia or pre-leukaemic and normal children.

Since there is no reason to suppose that I is correlated with P, except in so far as the trends in them might by chance coincide, on taking logarithms and expanding

$$\log_{10}L = \log_{10}(1-k\overline{P})-\log_{10}(1-\overline{P}) - 0.43429 \left[k/(1-k\overline{P}) - 1/(1-\overline{P})\right] (P-\overline{P}) + T + e$$

where $\overline{P}$ = mean value of P
T = trend in $\log_{10}I$ and can be represented by a low order polynomial in time
e = variation about trend in $\log_{10}I$ and is <u>independent</u> of P.

So, in the multiple regression of $\log_{10}L$ on P and low order powers of time, the coefficient of P is $0.43429 \left[k/(1-k\overline{P})-1/(1-\overline{P})\right]$ and this may be estimated by the usual multiple regression techniques, hence k can be found.

No allowance was made for the fact that the older children had had a slightly longer time in which to die from pneumonia while incubating leukaemia than the younger children. But even ignoring this factor, the leukaemia blocking effects of pneumonia deaths were clearly much more marked for the older than for the younger children. For the values of k for the two age groups showed that pneumonia death rates for pre-leukaemic children were 36 times higher than normal for children who would otherwise have died from leukaemia between 2 and 4 years of age, and only four times higher than normal for children who would otherwise have died from leukaemia before the age of 2 years.

Since these findings are difficult to explain unless pre-leukaemia and leukaemia are the result of a continuous process with important side-effects on haemopoietic tissues, we tentatively suggest that other side-effects should be observable in populations whose members live in conditions which face haemopoietic neoplasm to compete not only with acute responses to bacterial infections but also with lasting effects of parasitic infections. Evidence that spleen and lymph node blocking effects are incurred as a result of malaria, kalazar, or other parasitic infections is purely circumstantial, but it includes (1) the rarity of lymphatic leukaemias in China, Japan, Malaya and India (Segi and Kurihara, 1964; Wells and Lau, 1960; Muir, 1964), (2) the anatomical distribution of the tumours found in cases of African lymphoma (i.e. jaws, eyes, ovaries, etc.) (Burkitt, 1962), (3) the geographical distributions of those cases and their tendency to "drift" (Pike et al., 1967), (4) the fact that the commonest type of juvenile neoplasm is lymphoma in the tropics (Haddow, 1963) and leukaemia in Europe and North America.

References

Burch, P. Natural and radiation carcinogenesis in man. I. Theory of initiation phase. <u>Proc. R.Soc.</u> (Biol.), <u>162</u>, 223-239, 1965.

Burkitt, D. A tumor syndrome affecting children in tropical Africa. <u>Postgrad. Med. J.</u>, <u>38</u>, 71-79, 1962.

Doll, R. In <u>Current Researches in Leukaemia</u>, edited by Hayhoe, Cambridge, Cambridge University Press, p. 280, 1965.

Haddow, A.J. Age incidence in Burkitt's lymphoma syndrome. <u>E. Afr. Med. J.</u>, <u>41</u>, 1-6, 1963.

Hewitt, D. Some features of leukaemia mortality. Br. J. Prev. soc. Med., 9, 81-88, 1955.

Hewitt, D. Leukaemia mortality in infancy. New Engl. J. Med., 270, 932-935, 1964.

Muir, C.S. Proc. Eighth Int. Conf. Soc. Geog. Pathol., Basel, Karger, 1964.

Pike, M.C., Williams, E.H., and Wright, B. Burkitt's tumour in the West Nile district of Ugandi, 1961-1965. Br. Med. J., 2, 395-399, 1967.

Registrar-General, England and Wales. Statistical Reviews, H.M.S.O., London, 1911-1965.

Segi, M., and Kurihara, M. Cancer mortality for selected sites, Dept. of Public Health, Sendai, Japan, 1964.

Stewart, A.M. Aetiology of childhood malignancies. Br. Med. J., 1, 452-460, 1961.

Stewart, A.M., and Kneale, G.W. Changes in the cancer risk associated with obstetric radiography. Lancet, 1, 104-107, 1968.

Wells, R., and Lau, K.S. Incidence of leukaemia in Singapore, and parity of chronic lymphocytic leukaemia in Chinese. Br. Med. J., 1, 759-763, 1960.

Wise, M.E. Irradiation and leukaemia. Br. Med. J., 2, 48-49, 1961.

Dr. Bloom: It is well established that head circumference does not correlate well with brain size except in the extreme. Therefore, in the in utero exposed with many so-called small heads, one cannot use the term "microcephaly" which Dr. Miller wisely avoided, but which others use all too often. Therefore, we cannot, on the basis of head circumference measurements alone, draw any conclusion about the central nervous system effect in this group.

The second comment I wish to make is that head circumference must, to have any meaning, be considered in relation to body size. Even head circumferences which are two standard deviations below the mean may have little significance clinically.

My last comment is on the matter of transformation. The mechanism of transformation is poorly understood at present, though presumably it involves the incorporation of viral genetic material into the recipient cell genome with resultant mutation of the cell.

We do not understand why some cells, or the cells of some persons, seem to be particularly sensitive to this incorporation. We ought perhaps to understand this phenomenon somewhat better before applying it on a large scale to populations which we feel may be at risk in terms of malignant diseases. Transformation may well prove to be a fairly common finding in normal persons with no particular risk at all in terms of neoplasia.

CHAPTER XII

IMPLICATIONS AND APPLICATIONS OF RADIATION TOXICITY DATA TO OTHER ENVIRONMENTAL HAZARDS

Austin M. Brues

I have just come in from the suburbs, along a familiar drive by the Chicago River and drainage canal, past a large plant where the Sanitary District, it appears, converts water pollution into air pollution. As influenced by the frequent atmospheric inversions, this results in a dense cloud over the highway which blots out the noon-day sun, creating obvious automotive and pulmonary hazards and, no doubt, genetic and other subtle insults as well. Unlike a comparable radiation hazard, this is familiar and obvious, and is taken more as an annoyance and less as a threat. Along the same route a slightly more pungent but less stygian cloud marks the production of a large share of the city's electric power.

Some years ago an imaginative writer undertook to consider what would have happened in a world in which nuclear fission had been the customary source of power, and into which the combustion of fossil fuels had been introduced as an alternative and somewhat simpler technique.

According to the parable, the latter had attracted much public attention and engendered no small degree of alarm, and, being novel and spectacular, has been placed under rigid control and made the subject of intensive biological and medical research. Years passed while experimental fossil fuel plants were set up in remote localities, subject to approval by hazard committees and scrutinized by national and international authorities. Well-financed studies of the hazards of coal-tar and shale oil derivatives opened up important areas of physiology and biology, expanded our understanding of mutagenesis and carcinogenesis, and eventually led to a re-evaluation of radiation.

We find ourselves, in fact, pursuing this path in the reverse direction. In so doing, it is clear that the variety of environmental pollution hazards makes the task a much more complex one than confronted radiation research. I think, however, that much can be learned from the history of radiation toxicity about the philosophy of hazard evaluation and about empirical approaches to its control.

The earliest radiation protection standards were developed in response to the needs of radiological workers to protect themselves against types of damage that were known to exist, and were accepted as calculated risks, in patients treated for serious diseases. These standards embodied assumptions that were widely used in the practice of industrial hygiene, namely that safe levels of exposure to noxious agents can be defined, below which damage fails to occur or may be fully recoverable. One needs, therefore, only to look for minimal changes which appear temporary or trivial, and introduce a "safety factor" (usually a factor of ten). Erythema of the skin as seen in exposure to the sun, and leucopenia as seen in some infectious states, typified these trivial criteria of "minimal" radiation damage.

The production of malignant tumours of bone by radium was recognized in the 1930's, and again a "threshold" value was assumed and a factor of safety was introduced. When it was found, however, that radiation produced damage to the genetic material, the basic concept began to change; for in this case, it was unreasonable to suspect that this migh be a statistical result of chance damage to single molecular entities, and therefore have no effective threshold.

Along with the development of molecular and theoretical biology - to which radiation research has made no small contribution - it has been suggested that changes in the informational content of somatic cell nuclei may similarly have no lower limit, and that the rate of ageing may itself depend upon gradual irreversible loss of molecular information in individual cells.

There is still much to be learned in these matters. As regards cancer, the simplest assumption that can be made is that each single hit on some hypothetical site produces an equal probability of a malignant cell transformation. This single-hit hypothesis does not always appear to hold true even in the case of simple genetic mutation, and as regards carcinogenesis it seems to fail in the case of bone tumours and various other conditions although it has not been possible to rule it out in human leukaemia and thyroid tumours and in one or two instances of experimental cancer.

The fact is that no firm basis for a general model of carcinogenesis exists in our present stage of knowledge, and the situation seems to become less clear with recent trends in cancer research. The assumption of a linear or proportional relation between radiation and probability of malignant disease would suggest that the process is mediated by a single molecular event.

Many other models have been suggested which fit with a good deal of the available information. Some of these, built around radiation exposures, are based on the assumption that multiple "hits" are required, perhaps on the genetic equipment of a cell, or on several cells in proximity. In some cases their sponsors envisage that certain individuals may already harbour some mutational or other condition which may predispose them to tumour formation by establishing some of the changes that are otherwise provided by additional irradiation. Unfortunately the cliché is voiced, more often than not, that one must choose between a "linear" dose-effect relation and the existence of a true threshold below which irradiation is incompetent to induce a tumour. It seems fair to say that this rather general belief in a two-valued choice has stultified much of the thinking on this subject.

It might be worth while to consider some other known facts about carcinogenesis that deserve consideration. There is a great deal of knowledge implicating viruses as a causative factor in experimental animals. Yet tumours associated with viruses are in all or almost all cases focal, and this presupposes that other factors are quite necessary; perhaps biochemical, structural, or immunological factors necessary for the survival or transformation of infected cells. There is much evidence in the experimental literature that carcinogenesis may proceed through at least two discrete stages.

Then, again, there is growing appreciation of the fact that tumour cells differ in their surface properties and interconnecting relationships from non-neoplastic cells.

Possibly related to this is the growing knowledge of tumour immunology, which suggests that one stage in the malignant process may be the loss of a cell recognition character, and that this, under rare and special circumstances, may allow the propagation of a clone of cells with malignant properties. It has to be remembered that the only known, general property of the malignant cell is its communal behaviour within the organisms, and that past attempts to find a single common cell property have invariably met with frustration.

Another late or chronic radiation effect on the whole organism is an apparently non-specific enhancement of the normal mortality rate. The significance of this is hardly better appreciated than that of the normal enhancement which appears with the passage of the organism's life. Among the many theories of ageing one would envisage the systematic accumulation of particular properties of tissues; another, the random accumulation of molecular misinformation of all sorts in different somatic cells. A few experiments have even appeared to show a "conditioning" effect in which survival is improved during the middle part of life, possibly at the eventual expense of the final life-span. It can, of course, be useful to the survival of a species if its members respond to environmental stresses by better survival in the propagating period, and by their elimination beyond it.

Turning now from theory to practice, present evidence has accumulated to the point where it is no longer blandly assumed that there are safe or ineffective levels of radiation exposure. Once doubt is raised about the existence of a "threshold" one must consider the problem as one in which it is necessary to consider the balance between somewhat unknown individual risks against somewhat predictable benefits or needs. Therefore, there is a great deal of re-thinking in the evaluation of acceptable levels of radiation exposure.

In the matter of genetic risks this involves less consideration of individual exposures, provided the mutational load of the whole population, assuming a reasonable amount of mixing through generations, is kept at a low level. It may even be suggested that the normal mutational load, which provides the potential for diversification of a species as its environment undergoes change, might be especially advantageous in a time such as now, with environmental alterations, from one generation to the next, occurring so much more rapidly than in the past.

In the matter of somatic injury, particularly as regards cancer and ageing, the understanding has grown that a threshold cannot be assumed. It is now accepted that the professionally exposed person can be assigned a greater exposure limit than members of the general population. This, of course, has been disturbing to some who have relied in the past on the existence of a "safe" exposure level. This double standard has been rationalized in a number of ways, none of which is wholly satisfactory, but which add up to a suitable rationalization. First is, that employment in activities which involve some risk is generally adopted by free choice. Going along with this is the fact that in choosing one activity, one avoids another which has its own hazards. The radiologist is not likely to moonlight as a steeplejack - although, by free choice, he may elect to be an amateur mountaineer in his spare time. Either of these, of course, would grossly overshadow the risk of practising radiology.

The worker is, of course, subject to regular monitoring, while the general population is not, which confers a certain degree of protection as against the population in the vicinity of a nuclear establishment. And, finally, a small statistical hazard is not felt (because it is not detectable) unless it occurs in a large population. This is essentially a sophistic argument, but it raises a philosophical question that is going to have to be recognized in relation to other hazards that act statistically: is one more concerned about a small individual risk, or about a large absolute number of injured individuals? A 5% increase in the leukaemia rate, which has occurred many times in past years and for unknown reasons, would entail thousands of deaths a year, but would be impossible to detect.

Much attention has been given to the problem of global fall-out and its possible consequences; and although the maximum likely effect of it cannot possibly be detected, the more pessimistic extrapolations of what little we do know, have yielded large hypothetical numbers of injured individuals. The same arguments will become applicable to pollutants as the world becomes smaller and its population becomes larger and even more demanding of its resources and of their energy potential. The time is already here when we are called upon to compare the hazards of energy production by nuclear and by traditional sources; and there is indeed no background of knowledge about the traditional sources with which to compare that little we have learned about radiation.

Returning to the global radiation hazard, one way in which attempts have been made to derive an "acceptable" limit is based on our knowledge of the natural radiation to which all are necessarily exposed. Since this natural radiation level varies from place to place and is, in many populated areas, two or three times what it is in others, it has not generally been considered sensible to reduce the whole population exposure to limits much below the limits of normal variation.

Considering other hazards to the individual besides radiation we may think of some which are entailed in occupational choice, such as those afflicting the coal miner, and of those resulting from choice of the hazard itself, and in that instance the smoking of cigarettes is the prime example.

I have considered in a semiquantitative way how the cigarette hazard might be compared with the radium hazard, on which allowable exposure levels have been established. There appears to be a high correlation between cigarette consumption and cancer of the lung. One value which is based on the statistics of several countries among which the smoking habits vary, indicates that 1,200 cigarettes a year per person is associated with a yearly increment of about 50 cancers per 100,000 persons. This amounts to 2.4×10^6 cigarettes per cancer. This sounds like a large number, but is within an order of magnitude of the potential of a dedicated smoker.

Correlations also exist between radium deposited in the skeleton and the probability of resulting cancer in an individual. I will make an educated guess that 10 microcuries of deposited radium may be associated with about one cancer in 20 years. One cigarette then becomes comparable to about 10^8 radium disintegrations, or roughly one microcurie-hour. If the maximum permissible radium burden is then set at 0.1 microcurie-hour per hour, we should set a limit of one cigarette every ten hours, or 2.4 cigarettes a day.

The above is an "occupational" level, which would apply to persons who advertise cigarettes on television or to actors who are directed to smoke on stage. A reduction of this by ten would allow segments of society not exposed occupationally about two per week, and a further reduction by a factor of three might involve non-smokers in a smoking-car.

It is probably only in the case of medical benefits resulting from medical procedures can we talk sensibly of balancing the same kind of advantage and disadvantage in the same individual. One example of this that might be cited, is the routine roentgenologic examination of the thorax if done annually on persons above minimum cigarette-smoking age.

It may be possible to make an order-of-magnitude guess concerning the benefits to be anticipated from taking X rays of the chest every year, but if we are talking about males in their forties, it is probably not exaggerating to suggest that an annual chest plate on such an individual may have a probability of about 10^{-3} of revealing a small cancer of the bronchogenic tissue which would not otherwise have been detected until it reached a dangerous state. Then one has to reach for a figure representing the benefits accruing from that revelation, and for this I will guess that something like one-tenth of these individuals might be saved or might have a good portion of life saved. This brings the probability of a favourable result of an annual chest examination to 10^{-4}.

Now if the chest plate is taken with modern techniques, even the most pessimistic estimates that have been made about the probability of leukaemia induction from irradiation of that part of the bone marrow which is seen in the chest plate would indicate a probability of no greater than about 10^{-7} per examination per year for about ten years or a total probability of something in the order of 10^{-6}. Therefore, in this case I think it is possible to assume that, plus or minus an order of magnitude, the routine chest plate in the middle-aged male is a good thing to do by a factor of about 100.

I am happy that Dr. Stewart was able to attend this meeting, because the other example which I have taken to indicate a balance between the two factors is the effect of prenatal irradiation on the induction of childhood tumours in individuals irradiated in the later stages of gestation, and the possible benefit of that procedure to mother and child at the time of childbirth. In this instance it would appear that irradiation of about 10% of a three-year cohort of foetuses in England and Wales, who were subjected to this procedure, might have resulted in something in the order of 100 cases of childhood malignancy.

To estimate the balance one must explore whether the number of lives saved by that procedure was greater or less than this approximate figure. I would have to guess that the balance is much in favour of the procedure, but perhaps only if it is performed on the basis of a sound clinical indication rather than on a routine basis or for trivial reasons.

Now I would like to say a word about two very different kinds of hazards: I speak now of risks in general, which may result from insults other than radiation.

We have to distinguish between what I choose to call statistical hazards and what might be called physiological hazards. In the case of statistical hazards, as in the case of cancer induction, or as in the case of automotive deaths related to speed or condition of roads, an increasing risk means just this: it means an increase in the proportion of individuals who suffer completely while other individuals subjected to the same statistical hazard escape. The physiological hazard, on the other hand, is one in which a certain degree of exposure is required before any risk at all is incurred, or from which full recovery may occur, and which affect almost all equally exposed persons about equally. Perhaps sulphur dioxide or carbon monoxide might fall in this category. I hasten to say, however, that this may not be the case; and this exemplifies the fact that for the whole range of environmental pollutants, we are going to have to look for this distinction just as we have done in the past 40 years of radiation research.

There are, of course, grey areas in which both processes are involved, but basically, we have to distinguish between degrees of probability of serious damage on the one hand, and degrees of impairment of all those exposed on the other.

To return to radiation, a case in point, which has not been resolved, is the effect of radiation on the early human foetus, in contrast to the later human foetus which was more at issue in connection with leukaemia and childhood tumours.

If the early foetus is exposed to doses of radiation above 50 or 100 R, this would appear from available data to result in idiocy and microcephaly in a very considerable proportion of the population. The question has been raised, and we have at the present time no way of knowing the answer, whether this is a statistical hazard, so that if 10% of the individuals are affected following 100 R, one person in 1,000 might be affected by 1R in the same period of gestation. We might suppose that in this case the disability is due to destruction and inhibition of growth, or disarrangement of the order of cells, in a sensitive part of the developing cortex of the brain, in which case the effect is a matter of gradually increasing impairment with gradually increasing dose, but the best one can do at the present time is to theorize about pathogenesis. Both epidemiology and basic biology have a part to play in the solution.

Now a great many hazardous environmental agents besides radiation are carcinogenic and mutagenic. Some of them injure chromosomes visibly and this suggests strongly that they may contribute to general somatic cell damage, and may be considered as potential carcinogens and as agents tending to shorten life, even when direct evidence is lacking. Approaches of this sort will, therefore, become of increasing importance, and are likely to become popular in the entire field of chemical pollution at least, and possibly other environmental influences.

Some of the metals, for example, have traditionally been thought to be physiological hazards with a threshold of action. Lead is one of these, but lately it has been found that in large doses it will produce kidney tumours in the rat. Chromium and nickel, for example, are well-known carcinogenic hazards. Beryllium is a particularly interesting case since with the appearance of the so-called sporadic neighbourhood cases, persons at a considerable distance from plants giving off beryllium effluent, the type of hazard, or combination of hazards, becomes doubtful. This may be an example of a statistical effect which depends primarily on individual susceptibilities, or perhaps not.

Sunlight is a very well-documented instance of a statistical carcinogenic hazard. If one compares the northern and the southern United States, one finds the incidence of skin cancer, which occurs mainly on exposed areas, to increase by a factor of four as one moves south where the exposure to actinic rays becomes correspondingly greater.

Now I would like to refer to a thought that is unfortunately becoming popular, that radiation research has accomplished its end, that we are fully familiar with radiation effects, and that it would be well to withdraw support from radiation research and put it into the next thing, which in this case is the study of other environmental hazards.

At the risk of seeming to have a paradoxical approach to this matter, I would like to suggest that radiation research, which offered so much in the past, still has a great deal to offer. What are some of the basic questions? I am not concerned now with the question of whether such-and-such a drug is mutagenic, whether such-and-such a chemical compound is carcinogenic. These are problems that have to be investigated *ad hoc* and in their own right, but what are some of the basic questions?

One basic question is: Which are the potentially non-threshold statistical effects? Genetic effects are generally evaluated on this basis. So are carcinogenic effects, but with a little less confidence because of the greater complexity of the process.

Secondly, what are the interactions between agents which produce these effects? To put it even more generally, between these agents and predisposing states? The physiological state of a tissue, the relation of injury to the cell cycle, and many other conditions are important here and are being actively studied with radiation.

Another question is how can we validly make quantitative comparisons between species? Differences in the action of chemical carcinogens are often rationalized on the basis of differences in metabolic handling of the agent by different species. It is probably on some basis such as this that certain dye intermediates produce cancer of the bladder in dogs and in man, but not in the small rodents so often used as test animals for carcinogens.

Another category of species differences seem to apply to radiation as well. It appears, from what is now known, that the larger species show a carcinogenic response to localized irradiation, not in relation to the number of cells at risk, but more nearly in relation to the irradiated fraction of the whole tissue at risk. This question which is conveniently studied with radiation as the test-insult, undoubtedly has quite general application.

I have only mentioned three rather obvious examples of our lack of some very fundamental knowledge about the action of various noxious agents. Radiation is a particularly favourable subject for the study of these things because exposures can be measured, timed and localized quite precisely and because there is a great deal of possible control over the distribution of energy deposition not only on the gross level, but on the molecular level.

I conclude that further progress in subtle radiation effects will have wide and useful applications to the evaluation of a great many environmental hazards, and moreover that there are many basic questions which deserve a good deal more attention than they have been getting from experimental radiologists.

CHAPTER XIII

THE DEGRADATION OF OUR ENVIRONMENT

Lord Ritchie-Calder

I count it a privilege to be here and to participate in the last colloquium of the radiation series. The first, in May 1960, was on radioisotopes in man's environment and the second, a year later, was on public health and the problems of radioactive waste disposal. From these I was asked to produce the book, "Living with the Atom".

On that occasion, the night before we assembled, Dr. Rust took me onto the campus to Stagg Field and showed me the plaque: "On December 2, 1942, man achieved here the first self-sustaining chain reaction and thereby initiated the controlled release of nuclear energy."

I remember Dr. Rust saying to me on that occasion, rather sadly, "We don't know whether that is a boast or a confession".

It was symbolic of the crisis of conscience that followed the cataclysmic release of atomic energy which created the deep scientific concern about the biological consequences of that action. Listening to your deliberations today, I thought how far we have progressed since those early days when you here can discuss, as you have done with profundity and scientific objectivity, issues which were then loaded with political inhibitions.

I still remember certain difficulties we had at that time, when we were still bomb-testing. It was almost treason to suggest, as you well know, the kind of things that might follow from the bomb tests. And most of us taking part in these deliberations were, as Dr. Alice Stewart has said here, regarded as dangerous left-wing politicians.

It was, after all, the bomb which precipitated not only fall-out but the intensive research work which has gone on ever since. While appreciating the value of such studies, I am reminded of an occasion during the First World War, when Mr. Winston Churchill had a quarrel with the Government. He went into retirement and then out to France as a colonel in the Royal Scots, and into the trenches.

He was not there very long, a few months, before he came back. He then spoke in the House of Commons and he told his colleagues that he was very grateful for the experience of being in the front lines, because it cleared his mind. Mr. Arthur Balfour retorted that he was very glad that his Right Honourable friend's mind had been cleared, but he thought a world war was a very expensive way of doing it.

I think, in retrospect, that the bomb was a pretty expensive way of starting you on your research.

Now, I am talking beyond, if you like, the point which Dr. Brues has just been discussing. I am putting radiation hazards into a context of all the hazards throughout the world with which we are now confronted. Environmental risks have been with us for a very long time, but the trouble is that the speed of change has now been accelerated.

Since 1945, at Alamagordo, we have in the world experienced four epochal revolutions: first, the atomic age; second, the computer age; third, the space age; and, now the fourth which is now developing rapidly, and is what I would like to call the DNA or genetic engineering age.

All of this has happened in the lifetime of the protesting students of today. I have a great deal of sympathy with them in the sense that they have had to envelope, as it were, all of these changes and, indeed, accept them in a way which their elders find it very difficult to grasp. We older people are still trying to explain to ourselves why these things happened. The young take them completely for granted.

When Astronaut White stepped out of his space capsule and "walked" across the continent of America from Florida to California in 25 minutes, not one single member of the new generation was in the least surprised. They reasoned that you just hire an engineer and he propels you at 17,500 miles an hour into space. They did know something about Newtonian physics. They did not expect him to fall down.

I want to deal with the wider issues, and just point out several examples of how casual things have become because we have not had the same sort of concern as we have developed about atomic energy and radiation hazards.

Recently in a London suburb a thief walked out of a place, where they make nothing more lethal than "pop" records, with a container. It was the size of a jerry-can. It was quite a nice container. It has even been suggested that he only wanted the container. He did not have to evade elaborate security precautions. There were none. He did not have to break into a vault. The container was not locked away. He just walked out with enough cyanide in the container to kill half the population in Greater London.

The London police in their television appeals to the thief and their "loud-hailer announcements, asked him, very politely, not to pour the contents down the drains. It was on the news bulletin that night; it got a back page reference in the newspapers the next day. I still do not know what happened. If the police recovered it, they did not tell us, or, if they tried to tell us, the news media did not bother to report it. If they have not recovered it, presumably, someone still has enough cyanide to kill half the population of London.

Another example: a research worker in a British microbiological station died of a bacterial agent which he had "invented". He had produced a mutant organism agair which no natural immunity in man existed. And a famous scientist half in jest said to me at the time, "Thank God he did not sneeze. He could have produced a world epidemic."

Twenty-seven years ago, British scientists carried out biological tests on the Island of Gruinard off the north-west coast of Scotland. They sprayed the island with a specially virulent form of anthrax. That was when, according to Dr. Gordon Smith, Director of the United Kingdom Microbiological Research Establishment, the authorities decided that microbiological warfare was, in fact, a practical possibility. That was 27 year ago. The island is still uninhabited and without livestock. It will, according to Dr. Smith, remain so for another 100 years because the anthrax bacillus will persist that long. We have had sporadic outbreaks of anthrax on the north Scottish mainland since that time. Rightly or wrongly, it is called "Gruinard anthrax" by the Scottish veterinarians.

And we can recall what happened at the Dugway Proving Grounds in Utah where the experiments with a new nozzle for the dissemination of nerve gas led to the death of 6,000 sheep on ranchlands 30 miles away.

We have read quite recently that it has been proposed to fill up old ships with obsolete chemical warfare materials, which the United States authorities would then sink in the Atlantic. Britain's stock-pile of World War II chemical weapons was so disposed many years ago, about 100,000 tons, some off the west coast of Ireland and some in the Bay of Biscay. Captured German chemical warfare stocks, tens of thousands of shells, for example, were sunk in the Baltic and later in the Atlantic.

My most recent television appearance was on a British Broadcasting Company programme called "Muck Today; Poison Tomorrow". We showed the devastation that occurred around a brickworks: dead orchards and cattle staggering to their death with fluoride poisoning. We pictured the killing fumes from the chimney-stacks. We also viewed hospital wards with the victims of bronchial complaints from the fumes from the chimney-stacks of a chemical works - new irritants from a new process. We showed industrial detergents foaming in a river and being blown into a town and piling up like snow-drifts in the streets. Man's degradation of his environment.

We all know the story of Lake Erie, the unbelievable story of how the living waters of a great lake are dead or dying. In its struggle to neutralize the industrial effluents and the pickling acids of the steelworks, it gives up its oxygen. Its once rich fishing industry has been ruined. The anaerobic organisms have taken over. A Toledo industrialist said, "Don't blame us for the stink. It's these damned dead fish."

On 28 January 1969, I arrived in Santa Barbara, California. I had a heavy writing assignment ahead of me, but I had the anticipatory comfort that my wife and I would have the use of a cottage right on Miramar Beach, which some of you may remember, and I mean "remember", as one of the loveliest of all the California beaches. The day we arrived was the day of the oil leak from the offshore drilling. I took it as a personal affront.

For the last two years I have been involved in the House of Lords and elsewhere with the consequences of the Torrey Canyon, the tanker which ran aground between the Scilly Islands and the coast of Cornwall.

Now, I think for our purposes, my purposes anyway, today, the circumstances of the wreck of the Torrey Canyon are apposite and it is also apposite to what happened to Santa Barbara.

The Torrey Canyon was built at Newport News, Virginia, for the use of a large oil company. It was taken to Japan and stretched to nearly twice its original capacity, by the insertion of a mid-section. It was registered under the Liberian "flag of convenience" and, for income tax purposes, was owned, with a sister ship, by a shipping company which is only, and I mean "only", a filing-cabinet in a lawyer's office in Bermuda.

The captain and crew were recruited in Italy. And just to complicate the situation still further, the Torrey Canyon, at the time of the disaster, was under charter to another oil company, part-owned by the British Government. It was, at the time of its accident, bringing 120,000 tons of Kuwait oil to Milford Haven in Wales. The ship was on a very tight schedule because the owner company in question had only hired it out for a very short time. It was essential that it dock at Milford Haven by a certain hour, 11.00 o'clock on a Saturday night, because so big a ship would have had to wait another five days for a suitable high tide. The captain, in order to make his scheduled arrival, took a short-cut between the Scillies and Land's End and impaled his ship on the Seven Stones.

The tanker began to spew oil in great slicks which drifted toward the holiday coasts of Cornwall.

After delays, due to attempts to salvage the ship and cargo, the tanker began to break up with the threat of its whole cargo drifting ashore. The British Government at this moment took very drastic measures. Bombers with high explosives and incendiaries went into action to try to rip open its decks and set fire to the oil still in the tanks.

Their attack was relatively successful. The ship sank, with what remained of the oil destroyed, but vast quantities had already escaped. The Navy, having failed to burn off the oil from the surface of the sea with incendiaries, then used detergents to emulsify the slick. This is a measure, I may say, which is unlikely to be repeated because it is a question whether the cure was not worse than the complaint, and whether the detergents were not as harmful as the oils, or even more so, to the marine life.

Harbours and shell fisheries had to be protected with booms and the damaged beaches had to be cleaned with detergents, with bulldozers, and with flame-throwers.

The effects of the Torrey Canyon sinking, weeks later, on the coast and fisheries of France, were even worse.

The costs and damage were enormous. The British and French Governments took steps to recover damages from the oil company trying to reach it behind its screen of the Liberian flag and the filing-drawer of the shipping company.

The self-same oil company received concessions for off-shore boring in the Santa Barbara Channel from the United States Department of the Interior. The drilling site was outside of the three-mile limit of the off-shore jurisdiction and drilling regulations of the State of California. The federal regulations are less strict than those of the State of California and even those were further relaxed in this case, to accommodate the oil company.

The main oil deposit is at 3,500 feet in the subsoil of the channel but there was a pocket of brown oil at a shallower level. The oil company wanted the shallow oil as a bonus. To get it, they needed to case the drill-hole down only to 300 feet instead of 500 feet which is required by federal regulations, so concession was made to them. They then continued their drilling down to the main deposit.

The oil was reached, and when the drill was withdrawn, the oil under pressure blew into the waters of the Santa Barbara Channel. With great difficulty, and after much havoc, the original leak was plugged. The Secretary of Interior, after public outcry, suspended all oil boring in the Santa Barbara Channel but was persuaded by his advisors that secondary borings at the site would reduce the pressure. This "hypodermic" operation triggered off a further uncontrollable seepage into fissures in the sea bottom and the seepage started all over again.

The white horses of the Pacific rollers came pounding in, the colour of molasses. The spray drenched the windows of our cottage with tarry oil. The beaches were smothered with goo, the consistency of tar, and became quite unusable.

There was a buoy, marking the navigation channel, just in front of our picture-window. I called it "Execution Dock", after the place at Wapping on the Thames where they used to hang pirates. But there was this difference, it was the execution of the innocents. The great diving birds, gleaming white in the sun, would swoop out of the sky after their swimming-food. They would surface, covered with oil. They would paddle around bewildered and struggle to the buoy. There they would stand on the buoy, stretching their pinions to try to unstick them. It was all symbolic, very symbolic. They looked like the emblem of the United States spread-eagled on the almighty dollar, dripping tar. They would flap helplessly and then, in a desperate effort to take off in flight, would plunge to their death by drowning. Thousands of birds died in this way.

Herds of seals on the island nature preserves died by suffocation. The effects on marine life and other creatures in this, one of the world's great migration routes, were inestimable.

I have recounted the Santa Barbara Channel affair at some length, because it was utterly reprehensible and because it shows the irresponsibility and fallibility of experts. And, indeed, it is the irresponsibility and fallibility of experts that put our whole environment at risk.

There was no question of scientific speculation, any more than there was financial speculation, because those off-shore oil deposits were well-known extensions of the landward oil fields. Indeed, it had been urged that the Santa Barbara Channel oil should be earmarked as a national oil reserve against a national emergency when the strategical need would justify its exploitation.

Against all arguments of amenities, the State of California had sanctioned off-shore drilling within its three-mile limit on the specious argument, if I may say so, that the levy on the oil would help to pay for nature conservancy.

The Federal permission, hustled through Washington, was even less defensible. Those operations in the Federal drilling sector were along the fissures of an earthquake belt, the off-shore cracks from the San Andreas Fault. Seismologists are currently predicting an imminent earthquake along this fault, bigger possibly, they say, than the great San Francisco earthquake.

Drilling in that fissured area could, as did happen, produce submarine seepage. The engineer for that drilling was well aware, in fact he admitted it at the inquiry, that the curtailment of the casing involved a definite risk of a blow-out. But he was the hired man. His warning could be and was ignored. There was no ethic in his profession to protect him, nor to compel him to intervene, for the public good.

Now, I cite these examples of irresponsibility, ignorance or avarice, which are exploiting our environment and prejudicing our posterity, as bleak consolation, without, I insist, any reprieve for those who are concerned with radiation hazards.

Imagine if any one of these instances had had a radiation damage analogy, and imagine what the public alarm and the outcry would have been. Imagine also what would have happened if that stolen cyanide, I mentioned earlier, had been, say, a radio-cobalt source which would have been dangerous to individuals but which would not have actually threatened half the population of London. There would have been road-blocks, monitoring squads and even door-to-door searches. There would have been screaming headlines and stern editorials.

If the Gruinard or the Dugway incidents had been nuclear instead of biological, there would have been a far greater outcry than there was. In fact, there was no outcry about Gruinard at all. There was a modest reaction to the Dugway incident.*

If the Torrey Canyon had been a nuclear-powered ship or if the Santa Barbara Channel leak had been seepage of a low-level, let alone high-level, radioactive effluent, we would have had an alarm comparable with the Palomaris situation, when the nuclear bomb fell into the waters off the coast of Spain.

No-one here would reject a proper concern about any radiation incident with real or potential dangers. But as one who has been actively encouraging such proper concern for the past 24 years, I am citing these examples of massive degradation of the environment to show that anything to do with radioactivity produces a public reaction out of all proportion to that created by any other circumstance. Something of which you are painfully aware.

When we were starting these colloquia in May 1960, the World Health Organization study group on the Mental Health Aspects of the Peaceful Uses of Atomic Energy, of which I was a member, had just finished its work. One of our conclusions was that apart from the supercharged emotions about the bomb, there was universal disquiet about atomic energy per se.

The group on that occasion, recognized that "the crust of our vaunted civilization was only eggshell thick and that confronted with the release of immeasurable power from the infinitesimally small atom, civilized man tend to cower, like his Neanderthal forefathers, in the dark caves of his own emotions." As we said on that occasion, "We are back in the childhood of mankind".

The elemental Gods which primitive man had to appease had become radioactive.

The partial test-ban agreement has given a degree of reassurance. But strangely enough, and this is the irrationality of the whole thing, the Chinese and the French fall-out do not seem to be so bad. Our emotions, you see, do not quantify. The fall-out is not ours, so our guilt sense does not magnify it.

The WHO group recognized that fall-out was one of the main disturbing factors.

---

* In November 1969, the President of the United States of America announced that the United States would not under any conditions engage in germ warfare and would destroy its stock-piles of germ warfare weapons. The campaign by Rep. Richard McCarthy and the study by the National Security Council were stimulated by the Dugway accident. The statement by the President resulted from that study.

It was just the idea that all fall-out, apart from its nature (the psychologists on that occasion identified it with the primitive oral-anal response, breast-feeding and excretion) was psychologically identified with body waste.

I remember the chairman, a psychiatrist, saying, as we read all these clippings from the press of the world about the Windscale accident, "All the editors must have been breast fed".

Now, those who try to establish facts by research and by measurement are likely, and very properly, to become impatient with nuclear mythology, but as we agreed in early colloquia of this series, the folk lore was, and still is, a fact to be taken into account, and I would add, it is not wholly reprehensible.

It has, however much it seems unreasonable at times, encouraged prudence which has made peaceful atomic energy the safest of all industries in the world. It reminded scientists and the practitioners of Claude Bernard's counsel over a century ago: "True science teaches us to doubt and in ignorance to refrain."

So, in this field of atomic energy, of nuclear proportions, we have edged forward, confirming each step with the caution of someone using a mine detector in an uncharted minefield. The on-cost to industry has been heavy and some would say that the precautions are excessive and unnecessarily burdensome, and, indeed, causing in many cases unnecessary delay in beneficial development. But I want to say this very emphatically, it is an error on the side of righteousness and it is a reproach to the other modern industries which have been recklessly indifferent about the degradation of the environment.

I remember, gratefully, the conference on radiation hazards organized by the United Nations agencies (World Health Organization, Food and Agriculture Organization, and the International Atomic Energy Agency) in Geneva several years ago. Many of the participants argued that, in terms of the total environment and of the total population, there was and should be no maximum permissible dose; that is to say that, in principle, no radiation exposure was permissible in the sense that, in the event of an incident or an accident, we might console ourselves by saying that, "There is no need to worry until the level reaches so-and-so".

Dr. Brues has pointed out, these measurements of safety are valid, but what was involved here was that the only consideration should be that the atmospheric radiation should be returned to natural levels as quickly as possible. Now, that is a very important attitude. Think how much better off we, and indeed posterity, would be if that kind of attitude had been applied to the contamination of the environment by the effluents and fumes and wastes of other industries. Dr. Brues has given us an excellent analogy of the coal industry if it had followed instead of preceded the nuclear industry.

In contrast to what has happened in the nuclear field, the attitude in much of industry has been, "Let's see how long we can get away with it". And when the damage has been done, often irreparably, the public authorities have had to step in, belatedly and ineffectively, with laws and regulations. The principle of "Innocent until proved guilty" should not apply here. It should be incumbent on any industry, as it is on the atomic industry, to prove, in advance, that any new factors which they are introducing into the environment are innocent.

We should not have to wait until smog has well passed the "maximum permissible" dosage of chemical pollutants to bring in laws compelling automobiles to consume their own combustion wastes. I was appalled recently while sitting in the House of Lords, to hear a minister say, "In Britain at least there is no substantial evidence that the exhaust from motor cars is a serious danger". Now, of course, next year we will put it in our regulations. We have to, because the Americans have said we will not be able to sell our cars unless we do. In that respect you are ahead of us here.

We should not have to wait until rivers and lakes are hopelessly polluted before compelling industries to do something about their noxious effluents and then be told that preventive or corrective measures will be so costly that industrial products will be non-competitive or priced out of the market. That, indeed, is what we have all been told in Britain, whenever we try to impose conservation measures, or to say we should be doing something about our fumes or liquid effluent and so on. We are always told that, "If you impose that restriction, you will price us out of the market. Our competitors are not controlled by these conditions".

In the nuclear-based industries, the social costs have been a built-in factor from the start and, although there have been grumblings, the economics of the industry have taken them into account and, since the precautions are internationally established, the element of unfair competition has, to that degree, been reduced. Here again, the nuclear industry has set an example to other industries which ought to be governed by international standards since, in the terms of which I have talked, the massive pollution of the biosphere is no longer a matter of local or national concern. The effects are universal and affect everyone, everywhere.

Let us take an example. At the United Nations Science and Technology Conference in Geneva in 1963, we took stock of the effects of industrialization on our total environment so far.

The atmosphere is not only the air we breathe; it is also the envelope which protects living things from harmful radiation from the sun and from outer space. It is also the medium of the climate, of the winds and of the rains. And those, in turn, are inseparable from the hydrosphere including the oceans, covering seven-tenths of the globe, with their currents and evaporation; from the biosphere, with the plants and their transpiration and, in terms of human activity, concerned with the minerals mined from the lithosphere, the rock crust.

Millions of years ago the sun encouraged the growth of the primeval forests which became our coal and the organic growth in the seas which became our oil. Those fossil fuels have been locked away for eons of time, but they have been extracted by man and put back into the atmosphere from the chimney-stacks and exhaust-pipes of modern engineering.

By burning fuel, human activities have affected the atmosphere. About 6 billion tons of carbon are mixed with the atmosphere every year. During the past century, industrialization, by burning fossil fuel, has released more than 400 billion tons of carbon which have been artificially introduced into the atmosphere. The concentration in the air we breathe has been increased by about 10%, and, if all the known resources of coal and oil were burned, the concentration would be ten times that.

This is something more than a public health problem, more than a question of what goes into the lungs of the individual, more than a question of smog. This carbon, in excess of what might be called the natural background, can affect the climate in two different ways: the carbon monoxide and dioxide can modify the sun's rays. The carbon cycle is a self-adjusting mechanism. Carbon dioxide is, of course, indispensable to plants and is, therefore, a source of life. But there is a balance which is maintained by excess carbon dioxide being absorbed into the sea.

The excess is now, and has been for a long time, taxing the absorptive capacity of the sea and is disturbing the heat balance because of what is known as the greenhouse effect. A greenhouse lets in the sun's rays, but retains the convection heat. The carbon dioxide does just that. It keeps the heat at the surface of the earth and, in excess, modifies our climate.

It has been estimated by some that with the present rate of increase of carbon dioxide, 6 billion tons a year, the mean annual temperature of the earth will increase by 3.6 degrees Centigrade in the next 40 years. I repeat, the mean annual temperature. Experts may argue about the time factor, as to whether it is 40 years or not.

Certain effects, however, are already apparent not only in the industrialized northern hemisphere, but in the southern hemisphere. The north polar ice is thinning and shrinking. The seas, with their blanket of carbon dioxide, are changing their temperature, with the result that the marine life, plant life, etc. is increasing and transpiring more carbon dioxide. One of the manifestations of this is the migration of the whitefish farther and farther up the Baffin Straits, because it is warming up. With this combination, as I say, fish are migrating and even changing their latitudes.

On land the snow-line is retreating, the permafrost line in Siberia, as well as in the Western hemisphere, is being altered and the glaciers are melting. And, indeed, on a long stay I had in the Arctic it seemed unquestionable that even the depth of the permafrost is now being affected.

In Scandinavia, land which was perennially under snow and ice, at least as far back as the days of Eric the Red, are melting and the arrowheads of over 1,000 years ago, when the black earth was last exposed, have been found.

The melting of the sea ice will, of course, not affect the sea level, because the volume of the sea ice is the same as the water it displaces, but the melting of the land ice, the ice caps and glaciers, in which such vast amounts of water are now locked up, will introduce additional water to the oceans and raise the sea level. And this is happening, incidentally, recognizably in Antarctica where, of course, you have two-and-a-half-mile-deep ice caps.

The rivers originating in glaciers and permanent snowfields will increase their flow and if the ice dams, such as are in the Himalayas, break, the results in flooding will be absolutely catastrophic. In this process over the world, the climate will change with increased precipitation and in some areas also aridity of now fertile regions.

I know that we are all weather prophets and have our pet theories, including, you remember, the widely held theory that freakish weather was caused by the H-bomb tests. We are all prophets but we do not have to look 40 years ahead nor be screwballs or cranks to recognize that our weather is at least becoming increasingly eccentric.

We can be cosmically indignant and say that was because of our meddling with the magnetic forces by exploding the Rainbow Bomb in the Van Allen Belt, or you may watch the take-off, the landings or the stack-up of jet aircraft at O'Hare Field or Kennedy Airport or Heathrow in London and watch the black exhausts and the jet trails and think of all the jets criss-crossing the country and the continents.

You can cite the uncombusted waste of those jet engines or you can consider the condensation trails. You should remember what we have learned from artificial precipitation projects and realize that supersaturated clouds only need nucleation points, tangible toeholds, to change into rain and that, of course, happens with the jet trails. And we take for granted that our air transport operations must be influencing, to some degree, the pattern of precipitation. Add to that, of course, the rocket trails as well.

When I was asked to talk on the degradation of the environment, I was cast in a role that has now become my regular role, the prophet of woe, the man with the sandwich board who goes around saying, "Beware the wrath to come", because the despoilers, the degraders, are the many people of our planet. There are too many already and inescapably there will be twice as many in 30 years time - at least twice. It is a biologically committed figure. Half the population of the world is now under 15 years of age and, even if they oblige us in our international family planning programme, by only having two or three children, they would certainly give us around double what we have now.

Kingsley Davis has shown that on present trends there will be over 15 billion people in the world on present trends. We may vary these trends; we hope we can. That is to say there will be 15 billion people in the world, five times as many as the figures for our humanly degraded world of today, in which two-thirds of the world's population are denied nutritionally adequate food, or housing, or human dignity. That 15 billion will eventuate within the lifetime of a child born today and, again on present trends, unless we do something about it, will all be living in cities: Ecumenopolis, World City of which Boswash, the built-up area from Boston to Washington, and Sansan, stretching from San Diego to San Francisco with Route 101 as its Main Street, and Chorleans, from Chicago to New Orleans will be its suburbs.

Within that urbanization, you realize all the implications, everything we are talking about: the wastes, the extravagant use of resources and everything else.

Now, as a professor of international relations, I am a paid optimist. I have to be optimistic or I would go mad. But while I believe that human ingenuity can find the answers, and I truly think it can, do not quote me too loudly because every time I say we can feed 7,000 million people quite adequately by the year 2000, the Vatican quotes me.

I am compelled to say that the present misdirection of human talent and the anarchy of science and technology qualify my optimism. I know I am ungracious and soured and a square when I question the wisdom of the Space Programme. I am not, in this context, discussing the expenditure nor am I suggesting that you can take the hardware of the programme and turn it into food for the starving millions, but I do say a crash programme of this kind diverts human ingenuity from tackling the problems of this planet; it is, in fact, redirecting brains which would be better used, if they applied themselves to the pressing human problems, in a crash programme in terms of world needs.

More directly, in terms of our terrestrial environment, and I repeat terrestrial environment, have we provided against the risks? When the International Geophysical Year first showed the possibility of artificial satellites, the International Council of Scientific

Unions set up a thing called CETEX. That is not a headache powder nor a foundation garment. It is the committee to deal with Contamination by Extra Terrestrial Exploration. It was a scientific vigilance corps to see that man's intervention in space did not foul up scientific observations.

Well, you know, since then we have had the obscenity of the copper filings scattered in space and the effrontery of the Rainbow Bomb produce an artificial aurora borealis just for the hell of it. I might add that every cosmologist and every geophysicist of any reputation in the world protested against the Rainbow Bomb and no attention was paid to them.

CETEX from the outset warned about the biological risks. I remember writing an article pointing up the warnings that CETEX was trying to convey. I pointed out that the moon was a celestial grand piano gathering cosmic dust with no winds to disturb it. I recalled the suggestion of Arrhenius that dispersed through the universe might be (were, according to him) biotic spores which in congenial circumstances might develop on the planets. But on the moon there would also be pre-biotic dust, that is to say the essential elements of life without DNA or RNA codes to organize them.

Now, let us see what happens. An earthling arrives on the moon and sneezes. (You notice also we have not succeeded in getting a sneezeless astronaut.) His DNA triggers off a life process. Oh, it does not lead to anything as spectacular as a quasi-man or a lunar violet; it could just be a slime crawling over the face of the moon and turning it into gorgonzola cheese.

I know in space medicine such possibilities are considered and, as far as possible, taken care of, but I do hope, and I say this very earnestly, I hope that in the space programme and beyond the space programme, not just in space medicine for the programme, that people are sitting down as you have been sitting down for the last few days and are considering in advance what they may be doing.

Do not forget, this is the important thing, that the passage to the moon is a two-way passage. Remember the lesson of the rabbit and the prickly pear in Australia. Or the story of thanet grass and the Colorado beetle.

In "Nature", Dr. Alexander of the Laboratory of Soil Microbiology at Cornell University issued a salutary warning, or at least put it in scientific terms which many of us have been trying to put in general terms, "The possible contamination of earth by lunar or martian life". He reminded us of how little we knew about the contacts that the astronauts and their machinery would be making or about the materials they would be bringing back. He mentioned the recent conference at which the participants had agreed that, while life as we would recognize it may not exist on the moon, "the possibility of extraterrestrial life and the concomitant possibility of back contamination must be presumed to exist". And he said that that was the unanimous finding of this conference. And indeed the likelihood is specifically recognized in the quarantine arrangements that NASA made for the returning astronauts.

The crew and their vehicle remained sealed after it arrived at the lunar receiving laboratory at Houston. But, quarantine against what? What is the incubation period of a lunar bug?

As the Deputy Surgeon General of the U.S. Public Health Service has said,

"We must make an arbitrary approach to quarantine but must also recognize that quarantine is a crude concept and a crude approach to a problem of this sort. I would not feel safe in putting much faith in it as a security method". I would agree.

You may recall how H.G. Wells, all those years ago, wrote "War of the Worlds" in which his Martians had practically taken the earth over and they all died of common cold or at least the unfamiliar germs of the earth's atmosphere.

As Dr. Alexander reminded us in the article in "Nature", if there are spores or micro-organisms on the Moon or Mars, they are adapted to extremes of environment and would have a rare persistence in the banana belt of the more moderate earth and might develop even more profusely. The quarantine precautions of the apollo landings seem to be reassuring on this score.

I know what some people say, and they say it to me all the time. "If we listen to you and all your cautions, we would never do anything."

I am not trying to start trouble. I am sorry but I am only repeating what Claude Bernard enjoined: "True science teaches us to doubt and in ignorance to refrain." In the idiom of modern circumstance and with an urgency in a world of technicological change, (I do not say "scientific" impetuosity) this becomes all the more important. I repeat, the technological rapidity of change is one of the elements with which we have got to deal. The stakes are much too high for us to be complacent.

Now, this becomes agonizing to me, who has spent most of my adult life as a cheer leader for science and technology. It becomes far more agonizing when the risks are involved in doing good, or what appears to be benevolent development.

I have travelled something like 2.5 million miles in the past 20 years, mainly for the United Nations and its specialized agencies, trying to see how science and technology can be used for the well-being of the scientifically and technologically underprivileged people of the earth. In one area, we have been dramatically successful. With sulpha drugs, antibiotics and DDT, we have reduced the epidemics of killer diseases and since they were rampant in the poorer countries, it was just a relative success. Death control improved the expectation of life, but it had a staggering effect.

For example, the expectation of life of a girl baby born in India in 1946 was 27. Today it is 48, still well below the life expectancy in the advanced countries, but significantly covering the whole of her reproductive life span. So she just goes on having babies and we now have the world's population increasing at a fantastic rate. I do not believe, ladies and gentlemen, that there is a great orgy of procreation going on. Couples are not having more children, more children are surviving, and they are surviving to have more children.

Now, I have believed, and I still believe, that the wit of man can redress the balance, given reasonable family planning and the application of science to the problems of food supply. I used to go around, glibly saying, "Give us the agricultural equivalent of DDT". By that, I meant that we had an insecticide which coped with the insect-borne diseases. WHO, UNICEF, and AID moved in and all that was necessary to reduce the death rates was the co-operation of illiterate peoples in allowing the spraying and the like, and not a long, slow haul and elaborate social services and public education.

What I was wanting in asking for the agricultural equivalent of DDT was something, some break-through in agriculture, which would spectacularly increase food yields, techniques which peasant peoples would recognize and co-operate in. I think we have got it. I think we have got it in the high-yielding Mexican wheats and the IRI, International Rice Institute, rice strains.

On paper, and statistically, we have solved the food problem of India.

I want everyone to know, including the Indians, that everyone is going hell for leather for this manifest improvement. I want them to realize what is involved. The yields will depend on heavy irrigation, heavy use of fertilisers and very heavy applications of pesticides. The last are essential because, if every plant is a perfected strain, a single virus could destroy the lot. Heavy irrigation means that the plantings will be confined to the river plains. The Plains of the Ganges will become the Indian prairies. If the fertilizers are not properly managed and the pesticides are indiscriminately, or ignorantly applied, the wash-offs in the monsoons will be terrific, with unpredictable ecological consequences in the river and oceanic systems. I mooted this in a recent television programme and the industrial chemist who was participating in the programme just ridiculed the idea and said, "It will be all right if only they read the small print on the containers".

Now, I have cited all these other problems other than radiation hazard, other aspects of the degradation of the environment as a supplement to your discussions, not just to comfort those engaged in nuclear precautions, not to comfort you by saying there are other nightmares, other forms of nightmares, and certainly not suggesting that in any way we should curtail what is being done in radiation health science. But to suggest seriously that after the cataclysmic release of nuclear energy as a bomb, with all its military and political consequences, and after the return to sanity after the test ban, the tentative handling of nuclear energy is highly creditable, very creditable. Claude Bernard would have approved.

It has been a case of going into the most dangerous minefield mankind has ever known, with a mine detector and carefully establishing every foothold. I do ask you, as an outsider, do not be afraid of well doing, do not give up and do not relax vigilance because the penalties of ignorance and avarice, which are the components of pollution, means more pollution and no less than the forfeit of the future of mankind.

SUBJECT INDEX